Dr. Mark Stengler's

NATURAL HEALING ENCYCLOPEDIA

625R0006C5

Table of Contents

Part III: Heart and Blood

Part IV: Energy and Fatigue

Part V: Weight Loss

Part IX: Immune System

Part X: Men and Women's Health

Part XI: Dr. Stengler's Urgent Health Warnings

Part XII: Dr. Stengler's Top 19 Healing Secrets

PART I

Pain

Natural Pain Relievers
That Really Work

For most people, prescription and over-the-counter (OTC) pain relievers are fine for occasional use, but they carry increasing risks the longer they are taken.

Aspirin and other nonsteroidal anti-inflammatory drugs (NSAIDs), such as *ibuprofen* (Advil), *naproxen* (Aleve) and *ketoprofen* (Orudis KT), can cause digestive problems, including internal bleeding. *Acetaminophen* (Tylenol) is potentially toxic to the liver and kidneys after months of use. Prescription drugs that contain either barbiturates, such as phenobarbital (Solfoton), or opiates, such as oxycodone (OxyContin), are potentially habit-forming.

These are some of the reasons why many people are turning to natural pain relievers—vitamins, minerals, herbs and homeopathic remedies (highly diluted natural substances made from plants, minerals and animal products).*

Natural pain relievers aren't as strong as pharmaceutical products, so they may not work as fast. But because they are less toxic, they typically are much safer over the long run, especially for treating chronic pain.

*Even when a natural remedy (or drug) effectively relieves pain, it is important to discover and treat the underlying cause. Consult your doctor, especially if muscle or joint pain or other symptoms worsen.

Both drugs and natural pain relievers block the body's pain signals, but natural remedies also enhance the body's own recuperative power to repair injured tissue and fight disease. *My favorite natural pain relievers...*

Arthritis and back pain

• **MSM** (Methylsulfonylmethane). This compound, which occurs naturally in living organisms, acts as a potent anti-inflammatory. It reduces muscle spasm and slows down the overactive nerve impulses that may cause this condition.

Because most back pain is the result of muscle spasm and inflammation, MSM often brings lasting relief and can prevent future episodes. In addition, it has been shown to ease the pain associated with fibromyalgia and osteoarthritis.

Typical dosage: For preventive purposes (for arthritis, chronic back pain, fibromyalgia, etc.), take 1,000 to 2,000 mg daily, indefinitely. For relief of acute pain, the effective dose depends on individual factors, such as weight and age. Start at 3,000 mg per day and increase in increments of 1,000 mg every two to three days, until you experience relief or reach 6,000 mg daily.

Helpful: Take MSM with food to minimize digestive upset.

• **Boswellia**. This herb, which is widely used in Ayurvedic (Indian) medicine, is another anti-inflammatory that treats both rheumatoid arthritis and osteoarthritis. A review of 11 German studies found that boswellia brought substantial benefits to 260 people who had not responded to conventional medical treatment. Most were able to curb their intake of anti-inflammatory medication.

Typical dosage: 1,500 mg of a standardized preparation (containing 60 percent to 65 percent boswellic acid), three times a day for six weeks. For long-term use, reduce the dosage to 750 mg, three times a day.

• **Rhus toxicodendron**. This homeopathic remedy, derived from poison oak, is particularly helpful for rheumatoid arthritis or osteoarthritis pain that is worse in the morning and improves with motion and activity… or that flares up before a storm or in damp weather.

Typical dosage: For long-term use for chronic pain, take a 6C potency pellet, two to three times daily.

Injury

• **Arnica**. When pain is the result of a bump or bruise, this homeopathic remedy is extremely effective, sometimes within minutes. It is also very helpful for muscle soreness after overexertion.

Typical dosage: Dissolve two 30C potency pellets under your tongue every 15 minutes for a total of up to three doses per day, until the pain goes away.

Arnica is also available as a cream or tincture. Apply it directly to the painful spot.

• **Rhus toxicodendron**. This homeopathic remedy, also used for arthritis, is ideal for strains and sprains. Besides relieving pain, it speeds recovery.

Typical dosage: Dissolve a 30C potency pellet under your tongue, two to three times daily for two days.

• **Bromelain**. This protein-dissolving enzyme is found in pineapple stems. It effectively reduces the swelling and bruising that cause pain for days after injury. Bromelain breaks down the blood clots that form as a result of physical trauma, restoring circulation and healing damaged tissue.

Typical dosage: 500 mg, three times daily between meals. Look for a bromelain preparation standardized to 1,600 MCU (milk-clotting units) per 500 mg.

Caution: Bromelain has a slight blood-thinning effect. Check with your doctor before taking it if you're on blood-thinning medication, such as warfarin (Coumadin).

Nerve pain

• **Capsaicin**. A potent compound found in cayenne pepper, capsaicin apparently blocks the messenger chemical substance P from carrying pain signals along the nerves.

It can be highly effective against the often severe pain of shingles (herpes zoster). Capsaicin also relieves diabetic neuropathy, the pain that develops usually in the legs and feet of diabetics because of nerve damage.

Typical dosage: Apply a cream that contains 0.025 percent to 0.075 percent capsaicin extract to the painful area, two to four times daily.

What Relief!
Natural Ways to Curb Your Pain

Not long ago, a 60-year-old woman came to my office suffering from severe arthritis pain in both hands. I gave her a bean-sized dab of a homeopathic gel that she applied directly to the skin on her hands. After a few applications in the span of 30 minutes, her pain was reduced by 90 percent. She did not need to apply the gel again for two weeks.

I witnessed a similar result with a retired National Football League player. He had severe chronic hip pain from past injuries. With one application of the gel, his pain was relieved by 70 percent for two full days.

The relief that these people experienced has given them each a new lease on life. *But here's the best news*—unlike pharmaceutical pain relievers, which often cause gastrointestinal upset or damage to internal organs, natural therapies can reduce pain without adverse effects.

What are you taking for pain?

Most Americans take too many pharmaceutical pain relievers. An estimated 175 million American adults take over-the-counter (OTC) pain relievers regularly. About one-fifth of Americans in their 60s take at least one painkiller for chronic pain on a regular basis.

There has been a lot of news about the life-threatening risks of anti-inflammatory medications such as *rofecoxib* (Vioxx) and *celecoxib* (Celebrex), two pain relievers that had been heavily prescribed by conventional doctors to treat the chronic pain of arthritis and similar conditions. Vioxx was pulled off the market by its manufacturer, Merck, following research that linked it to increased risk of heart attack and stroke. Celebrex now carries warnings about adverse effects, such as increased risk of cardiovascular thrombotic events, heart attack and stroke. Abdominal pain, diarrhea, skin reactions and *edema* (water retention) may also occur.

Of course, pain-relieving drugs can be a blessing in the event of injury, severe acute migraines or diseases, such as terminal cancer. A number of years ago, when I had a wisdom tooth extracted, I received a local anesthetic. Afterward, I went to an acupuncturist for pain relief so I wouldn't need any painkillers. For about one hour after the acupuncture, I was fine—but then the pain-relieving *endorphins* wore off. I tried a few natural remedies, but when the pain became excruciating, I resorted to the OTC pain reliever *acetaminophen* (Tylenol). That did the trick.

But many people use painkillers on a regular basis for several months or even years, which increases the risk of dangerous side effects. For instance, people who rely on acetaminophen increase their risk of developing stomach ulcers, liver disease and kidney disease. If you regularly take Celebrex or an OTC *nonsteroidal anti-inflammatory drug* (NSAID), such as aspirin or *naproxen* (Aleve), you run the risk of kidney and stomach damage. Regular use of NSAIDs also increases risk of heart attack, according to the FDA.

Better results, fewer risks

Before you take any remedy, it's important for your doctor to identify what is causing your pain. Remember, pain is your body's distress signal that something is being irritated or damaged. Sometimes we protect ourselves by reacting instinctively. If you touch something hot, for example, you eliminate the pain by quickly pulling back your hand.

But what if your back hurts? You may need a pain reliever—but back pain also can be a signal that you're harming your body by bending or sitting the wrong way. You may need to address the underlying cause to prevent further injury. Pain receptors are found in the skin, around bones and joints—even in the walls of arteries. If a muscle is torn, for example, a pain signal is released from fibers in the shredded tissue.

In light of the dangers from prescription and OTC drugs, what safe alternatives are available to you? There are many natural supplements that I recommend.

Nature's pain relievers

If you take prescription or OTC pain medication, work with a naturopathic physician, holistic medical doctor or chiropractor who will incorporate natural pain fighters into your treatment regimen. With his/her help, you may be able to reduce your dosage of pain medication (natural pain relievers can be used safely with prescription or OTC pain-killers)—or even eliminate the drugs altogether.

All-natural pain-fighting supplements are even more effective when they are combined with physical therapies, like acupuncture, chiropractic, magnet therapy or osteopathic manipulation (a technique in which an osteopathic physician uses his hands to move a patient's muscles and joints with stretching, gentle pressure and resistance). *Physiotherapy* (a treatment that utilizes physical agents, such as exercise and massage, to develop, maintain and restore movement and functional ability) also is helpful.

Here are—in no special order—the best natural pain relievers, which can be taken alone or in combination…

• **White willow bark extract** is helpful for headaches, arthritis, muscle aches and fever. In Europe, doctors prescribe this herbal remedy for back pain, and recent research supports this use. One study conducted in Haifa, Israel, involved 191 patients with chronic low-back pain who took one of two doses of willow bark extract or a placebo daily for four weeks. Researchers found that 39 percent of patients taking the higher dose of willow bark extract had complete pain relief, compared with only six percent of those taking a placebo. The participants who benefited the most took willow bark extract that contained 240 mg of the compound *salicin*, the active constituent in this herbal remedy. (Aspirin is made from *acetylsalicylic acid*, which has many of the chemical properties of salicin.) However, aspirin can cause gastrointestinal ulceration and other side effects, including kidney damage. Willow bark extract is believed to work by inhibiting naturally occurring enzymes that cause inflammation and pain.

I recommend taking willow bark extract that contains 240 mg of salicin daily. In rare cases, willow bark extract can cause mild stomach upset. Do not take willow bark if you have a history of ulcers, gastritis or kidney disease. It also should not be taken by anyone who is allergic to aspirin. As with aspirin, willow bark extract should never be given to children under age 12 who have a fever—in rare instances, it can cause a fatal disease called *Reye's syndrome*. Willow bark extract has blood-thinning properties, so avoid it if you take a blood thinner, such as *warfarin* (Coumadin). For low-back pain, you may need to take willow bark extract for a week or more before you get results.

• **Methylsulfonylmethane (MSM)** is a popular nutritional supplement that relieves muscle and joint pain. According to Stanley Jacob, MD, a professor at Oregon Health & Science University who has conducted much of the original research on MSM, this supplement reduces inflammation by improving blood flow. Your cells have receptors that send out pain signals when they're deprived of blood. That's why increased blood flow diminishes pain.

MSM, the natural compound found in green vegetables, fruits and grains, decreases muscle spasms and softens painful scar tissue from previous injuries. A double-blind study of 50 people with osteoarthritis of the knee found that MSM helps relieve arthritis pain.

Start with a daily dose of 3,000 mg to 5,000 mg of MSM. If your pain and/or inflammation doesn't improve within five days, increase the dose up to 8,000 mg daily, taken in several doses throughout the day. If you develop digestive upset or loose stools, reduce the dosage. If you prefer, you can apply MSM cream (per the label instructions) to your skin at the painful area. This product is available at health-food stores and works well for localized pain. MSM has a mild blood-thinning effect, so check with your doctor if you take a blood thinner.

• **S-adenosylmethionine (SAMe)** is a natural compound found in the body. The supplement is an effective treatment for people who have osteoarthritis accompanied by cartilage degeneration. SAMe's ability to reduce pain, stiffness and swelling is similar to that of NSAIDs such as ibuprofen and naproxen, and the anti-inflammatory medication Celebrex. There's also evidence that SAMe stimulates cartilage repair, which helps prevent bones from rubbing against one another. A 16-week study conducted at the University of California, Irvine, compared two groups of people who were being treated for knee pain caused by osteoarthritis. Some took 1,200 mg of SAMe daily, while others took 200 mg of Celebrex. It took longer for people to get relief from SAMe, but by the second month, SAMe proved to be just as effective as Celebrex.

Most patients with osteoarthritis and *fibromyalgia* (a disorder characterized by widespread pain in muscles, tendons and ligaments) who take SAMe notice improvement within four to eight weeks. Many studies use 1,200 mg of SAMe daily in divided doses. In my experience, taking 400 mg twice daily works well. It's a good idea to take a multivitamin or 50 mg B-complex supplement daily while you're taking SAMe. The vitamin B-12 and folic acid contained in either supplement help your body metabolize SAMe, which means that the remedy goes to work faster.

• **Kaprex** is effective for mild pain caused by injury or osteoarthritis. It is a blend of hops, rosemary extract and *oleanic acid,* which is derived from olive leaf extract. Rather than blocking the body's pain-causing enzymes, these natural substances inhibit pain-causing chemicals known as *prostaglandins.*

In a study sponsored by the Institute for Functional Medicine, the research arm of the supplement manufacturer Metagenics, taking Kaprex for six weeks reduced minor pain by as much as 72 percent. I recommend taking one 440 mg tablet three times daily. Kaprex is manufactured by Metagenics (800-692-9400, www.metagenics.com), the institute's product branch. The product is sold only in doctors' offices. To find a practitioner in your area who sells Kaprex, call the toll-free number. Kaprex has no known side effects and does not interact with other medications.

• **Proteolytic enzymes**, including *bromelain, trypsin, chymotrypsin, pancreatin, papain* and a range of protein-digesting enzymes derived from the fermentation of fungus, reduce pain and inflammation by improving blood flow. You can find these natural pain fighters at health-food stores in products labeled "proteolytic enzymes." Take as directed on the label. Bromelain, a favorite of athletes, is available on its own. Extracted from pineapple stems, bromelain reduces swelling by breaking down blood clots that can form as a result of trauma and impede circulation. It works well for bruises, sprains and surgical recovery. If you use bromelain, take 500 mg three times daily between meals.

Repair is a high-potency formula of proteolytic enzymes that I often recommend. It is manufactured by Enzymedica (to find a retailer, call 888-918-1118 or go to www.enzymedica.com). Take two capsules two to three times daily between meals. Do not take Repair or any proteolytic enzyme formula if you have an active ulcer or gastritis. Any enzyme product can have a mild blood-thinning effect, so check with your doctor if you take a blood thinner.

•**PainMed** is the homeopathic gel that gave such quick relief to the patients I described at the beginning of this article. It is remarkably effective for relieving the pain of arthritis, muscle soreness and spasms, sprains, strains, stiffness, headaches (especially due to tension) as well as injuries, including bruises.

PainMed is a combination of nine highly diluted plant and flower materials, including *arnica, bryonia, hypericum* and *ledum*. Like other homeopathic remedies, it promotes the body's ability to heal itself. A bean-sized dab works well for anyone who has pain. It should be spread on the skin around the affected area. Following an injury, use it every 15 minutes, for a total of up to four applications. As the pain starts to diminish, apply less often. Do not reapply the gel once the pain is gone. PainMed does not sting, burn or irritate the skin. It is clear, has no odor, does not stain and dries quickly. Because it has so many uses and works so rapidly, PainMed is a good first-aid remedy to have on hand. To order, contact the manufacturer, GM International, Inc., (800-228-9850, www.gmipainmed.com).

Touch These Points—And Heal

There are pressure points on your feet, hands and outer ears that can help you relieve stress and ease health problems. That's the goal behind reflexology, a noninvasive healing technique that was introduced in the 1900s. You can perform it on yourself or a partner. To get you started, I spoke to reflexologist Bill Flocco, director and founder of the American Academy of Reflexology (www.american academyofreflexology.com). Give this technique a try—and enjoy the pain relief and deep sense of relaxation it can bring.

Reflexology is based on the idea that disease or injury in one part of the body can cause a buildup of substances that irritate nerve endings in reflex points in the feet, hands and ears. Thus, reflexing—applying pressure and gentle manipulation at points on the feet, hands and ears—corresponds to and helps specific areas of the body.

Example: The "reflexes" in the fingers and toes correspond to the head and neck.

For best results: Practice reflexology at least twice a day, at least four times weekly. Work on each reflex point or area for about five to 10 minutes. Sometimes relief occurs fairly quickly, or it can take several days, weeks or longer for reflexology to help. (Don't worry if you apply pressure to the wrong spot. You won't harm yourself.)

Caution: If pain is related to a medical condition, seek help from a physician.

How to help common complaints…

For each ailment, you can apply pressure to the hands, ears or feet for relief. Several of these reflex points are described here.

Jaw pain

This exercise helps *temporomandibular joint disorder* (TMJ). With the tip of your index finger, locate the small flap of cartilage at the top of the earlobe. Then move your finger about half an inch toward the back edge of the ear. Place the tip of the thumb behind the ear at this point, and with the index finger on the front, squeeze gently, applying firm, but not painful, pressure. Apply pressure to both ears at once.

After you have completed the ear reflexology, do it on your feet. While seated, place the left foot on the opposite knee. With the left hand, grasp the big toe and apply pressure with the tip of the thumb to the widest part of the big toe in the area closest to the second toe. Switch legs and repeat.

Shoulder pain

Locate the area of the ear slightly above the one addressed for jaw pain. Place the pad of the thumb on the back of the ear at that spot and the index finger in front. Working on both ears at once, gently squeeze and hold.

Lower back pain

Find the area just above the wrist on the thumb edge of the left palm. Grasping from behind with the fingers of the opposite hand, apply gentle pressure to this point with the tip of the thumb. Gently roll the tip of your thumb while applying pressure. Switch hands and repeat.

Reduce urinary frequency

Repeating this exercise four to six times daily might greatly reduce the number of times you urinate at night. Sitting, place your left foot on your right knee. Find the spot on the inner edge of the left foot that is in a direct line below the ankle bone, where the inner side of the foot and the sole of the foot meet. Using your right thumb, apply pressure at this point. Gently grasp and stabilize the left foot with the fingers on the right hand while you do this. Repeat on the opposite foot.

Blood Clots and Leg Pain

Carolee, a 61-year-old teacher of preschool, had been a patient of mine for the past year. With the help of dietary changes and nutritional supplements, we had made great strides in reducing her weight and controlling her chronic sinusitis and coughing. Unexpectedly, she began experiencing severe pain in her lower right leg during a vacation overseas. Her family took her to a clinic, where blood tests and an ultrasound were performed. The doctor suspected she had *thrombophlebitis* (blood clots in the veins of her legs). Left untreated, this condition can allow clots to travel from the leg and lodge in the blood vessels of the heart or brain, triggering a heart attack or stroke. However, the ultrasound and blood tests came back normal, and Carolee was diagnosed with *phlebitis* (inflammation of the vein) and given *acetaminophen* (Tylenol) for the pain. A week later, she returned to the US and came to my office because she was experiencing a stiff right calf muscle.

Because the results of her ultrasound were normal, I diagnosed Carolee as having *chronic venous insufficiency*—poor blood flow through the veins of the legs. At the time she had severe pain, there was stress on her circulatory system because she was still somewhat overweight, had taken a long flight (which can impede blood flow), walked more than she usually did and may have been mildly dehydrated. She probably had been suffering a degree of poor circulation for some time, but the symptoms manifested because of the excessive walking she did on her vacation. Poor blood flow could have contributed to the recent stiffness in her calf muscle.

Even though her ultrasound was normal, I was concerned about blood clots, so I recommended *nattokinase*, a protein-digesting enzyme capsule that improves circulation through blood vessels and breaks down clot-forming proteins. I also asked her to start taking an herbal formula containing *horse chestnut extract* (made from seeds of the horse chestnut tree)… *butcher's broom root extract* (a shrub from the lily family)… and *gotu kola leaf extract* (a perennial plant native to India, China, Australia and parts of South Africa). Horse chestnut and butcher's broom improve the function of vein valves, so that they prevent the backflow of venous blood. Gotu kola strengthens vein walls, so that they do not distend and pool blood. Carolee had access to a whirlpool tub, so I recommended that four times each day she alternate sitting on the side with her legs in the whirlpool for two minutes and putting her legs in the nearby pool's cooler water for 30 seconds. Alternating hot and cold and the massaging action of the whirlpool improves circulation. Exercise and elevation are recommended for people who don't have access to whirlpools.

Carolee reported great improvement within one week and had no remaining symptoms one month later. She continues to take the supplements to prevent the problem from recurring.

Get Rid of Your
Back Pain Forever

If you've tried everything and still aren't getting relief from back pain, take a lesson from a professional golfer. Two years prior to seeing me, he was ranked in the world's Top 50 golfers and on the PGA's Top 20 earnings list. He was on top of the world—until his back started bothering him.

At first, he thought nothing of it—merely employing ice and heat packs and popping Advil, but the pain wouldn't subside. It got so intense that he started dropping out of events or stopping in the middle of tournaments.

He went to the top sports doctors in the country. He saw orthopedic surgeons, chiropractors, *physiatrists* (MDs who do physical therapy) and acupuncturists. He had tests—X-rays, CT scans and MRIs.

They all yielded the same answer: There was nothing structurally wrong with his back—no narrowed discs, torn muscles, sprained ligaments—none of the usual causes of back pain from sports injury.

Determined to "tough it out," he continued playing while taking painkillers, going for chiropractic adjustments, and even getting injections. Nothing helped. The pain got worse and worse, and so did his ability to play golf. His scores suffered, and he went from playing 30 events per year to just eight. Within a few months, the pain became so excruciating that he could not even swing a golf club. Reluctantly, he dropped off the tour, and it looked like his career was over.

Then a friend told him about my clinic. I sensed his exasperation, but the more he described his mysterious ailment, the more confident I became that I could help him. He exhibited the classic symptoms of a hormonal imbalance—specifically a deficiency in cortisol (produced by the adrenal glands).

Cortisol is best known as the hormone your body makes under stress, but cortisol is much more. One of its primary tasks is to regulate inflammation. If you don't have enough cortisol, inflammation can escalate to cause immense pain.

What causes cortisol deficiency?

With today's go-go lifestyle, people are under constant stress, so their adrenal glands must work overtime to pump more hormones. Strong glands produce plenty of cortisol, but when adrenals become fatigued from too much stress, cortisol production decreases. From day to day, month after month, year after year, the adrenal glands can weaken.

Low cortisol levels are often accompanied by a deficiency in other hormones produced by the adrenals, such as *DHEA*. It's instrumental in helping your body heal from injuries, like the microscopic muscle tears you would get from repeatedly swinging a golf club! The good news is that in the vast majority of cases, adrenal fatigue is not permanent, and neither is the back pain it causes. Simply take the proper remedies to strengthen your glands and give them time to rest and rebuild.

So what happened to the golfer? After confirming the diagnosis with tests, I prescribed the herbs *rhodiola* and *Siberian ginseng*, plus some glandular extracts. I also put him on low-dose DHEA and minute doses of cortisol to take some strain off of his glands and regulate his hormonal levels while his adrenals healed. Within a few days, he was reporting less pain. Six weeks later, he was practicing again, and three months later, he made his comeback—playing in two PGA tournaments back-to-back!

His story is dramatic, but by no means unique. You don't have to be a famous athlete to suffer from adrenal fatigue; I've successfully treated well over a thousand patients—primarily age fifty and over. So if your back pain's resistant to the usual treatments, have your cortisol and DHEA levels checked. *If standard saliva, blood or urine tests indicate deficiencies, discuss the following remedies with your practitioner...*

• **Rhodiola rosea**—500 mg standardized to contain three percent to five percent of *rosavins* twice daily before meals.

• **Adrenal glandular extract**—250 mg, two to three times daily, before meals.

• **Ashwagandha**—250 to 500 mg of a standardized product daily before meals.

• **Pantothenic acid**—500 mg, three times daily with meals, along with a 50 mg B-complex or multi-supplement containing the remaining B vitamins.

• **Vitamin C**—1,000 to 2,000 mg twice daily.

• **DHEA**—Five to 15 mg for women, or 15 to 25 mg for men, daily with breakfast.

• **Cortisol**—2.5 to five mg three-to-four times daily.

Noisy Knuckles and Joints

I sometimes hear from patients who complain about loose joints that crack loudly. Joints that crack usually are not painful but can cause embarrassment—during a business meeting, for example. Joint fluid contains oxygen, nitrogen and carbon dioxide gases, which are released rapidly when the joint is stretched, resulting in a pop. Your ligaments may have gotten too lax, so the bones are not held together tightly. My patients have achieved great improvement using the homeopathic remedy *Calcarea fluorica* (at health-food stores), which provides calcium fluoride (at nontoxic levels) to tighten ligaments. Select a brand labeled "6X potency." Dissolve five tablets in your mouth, three times daily, for eight weeks or until popping subsides.

Another cause of joint cracking is dehydration of the *cartilage* (tough, elastic tissue that covers the ends of bones)—so bones no longer slide over one another smoothly and silently. To increase lubrication, take daily fish-oil supplements (do not use if you take a blood-thinning drug). Choose a product with a combined total of 1,000 mg of *eicosapentaenoic acid* (EPA) and *docosahexaenoic acid* (DHA). Within two months, this should rehydrate your joints, minimizing the snap, crackle and pop.

The Shocking Hidden Cause of Your Chronic Pain and Muscle Weakness… And the Simple Solution to Feeling Like Yourself Again

Do you suffer with unexplained pain and weakness? Or maybe you've even been diagnosed with fibromyalgia, but you're wondering what caused the condition in the first place? Well, it turns out that the answer may lie in, of all places, your neck.

Let me explain…

A common, but often overlooked, cause of fibromyalgia is an underfunctioning thyroid gland, or hypothyroidism. In fact, simply boosting your thyroid hormone levels may be the solution to resolving your pain and muscle weakness once and for all.

The metabolism cataclysm

The surprising link between the thyroid gland and fibromyalgia… and similar pain-related conditions… lies in metabolism, or the process that your cells use to convert food into energy. Every single cell in your body requires thyroid hormone to produce energy known as ATP. When your cells don't produce enough ATP it causes the release of pain signals.

But when enough thyroid hormone is delivered to your cells it allows the energy factories, known as mitochondria, to burn fuel for energy more efficiently.

A study in the journal *Thyroid Science* found that the metabolic rate (burning calories at a resting state) was 33 percent lower in people who have fibromyalgia.[1] A lower metabolic rate can lead to increased pain for people with fibromyalgia as well as fatigue, weight gain, depression, constipation, and headaches. In addition, research has shown that almost a quarter of all people with fibromyalgia have low thyroid. I happen to think that number is low. In my own practice I've found that the vast majority of my patients with fibromyalgia have some degree of low thyroid.

Know these signs and symptoms of low thyroid

- Anxiety
- Arthritis
- Asthma
- Allergies
- Brittle nails
- Cold hands and feet
- Eyebrow loss (especially outer one-third)
- High cholesterol
- Heart palpitations
- Hair loss and thinning
- Dry skin and hair
- Poor memory
- Infertility
- Headaches
- Depression

- Fibromyalgia
- Low libido
- Low body temperature
- PMS
- Fluid retention
- Raynaud's phenomenon
- Carpal tunnel syndrome
- Anemia
- Slow healing
- A puffy face
- Hoarse voice
- Muscle aches, tenderness, and stiffness
- Muscle weakness
- Heavier than normal menstrual periods

Tricky thyroid testing

The truth is most people with an under-functioning thyroid never get properly diagnosed. And, of course, without a proper diagnosis they never get treated for their low levels. If those low levels happen to be at the heart of *your* fibromyalgia symptoms—but you've never actually been diagnosed—you probably haven't had much luck in reducing your pain and muscle weakness.

The trouble lies in the testing. Most doctors rely on an inexpensive blood test known as the thyroid stimulating hormone or TSH test. A gland in your brain called the pituitary releases this hormone when it senses your blood levels of thyroid hormones are getting low. TSH stimulates your thyroid to produce more thyroid hormone.

An optimal TSH range is 0.5 to two (common reference range is 0.5 to 4.5 µIU/mL). However, as it turns out, TSH is not a very sensitive marker to identify if thyroid hormone is low *in* your tissues. In other words, a normal TSH test result doesn't necessarily mean that you don't have thyroid problems. The results can be misleading. But, unfortunately, many doctors don't keep up with the scientific literature and they're simply unaware of how limited the test really is. So the TSH remains the "gold standard" for many docs, and a lot of patients go undiagnosed as a result.

Your thyroid gland produces two main thyroid hormones, known as Free T4 (free thyroxine) and Free T3 (triiodothyronine). The term "free" refers to the *active* form of these hormones because most hormones that circulate in the blood are bound to a protein carrier and are inactive.

A good level of Free T4 is 1.2 ng/L or higher (common reference range is 0.8 to 1.8 ng/L). A good value of Free T3 is above three pg/mL (common reference range is 2.3 to 4.2 pg/mL). In general the higher the Free T3 the better you feel. This is because T3 is the most active thyroid hormone in your body and good levels mean better cell energy production and less pain.

Clearly your Free T4 and Free T3 levels are important indicators. But there's more to the story. Instead of measuring the amount of FREE thyroid hormones *within* your cells the test measures the amount of circulating thyroid hormones in your blood. But the amount of circulating thyroid hormones in your blood is not a good indicator of how much of the free thyroid hormones there are *inside* the cells.

You see, the circulating hormones still have to cross cell membranes and get into your cells to have activity. This means a test can say you have normal blood thyroid hormone levels, but you may still have low levels in the cells where it *really* counts. And to complicate matters even further your cells can become resistant to thyroid hormone. This is similar to people with type 2 diabetes when their pancreas produces enough insulin, but the cells do not readily accept this hormone that transports glucose into the cells. So ultimately one can have low thyroid function that's not detectable with a blood test!

There are a number of things that can contribute to your cells becoming resistant to thyroid hormones. Among them are...

- Chronic stress
- Chronic illness
- Genetic abnormalities
- Autoimmune thyroid
- Chemicals that interfere with cell thyroid receptors including:

Polychlorinated biphenyl (PCB): Chemicals that are no longer used, but still are in the environment. They were used for consumer items

---

Nutrients you need to convert T4 into T3

• Iodine	• Zinc	• B2	• B12
• Selenium	• Vitamin A	• B6	

Note: The herb ashwaganda can help with this conversion process.

including electrical equipment, fluorescent lights, plastics, and more.

Polybrominated diphenylethers (PBDEs): A class of toxic chemicals in wide used as fire retardants. They're found in common home items such as carpet, bedding, couches, and television screens.

Triclosan: An antifungal and antibacterial agent found in common household products such as toothpaste, mouthwash, cleaning supplies, skin care, clothing, and bedding.

Bisphenol A (BPA): An industrial chemical used in many hard plastic bottles and metal-based food and beverage cans since the 1960s.

Pesticides.

Drugs: Medications, especially those used for anxiety including diazepam (Valium), lorazepam (Atavan), and alprazolam (Xanax) have been observed to prevent T3 uptake.

Keeping tabs on your temperature

As strange as it may sound your average body temperature can play an important role in assessing your thyroid function. To figure out your average body temperature on several different days, at least three hours after waking up, take your temperature. Then take it two more times on each of those days about 3 hours apart. Average all of the numbers when you're done and if your average temperature is below 98.6°F then you likely have some level of low thyroid function.

T3-the superstar of thyroid therapy

There are studies that show that the T3 hormone is quite effective in reducing the muscle pain associated with fibromyalgia. In fact, approximately 75 percent of fibromyalgia patients improve with T3 therapy.[2,3] Under normal conditions… when everything is working as it should… your thyroid takes up iodine that you have ingested from your diet or supplements, and manufactures T4 and T3 hormone. Your liver and kidneys also use a number of different common nutrients (see the box above for a list of them) to convert T4 into the more active T3.

A high-potency multivitamin and mineral formula can supply most of your daily needs of these nutrients with the exception of iodine for patients who are deficient. You should work with a holistic doctor to make sure you have enough of these nutrients so that your body can manufacture the thyroid hormones it needs.

The importance of iodine

Estimates are that 70 percent of the world's population is low in iodine. Salt is the main source of the nutrient in the American diet, but many adults actively avoid it because of concerns about high blood pressure. However, the fact is, only up to 10 percent of people with high blood pressure actually benefit from cutting back on salt.

Iodine has many important functions in the human body, including the production of thyroid hormone. The recommended daily allowance for the nutrient in adults is 150 mcg. But, according to most nutrition-oriented doctors like me this is laughably low. To put things into perspective this is the same daily dose recommended by some veterinarians for a cat that weighs about 10 pounds!

In Japan, where they eat a lot of seaweed, the average person consumes around 13,800 mcg of iodine a day. You can increase your iodine intake with seaweed products, but you should always use caution because seaweed products may be contaminated with toxic metals such as arsenic. If you decide to eat more seaweed make sure they come from a reputable company you can trust that screens for heavy metal contamination. And remember supplementation with iodine above 500 mcg should be done only under a doctor's supervision.

I've had many patients ask me about the Skin Iodine Test as a simple way to measure your iodine needs. The test involves applying an iodine solution to the skin and observing how fast it disappears. The theory is that the speed at which the iodine disappears allows you to draw a correlation with low body iodine stores, since your body somehow wants to "suck up" the iodine through your skin.

Well I hate to be the bearer of bad news, but the Skin Iodine Test is based on shoddy science and doesn't represent your body's iodine stores at all. Guy Abraham, MD, studied this issue and found no value with this type of testing.[4] The fact is that 88 percent of iodine isn't normally absorbed by the skin. And besides, temperature and atmospheric pressure can affect skin absorption as well. Skip the Skin Iodine Test and check with your holistic doctor instead. He can order urine and blood tests to identify iodine deficiency.

Topping off your T3 with supplements

Many patients with fibromyalgia or chronic fatigue (both conditions have similar symptoms) respond well to supplements that boost T3 or direct T3 hormone replacement. If other holistic therapies such as improving your diet and supplementing with other helper nutrients haven't worked hormone supplements may be the answer.

T3 hormone supplements require a prescription and monitoring by a doctor. Many patients notice a significant improvement in muscle pain, mood, and energy within just two to four weeks of starting treatment. Signs you're getting too much T3 include a fast pulse, chest pain, heart palpitations, anxiety, and insomnia. These symptoms will go away once the T3 dose is reduced or stopped.

The best way to use T3 is in a sustained release formula twice a day since the hormone wears off so quickly in the body. I've seen patients benefit from as little as five mcg daily and all the way up to 150 mcg daily.

Unfortunately the majority of mainstream doctors… and even most endocrinologists… aren't aware of the research that shows how effective and safe T3 therapy is. If this is the case with your doc work with a holistic doctor instead to find out if T3 can help you. Statistically you have a 75 percent chance of benefitting. Great odds if you ask me.

T3 sustained release is available by prescription from a local compounding pharmacy. I offer this type of therapy at my clinic. If you are looking for a referral to someone who understands T3 therapy you can try the Association for the Advancement of Restorative Medicine (www.restorativemedicine.org) and the folks at Wilson's Temperature Syndrome (www.wilsonssyndrome.com).

Conquer Fibromyalgia Pain and Fatigue with This Potent "Vitamin Cocktail"

Chronic, wide spread muscular pain, sleep problems, and fatigue. If any of this sounds familiar you may be one of the over 5 million Americans that has fibromyalgia. And if you listen to the National Institute of Arthritis and Musculoskeletal and Skin Diseases you may just have to learn to live with it because, according to NIAMS, "Fibromyalgia can be difficult to treat." And they're right, if you're practicing conventional medicine. Prescriptions for pain medications and antidepressants are the mainstream medical approach and they can often provide mild benefits, but come accompanied by a host of potential side effects.

But imagine if there was a natural treatment that's highly effective for almost anyone suffering with fibromyalgia—as well as those struggling with chronic fatigue? Well, you can stop imagining; because such a therapy *does* exist, and I've witnessed it work time and time again over the years.

Increase energy production and reduce pain and fatigue

This targeted "miracle" treatment speeds key nutrients directly into your system using an IV. This special "vitamin cocktail" provides nutrients that help your cells increase energy intake an essential step for successfully treating fibromyalgia. You see, the more power the energy factories in your cells, known as mitochondria, produce the less pain signals your body creates. B vitamins, magnesium, and minerals such as potassium, chromium, calcium, and zinc all help provide the ingredients your cells need to generate the critical components that fuel energy, known as ATP.

By using an IV you can achieve at least ten times (some references suggest up to 100 times) the levels of these critical nutrients in your blood stream and cells as you could if you simply swallowed some pills instead. The goal is to flood your cells with these energy sparkplugs and let them do the rest.

Most fibromyalgia sufferers will notice improvement in their muscular pain and energy levels within one to two treatments. I usually have patients receive one treatment a week for five weeks. Almost everyone will notice great improvement within the five treatments. The IV therapy can then be continued at this point, or you can switch over to oral nutrients.

Thousands have successfully used modified Meyer's Cocktails

The classic intravenous formula that's been used by holistic doctors over the years is known as the "Meyers' Cocktail." It was pioneered by a medical doctor John Myers from Baltimore, Maryland. Myers used the intravenous formula for a variety of medical problems. His cocktail contained B vitamins, vitamin C, magnesium, and calcium.

Dr. Meyers passed away in 1984. Since then thousands of holistic doctors have been using modified versions of his formula. I too have tweaked the original formula over the years developing my own version which I call the "Energizer Formula." The following nutrients are diluted in a sterile bag of normal saline.

- B complex

- B12 (separate from the B complex)

- Folic acid (separate from the B complex)

- Vitamin C

- Calcium

- Magnesium

- Trace elements mixture including zinc, selenium, chromium, copper, and manganese.

I often follow up my "Energizer Formula" with a dose of the master antioxidant glutathione. The glutathione isn't mixed with the other nutrients to preserve its stability.

While the B vitamins, magnesium, and glutathione directly support energy production, the other nutrients help reduce inflammation and improve detoxification. As well, higher levels of magnesium reduce tight muscles and relax the nervous system.

The entire treatment takes about 30 minutes and, of course, this treatment should only be administered by a doctor trained in intravenous nutrient therapy.

Within just two treatments pain and fatigue improved!

A clinical trial published in the journal *Alternative Therapies* demonstrated just how effective this approach can be. Researchers used a modified Myers' Cocktail to treat a group of female fibromyalgia patients. All of the volunteers in the trial suffered with severe symptoms and reported a very poor quality of life as a result. They had all been living with their symptoms for at least five years and conventional medical treatments had failed.

The researchers administered weekly treatments of the cocktail to all of the volunteers. By week two, when the second cocktail was given *all* of the participants had a decrease in both pain and fatigue! And by the end of the 8 week clinical trial pain levels and fatigue had improved *significantly.*

There's no single cause for fibromyalgia. But the nice thing about the intravenous nutrient therapy is that it's well tolerated and helps the majority of patients with fibromyalgia, as well as those with fatigue, *regardless* of the cause. The concept is very simple increase energy production and you reduce body pain.

Identify and eliminate the problem at the source

While I like to use intravenous nutrient therapy with patients to help them get some immediate relief from the pain and fatigue my ultimate goal is track down the root cause of their fibromyalgia and fatigue. I typically use a combination of lab testing and good old-fashioned doctor detective work, evaluating each patient's unique symptoms. I find that some people have one main cause, while others have several.

Following are the most common root causes I have found:

• Hormone imbalance (particularly for fibromyalgia which mainly affects women)

• Sleep disorders (including sleep apnea)

• Allergies or Sensitivities to food, chemicals, and other environmental factors

• Toxins in the body such as toxic metals (lead, arsenic, mercury, and others)

• Poor digestion and detoxification

• Chronic infections

• Neurotransmitter (brain chemical) imbalance

- Blood sugar imbalance

- Nutritional deficiencies

- Emotional stress

- Poor circulation (hyper viscous blood)

- Poor stress management

- Autoimmunity

- Structural imbalances (particularly those with history of whiplash from motor vehicle accidents)

Once I track down the root cause, or causes, of a patient's pain and fatigue I can then create a comprehensive and individual plan for eliminating their problem at the source.

Fighting fibromyalgia one supplement at a time

Besides intravenous nutrients there are a number of other supplements I have found to be effective in treating fibromyalgia:

D-Ribose—this naturally occurring sugar improves energy production in all the cells of the body, including the muscle cells. A study published in the *Journal of Alternative and Complementary Medicine* found people with fibromyalgia and/or chronic fatigue syndrome supplemented with five grams of D ribose three times daily had significant improvement in energy, sleep, mental clarity, pain intensity, and well-being. A good starting dose is five grams three times daily blended in water and then after two to four weeks five grams twice daily works well as a maintenance dose. D-Ribose does not adversely affect blood sugar levels for people with diabetes or hypoglycemia.

Magnesium—important not only for energy production and detoxification but to keep the nervous system and muscles relaxed. I typically have patients supplement magnesium glycinate or a chelated form at a dose of 250 mg two to three times daily. If you have loose stools cut back on the dosage.

Methylsulfonylmethane (MSM)—a very effective and non-toxic supplement to relieve pain and stiffness of both the muscles and joints. A typical dose is 3,000 mg to 5,000 mg twice daily. Reduce the dose if you get loose stool.

5-hydroxytryptophan (5HTP)—used as an amino acid precursor to help the brain produce the brain chemical serotonin. Increased serotonin levels help reduce pain signals. It has been shown in studies to reduce fibromyalgia symptoms including pain severity, morning stiffness, and sleeplessness." Don't take this supplement if you are on psychiatric medications.

S'adenosylmethionine (SAMe)—known as "Sammy" this supplement has been shown to be effective for fibromyalgia. It acts as a "methyl donor" allowing a whole host of chemical reactions to occur in the body including the production of neurotransmitters such as serotonin. There have been two clinical trials demonstrating significant improvement in symptoms of fibromyalgia when compared to placebo.'

Work with your own doctor to determine which supplements are best for you. Also, as with any inflammatory condition, diet is important. You should be eating foods that fuel energy production and reduce inflammation, such as those found in the Mediterranean diet. Make sure to keep grains to a minimum, especially gluten containing varieties including wheat, barley, and rye. Simple sugars and alcohol increase inflammation so eliminate them from your diet. And be sure to keep red meat to a minimum.

This Common Drug—Not Old Age—Could Be the REAL Cause of Your Aching Painful Joints

If I had a dollar for every patient who has come to me complaining of joint pain after starting a cholesterol-lowering statin drug… well, let's just say I'd have a heck of a lot of dollars. Most of them arrive not only in pain, but frustrated too, since they've virtually been ignored by their cardiologists or prescribing physicians when they mentioned the problem. My solution is simple… stop the medication, and follow a naturopathic program designed to balance lipids and resolve the deeper causes of cardiovascular disease. As a result most of these patients not only begin to put heart disease in the rearview mirror, their joint pain starts to fade away too.

Study links statins to muscle and joint injuries

Since joint pain is a common statin side effect I wasn't at all surprised when a recent study, published in a major medical journal, concluded that statin drugs are associated with an increased risk of musculoskeletal injuries.[1] According to researchers, this includes an increased risk of dislocations, strains, and sprains. More specifically, they found that treatment with a statin was associated with a 19 percent increased risk of any type of musculoskeletal injury, a 13 percent increased risk of dislocations, strains, and sprains, and a nine percent increased risk of musculoskeletal pain.[2]

This was no small study either. It included 6,967 statin users and compared their symptoms to that of an equal amount of people who were not taking statins. Most of the treatment group (73.5 percent), were taking the statin drug simvastatin, known better as Zocor.

If you're on a statin and have been experiencing any muscle or joint symptoms you should try talking to your doctor about stopping the medication to see if your symptoms disappear. If you find that your concerns aren't being taken seriously it's time to find a new doctor. I recommend a naturopathic doctor who can help you resolve your cholesterol issues naturally with diet, exercise, and targeted supplements.

There are a number of tried and true natural lipid balancers that I've seen work successfully again and again over the years. Note that I use the word *balancers* since unlike the conventional medicine approach my goal isn't solely focused on suppressing cholesterol levels. I also target and correct for the underlying causes of heart disease including chronic inflammation, nutrient deficiencies, stress, genetics, medications, obesity, diet,

---

Potential statin side effects

- Abdominal cramping and/or pain
- Bloating and/or gas
- Constipation
- Diarrhea
- Difficulty sleeping
- Dizziness
- Drowsiness
- Flushing of the skin
- Headache
- High blood sugar (Type 2 diabetes)
- Infection
- Kidney damage
- Liver damage
- Memory Loss
- Mental Confusion
- Muscle aches, tenderness, or weakness (myalgia)
- Nausea and/or vomiting
- Rash

toxic metals and other pollutants, damaged or oxidized LDL cholesterol, and hormone deficiencies.

The ridiculously delicious cholesterol-busting diet

It seems a week doesn't go by without learning a new benefit of the delicious and heart-healthy Mediterranean diet. One of the more recent large studies included 7,400 people from the Mediterranean (mainly Spain) who were at high risk for heart disease with conditions such as high blood pressure and diabetes. Researchers compared two Mediterranean-style diets (one with an emphasis on extra virgin olive oil and the other with an emphasis on nuts like walnuts, almonds, hazelnuts) to that of a low fat diet (the standard American cardiology diet for heart-disease prevention).

The calorie count for both groups was controlled. And volunteers were randomly assigned to one of the three diet groups. Exercise and weight reduction were not part of the protocols.

The volunteers on the Mediterranean diets replaced red meats with white meats like chicken and ate three or more servings of fish each week. In addition, they ate three or more servings of fruit and two or more servings of vegetables a day and replaced used *extra virgin* olive oil which contains more vitamin E compounds and anti-inflammatory phytonutrients known as polyphenols.

Those on the low fat diet also ate three or more servings of fish or seafood a week and the same amount of fruits and vegetables. However, they were discouraged from consuming more than two tablespoons of vegetable oils a day, including olive oil.

The results were astounding. Overall, for those on the Mediterranean style diets, there was a 30 percent reduction in what's called "the primary endpoint," a combination of strokes, heart attacks, and deaths. In fact, the positive results that were seen were so compelling that the study was stopped early.[3] It's clear that at the very least we should be including extra virgin olive oil and nuts into our regular diet.

Super supplements for happy hearts

There are a number of natural lipid-balancing supplements that can help you reduce your cardiovascular risk without aching joints or musculoskeletal injuries coming along for the ride. Let's go over a few of my favorites that I routinely use with my own patients with great results.

Indian Gooseberry extract has been studied in humans and found to effectively balance lipid levels. Published research showed that Amlamax®, an extract form of Indian Gooseberry, taken at a dose of 500 mg twice a day for four months reduced total cholesterol by 17 percent, LDL cholesterol by 21 percent, and triglycerides by 24 percent. Good HDL cholesterol also rose by 15 percent.

Researchers found no differences in liver and kidney function tests as compared to those taking placebo.[4] Interestingly, animal studies show that this extract has something in common with statin drugs. Like statins, Amlamax® apparently suppresses an enzyme in the liver known as HMG CoA reductase that's needed to produce cholesterol. Yet unlike the drugs there haven't been any detrimental side effects found. This could be because as a natural food extract it's more compatible with human receptors than a synthetic drug, so the same kind of cell damage doesn't occur.

Omega 7 fatty acid is the new kid on the fatty acid block. Research at the world famous Cleveland Clinic, has shown that omega 7's can reduce total and LDL cholesterol, as well as triglycerides. The type of omega 7 that has been studied is a highly purified form extracted from fish called Provinal®. In an animal study Provinal® greatly improved plaque ridden arteries. Findings like these may be why leading doctors like Dr. Michael Roizen (co-author of *You: The Owner's Manual* with Dr. Oz) are so excited about the therapeutic potential of omega 7 and have recommend Provinal®, a rich supplemental source of the omega fatty acid.

Coenzyme Q10 (CoQ10) is a must for anyone concerned about cardiovascular disease and healthy lipid levels. One of the unique features of CoQ10 is that it reduces the *oxidation* of LDL cholesterol. As I've explained before, it's oxidation of cholesterol that triggers the inflammation and plaque formation in our arteries. One major medical journal published data showing that the oxidized LDL levels in patients who had heart attacks was about 3.5-fold higher than that of control subjects.[5]

Phytosterols are naturally occurring chemicals found in small amounts in foods such as fruits, vegetables, nuts, seeds, legumes, and other plant sources. Phytosterols are so effective at balancing cholesterol levels that even the FDA allows health claims on supplement labels to say that they can help reduce the risk of heart disease. These naturally occurring compounds work by inhibiting the cholesterol in your food from being absorbed into your digestive tract. I typically recommend 1,000 mg of phytosterols with each regular meal.

Fish oil is a great choice if you have high triglycerides. In fact, the patented drug form of prescription fish oil known as Lovaza® is specifically approved for this use. However you can spend a fraction of the cost by using high potency, good quality fish oil instead. The general dose is 3,000 to 4,000 mg daily of EPA and DHA.

Red Yeast Rice is my old stand by for those who have genetically high LDL cholesterol or for those who can't get their cardiologist off their back without lowering their lipid levels. It's been shown to significantly reduce the risk of heart attacks and other heart related events.[6] And unlike statins Red Yeast Rice hasn't been linked to joint, muscle, or liver damage.

Bergamot is an exciting, relatively new natural compound for lowering lipids. A twice daily dose of 500 mg of this food extract has been found to significantly reduce total cholesterol, LDL cholesterol, and triglycerides in just 30 days. At the same time, Bergamot increases good HDL cholesterol while lowering blood sugar levels.[7] This makes it a great choice for those who have both diabetes and cholesterol issues.

The Drug-Free Back Pain Solution

Few things are as frustrating as a visit to the doctor for back pain. According to conventional medicine there are only four ways to treat your pain... rest and wait, injections, heavy-duty pain medications, or surgery.

Before you know it you're locked into an endless parade of expensive doctor's visits filled with painful injections and prescriptions for toxic drugs that are likely to leave you strung out and addicted. Or you're stuck in a hospital bed recovering from a major operation praying that it was a success.

And do you want to know what the worst part is?

You may have been able to avoid it all.

Imagine a treatment for your chronic aching back or searing sciatica pain that doesn't require dangerous addictive pain medications or injections. A treatment that will not only help you avoid the surgeon's scalpel, but one that's so non-invasive that it doesn't even require anyone ever touching your body!

Because when you boil it down back pain is just like any other kind of pain and just like any other kind of pain it can be treated nutritionally. In fact, it only requires a couple capsules a day of a non-toxic ingredient that's already produced naturally in your body!

You'll be amazed at just how simple this solution is. I'll give you all the details on this nutritional pain breakthrough in just a few moments, but first let me shine some light on what's *really* going on back there when the pain kicks in.

Tracking down the real cause of back pain

They say misery loves company and if that's really the case, then you'll be happy to know that you're far from alone with your back pain. In fact, low back pain is the second most common reason for a visit to a doctor and for approximately five percent of the population it becomes a chronic problem.

One of the most common causes of low back pain is a degenerated disc. The lumbar discs have been compared to a jelly donut with a tough outer layer and soft, jelly-like material within. They act as "cushions" between each vertebra and they function like a shock absorber between the vertebral bodies when you move, twist, or lift.

Studies have found that by the age of 50, almost 95 percent of adults show some evidence of degenerative disc disease.[1] Degeneration of the disc makes it more likely to rupture or herniate which irritates the surrounding nerves leading to localized low back pain or the radiating pain that you find with sciatica.

But it turns out that it's what your discs are *made of* that could hold the key to reversing that back pain.

Knock out back pain, no injections no surgery

This mysterious substance isn't that mysterious at all. In fact, it's collagen.

Collagen is a very common substance in the human body. Composed of a chain of amino acids it acts like a sort of "glue" that provides the

A collagen supplement may be all you need to start reversing your back pain. But if you want to be more aggressive consider these additional back-supporting supplements:

- Methylsulfonylmethane (MSM) - 3,000 to 6,000 mg

- Glucosamine sulphate - 1,500 mg

- Chondroitin sulphate - 1,200 mg

building blocks of connective tissue as found in blood vessels, ligaments, tendons, and bones. It is also a primary component of skin, hair, and nails.

I've written to you before about studies that have concluded that collagen is great for both osteoarthritis and rheumatoid arthritis. It's also a great nutritional aid for the skin, hair, and nails—since they are all composed in part by collagen. But I've discovered over the years that collagen is also effective for both low back pain and the accompanying radiating nerve pain known as sciatica.

You see, collagen and another component found in collagen called hyaluronic acid (HA) are key components of your vertebral discs. They provide strength and elasticity. In addition, they help retain water in your discs creating a cushioning effect. But as you age the quality of the collagen inside your discs starts to fall.

A natural "prescription" for fast and permanent pain relief

Now before you run off and get yourself a bottle of collagen, you need to be sure you're getting the right form. The fact is, if you use the wrong kind you're wasting your money and you're not going to see the results you're looking for.

You see, regular collagen is too large of a molecule to be effectively absorbed in the digestive tract. But studies have been done that demonstrate absorption does occur with specially designed types of supplemental collagen. One well-studied form is Type 2 collagen, known as Undenatured Collagen Type II or UC II.

While there aren't any studies completed yet that look specifically at collagen as a treatment for low back pain, I have first hand experience using it with patients. I have found that it does work very well for people with degenerated discs that are causing low back pain and sciatica.

Take, for example, the experience of an 83 year-old patient of mine. After suffering with a lifetime of chronic lower back pain and sciatica she eventually found her way to my office. I advised her to start supplementing with 40 mg of UC II a day. Within just two short months she reported to me that her low back pain had retreated and her sciatica had all but disappeared. While I have heard it many times before, I was still amazed and thrilled her pain was alleviated by such a simple treatment.

You can get started on reversing your own degenerated disc pain today using a collagen supplement from your local health food store. Start with 40 mg of Undenatured Collagen Type II.

Be sure you're also drinking adequate purified water—at least 60 oz daily to keep your discs hydrated. And should you find that collagen alone isn't eliminating your pain fast enough chiropractic, acupuncture, physical therapy, and cold laser therapy are other non-invasive treatments that you can try.

If You Don't Want Stiff, Sore Joints Slowing You Down… You Owe It to Yourself to See This Discovery That Researchers Say Gives Twice the Joint Relief of Glucosamine and Chondroitin

What if there was a way you could help keep your knees healthy, strong and flexible for years to come? To help guard against daily wear and tear and keep them functioning well?

Same for your hips, shoulders, hands and joints?

What if it was safe, natural, and cost less than a dollar a day?

And what if it contained a powerful nutrient that was scientifically shown to give you twice the relief of glucosamine and chondroitin?

The secret to keeping discomfort at bay in your overworked joints is now easier than you think…

Skeptical? That's okay. But please hear me out. As a doctor, I only trust clinically researched ingredients. That's why in a moment, you'll read all about an eye-opening clinical study that documents how this natural phenomenon is far superior to glucosamine and chondroitin.

But first, I want you to know the shocking truth why so many popular supplements fall flat on their faces…

Many of my patients ask me, "Why is it that some natural joint supplements don't work for me?" Or, "Why do they help at first, then stop working?"

Important questions, especially if your joints feel like they're on fire after that long run… your knees creak… your shoulder feels like it's been in a deep freeze from an afternoon in your garden… or your hips hurt like crazy every once in a while.

Here's what I tell them, to their surprise…

The main reason a joint support supplement doesn't work or stops working is it fails to address the root causes of your joint problems.

Take glucosamine and chondroitin, for example. You may know they help support healthy joints by providing special proteins you need for healthy cartilage, joint fluid and tendons.

But as good as glucosamine and chondroitin are, we now know they don't address ALL of the "triggers"—such as inflammation or free radical attack. So you still hurt.

Some folks still suffer from occasional discomfort and stiffness because other formulas don't deliver the best combination of nutrients they need to be effective.

And still many suffer because other formulas are not manufactured to ensure the optimal efficacy of the ingredients… in fact, they may not work at all.

Well, these "solutions" weren't good enough for my patients. So I set out to find something better.

Now I'm pleased to report something that addresses ALL of these limitations. And it starts with UC-II® collagen…

A recent discovery that supports joint health, mobility and flexibility differently than glucosamine and chondroitin, and one study showed it can give you more than twice as much relief…

If you try to stay active you know what it feels like to suffer from stiffness and other nagging joint issues, especially the day after you exercise. You want relief based on researched results! And nothing I've seen has more solid scientific evidence and superior results than the extraordinary natural breakthrough, UC-II collagen.

Collagen is a natural protein—a major component of connective tissue that holds your joints together and provides elasticity so you can move easily. In addition, collagen is vital for cartilage production and repair.

The problem is, as you age, your collagen levels continue to decline… but when you take a clinically tested dosage of collagen—especially with a biologically available form of collagen like UCII— you can experience increased joint mobility and flexibility, like you enjoyed years ago!

In fact, NEW research shows that UC-II helps relieve overworked joints. Healthy volunteers who felt discomfort during and after activity took 40 mg per day of UC-II. An exercise test showed that the subjects were able to go longer without discomfort and recovered quicker from their post-exercise discomfort when compared to their baseline values. As an added bonus, they even experience greater range of motion in their knees.

Need more proof? You can imagine my excitement when I discovered another recent clinical study showed that UC-II outperforms glucosamine and chondroitin.

When I seek out new natural health solutions for my patients, I'm not easily impressed. I'm very picky, and I'm looking for outstanding results.

Well, I think I've found it in UC-II, and I'm not alone. In this double-blind study, subjects took either a daily dose of 40 mg of UC-II or a daily dose of 1,500 mg of glucosamine and 1,200 mg of chondroitin for 90 days.

Landmark Clinical Study Results

- More than TWICE as much improvement in comfort and flexibility in lower limbs reported by participants who took UC-II for three months rather than glucosamine and chondroitin

- More than DOUBLE the improvement reported by patients for everyday aches and pains with UC-II versus glucosamine and chondroitin

- UC-II patients reported more than three times better joint mobility after 90 days, than those taking glucosamine and chondroitin

- The results were clearly in favor of UC-II

If you're concerned about everyday wear and tear, getting twice as much support is like hitting the jackpot!

Why such remarkable results? Because it works on multiple levels to help aging joints.

First, UC-II is uniquely formulated in a patented, low-temperature process. This is unlike other forms of collagen where the manufacturing process alters the ingredient's molecular structure. Because of this cutting-edge process, UC-II is structurally superior, fast-acting and biologically available for superior joint support.

Then, UC-II works with your immune system to promote a healthy inflammatory response—again, something glucosamine and chondroitin don't do.

Add to that, UC-II provides the building blocks to healthy joint cartilage… and you have a totally unique, natural breakthrough that helps address your joint wear and tear delivers more relief for occasional joint stiffness and soreness.

For many of my patients, their relief is "off the charts!"

When patients at my clinic take UC-II, some tell me it doubles their overall improvement—to as much as 90 percent. Even better, you're invited to try the same UC-II my patients swear by—ound in my Joint Performance Plus formula.

To you, this can mean enjoying an active lifestyle, keeping up with the kids, perfecting your golf game or walking, shopping and dancing without having to worry about how you'll feel later.

It's a fact: My Joint Performance Plus formula would be a powerhouse if it only contained UC-II. But my team asked me to go one step further and issued this challenge: Could I pick the very best of the other nutrients I recommend to my patients for maximum support and combine them with UC-II into one revolutionary, natural formula? So I reviewed research studies, analyzed my patients' charts and confirmed their successes.

The result? A revolutionary six-in-one formula.

My vision for Joint Performance Plus was to bring together six of the most powerful nutrients for joint comfort and flexibility into one formula.

You may wonder, "Why should I take more than one nutrient for my joints?" Good question. My answer: Joint health is a complex issue, often with many different causes. The more causes you address, the more support you get!

Joint Performance Plus is the result of what I call "high-level healing"... what doctors like myself do.

That is, when treating patients I target the wear and tear that comes with age. Meaning, I often combine several nutrients for even greater, synergistic effect. And for the first time ever, all of the "best of the best" nutrients I give my patients for their occasional joint stiffness and discomfort are found in one single formula—and available to YOU.

As you'll see now, my formula, Joint Performance Plus, helps address all of the major causes of age-related discomfort and everyday aches to help you...

- form strong, healthy cartilage

- promote a healthy inflammatory response

- support flexibility

- reduce the breakdown of cartilage

- increase circulation

- inhibit joint-damaging free radicals

This is possible because, along with UC-II, this one-of-a-kind formula includes five more ingredients that give you the best joint support you've ever felt.

My Joint Performance Plus formula also includes a special form of turmeric—over 20 times more absorbable than ordinary turmeric

For centuries, natural healers in India have used the spice turmeric to help maintain healthy joints, and I've used it with good results at my clinic for years. Turmeric supports two aspects of joint comfort. First, as a powerful antioxidant, it quells joint damaging free radicals. Second, it even helps promote a healthy response to inflammation.

Yet there's a big problem: Ordinary turmeric is poorly absorbed by your body, so you have to take mega-doses to get the results you need. But my Joint Performance Plus formula includes a unique, highly absorbable form of turmeric—the only one I use.

This special form of turmeric is over 20 times more absorbable than typical turmeric—and that means more support for you! Plus I've included...

Grape seed extract with 20 to 50 times more joint-supporting antioxidant power than vitamin E and vitamin C. That's right, some people take vitamins C and E to neutralize free radicals, but these vitamins don't even come close to matching the antioxidant power of grape seed extract...

Grape seed extract has 20 times MORE antioxidant power than vitamin E and 50 times MORE antioxidant power than vitamin C.

And making sure you're getting enough antioxidants is one of the greatest things you can do to keep your joints healthy because they help neutralize the free radicals that can damage your joints.

What's more, grape seed extract can help improve circulation in the tiny vessels and capillaries that deliver critical nutrients all over your body, including your joints, so you can get even more relief.

Yet my Joint Performance Plus is even more powerful with ginger-root powder to help ease stiff joints and aid absorption of all the nutrients in this formula...

Ginger has long been prized and praised for centuries for easing stiffness and helping keep joints loose and comfortable. But ginger also improves your digestion, to help you better absorb all of the unique relief-giving nutrients in this formula. This is especially important if you're concerned about digestive reactions to supplements.

Plus, I've included pomegranate extract, with far more antioxidant clout than other super fruits, to help keep your joints strong and healthy...

Pomegranate, one of the oldest cultivated fruits in the world, has superior antioxidant strength for suppressing free radicals. But don't just take my word for it. Its ORAC level (a test developed at Tufts University that measures how effectively an antioxidant absorbs free radicals) is 10,500, for 3.5 ounces of the fruit which is more than twice as much as blackberries... three times more than blueberries... and nearly four times more than red raspberries.

In addition, pomegranate extract has been shown in vitro to help block the inflammatory molecule that plays a key role in cartilage breakdown.

Finally, my exclusive Joint Performance Plus formula includes a highly purified form of MSM that helps support strong, flexible and healthy joints!

MSM is the natural sulfur compound that can play a big part in helping you keep healthy connective tissue and joints. Joint Performance Plus includes a form of MSM superior to any other I've seen. It's distilled (which makes it purer), not crystallized, like typical MSM.

Even more important, an in-vitro study at the University of California report that the very same form of MSM found in my formula helps protect your cartilage from joint damaging enzymes that could cause wear and tear.

The best news of all… For the first time, you can order my Joint Performance Plus and get the exact same nutrients I give my patients for superior results. There's no other formula I stand behind that's as potent as Joint Performance Plus—in fact, it's the best joint support you've ever felt—and we guarantee it or your money back!

To order Joint Performance Plus, visit www.besthealthnutritionals.com or call 1-800-539-1447 and mention code G653PC02 to receive an exclusive 20 percent discount. As a loyal *Health Revelations* reader, you are always covered by Dr. Stengler's "Anytime Guarantee." If you're not completely satisfied for ANY reason at all—at ANY time—return the unused portion for a FULL refund, less shipping, even if you're on the last capsule in the bottle! No questions asked, and no explanations needed.

PART II

Cancer

Wheat Germ Extract:
A Promising New Cancer Fighter

Wheat germ was one of the original health foods. The "germ" is the most nutritious part of the wheat seed. Today fermented wheat germ extract (FWGE) is showing promise as a potential breakthrough for treating cancer patients.

The evidence: A number of cell, animal and human studies support the use and benefits of FWGE as an adjunct therapy, meaning one that is used as part of a broader treatment program.

• **Colorectal cancer**. A study of 170 patients who had received conventional treatments for colorectal cancer found that those who also took nine grams of FWGE daily for six months had less risk of developing new cancers. The cancer spread among only eight percent of the patients receiving FWGE, compared with 23 percent of those getting only conventional treatment.

• **Oral cancer**. Researchers compared 22 patients with oral cancer who took FWGE with 21 patients not receiving the supplement. FWGE reduced the risk for cancer progression by 85 percent.

• **Melanoma**. For one year, FWGE was given to 22 patients with advanced (stage 3) melanoma, and their progress was compared with 24 similar patients not receiving FWGE. Patients taking FWGE were half as likely to die from melanoma during this time.

• **Chemotherapy-induced infections**. Researchers studied 22 children and teenagers with different types of cancer. The 11 children who received FWGE had significantly fewer infections and fevers while they received chemotherapy.

• **Animal studies**. Numerous studies suggest benefits from FWGE for leukemia as well as breast, ovarian, gastric and thyroid cancers. In one study, laboratory rats received both FWGE and vitamin C in the treatment of lung, skin and colon cancers.

The combination prevented the cancer from spreading, but vitamin C alone did not. In another study, FWGE worked better alone than it did with vitamin C to treat kidney cancer.

How it works

FWGE appears to work by starving cancer cells of glucose, prompting their death... and by enhancing immune cell activity. Wheat germ contains chemicals that seem to have anticancer properties, and fermentation increases their concentration.

Note: FWGE is very different from the regular wheat germ you can buy at health-food stores. It comes in a powder and is sold in health-food stores and online.

Good brands: Avemar (www.avemar-alternativetherapy.com) and OncoMar (800-647-6100, www.xymogen.com).

My advice

If you would like to begin taking FWGE, check with your physician about incorporating it into your treatment program.

I recommend one packet a day, which equals nine grams. You can mix it into a glass of cold water and then drink it—or substitute a non-citrus juice, such as apple or cranberry (citrus can deactivate FWGE's active ingredient).

FWGE is not cheap—it costs about $160/month—but I think the expense is worth it, given the early indications that it may improve cancer survival rates.

Good news: FWGE is generally safe, and any side effects, such as diarrhea and flatulence, occur only occasionally.

Foods and Supplements That Prevent Cancer

If you are confused about whether certain vitamins, supplements or foods can prevent cancer, you're not alone. The results of several recent studies have been conflicting and perplexing—which is why this topic has raised questions for consumers as well as members of the health-care and research communities.

What you need to know: Cancer is not a single disease, and it can have many different causes. That makes it virtually impossible for any one nutrient to protect against all types of cancer. In fact, studying whether single nutrients reduce the risk for cancer often is like looking for a magic bullet—more wishful thinking than good science.

Nothing can absolutely guarantee that you'll remain cancer free. However, good nutrition and a healthful overall lifestyle—not smoking, not abusing alcohol, limiting exposure to pollutants, eliminating food additives, exercising and controlling stress—can lower your odds of developing cancer. Here are my top five foods and top five supplements that definitely can lower your long-term risk of getting cancer.

My top anticancer foods

Consume a diet that emphasizes a variety of fresh, natural and minimally processed foods. Include a selection of vegetables, some fruits (such as berries and kiwifruit), fish, chicken (free-range or organic), legumes, nuts and modest amounts of healthful starches (such as sweet potatoes and whole grains). Eat healthfully—and you will lay the foundation for everything else that you can do to lower your long-term risk for cancer.

My favorite anticancer foods…

• **Broccoli**. Cruciferous vegetables are my top anticancer food, and broccoli heads the list. It is rich in *sulforaphane*, an antioxidant that helps the liver break down and destroy cancer-causing toxins. Sulforaphane also increases the activity of liver enzymes that help to get cancerous substances out of the body. (Sulforaphane is available as a supplement, although I recommend people get this phytonutrient through food.) Even better, broccoli sprouts contain 50 times more sulforaphane than that found in regular broccoli. Broccoli sprouts also have been shown to fight *H. pylori*, a type of bacteria believed to cause stomach cancer.

Advice: Eat one-half cup of raw or lightly steamed broccoli daily. (Boiling reduces its nutritional value.) Add some broccoli sprouts to your salads or sandwiches.

• **Tomatoes**. This fruit is rich in lycopene, the antioxidant that gives tomatoes their red color. Studies have found that tomatoes reduce the risk for prostate cancer—and also might reduce the risk for lung and stomach cancers.

Advice: Consume cooked tomatoes or tomato sauce. Lycopene is best absorbed from cooked tomatoes because cooking breaks down the fiber in the tomatoes. A little fat (e.g., olive oil) also enhances absorption. Include one serving of tomato sauce (one-half cup) in your diet several times a week. Watermelon and guava also contain a lot of lycopene.

• **Cold-water fish**. Salmon, sardines and trout are rich in healthy omega-3 fats—specifically *eicosapentaenoic acid* (EPA) and *docosahexaenoic acid* (DHA). EPA and DHA have potent anti-inflammatory benefits. Low intake of these fats appears to be a factor in breast, colon, pancreatic and stomach cancers.

Advice: Eat cold-water fish at least once or twice a week, or take a fish oil supplement daily that contains one gram of EPA and DHA. Or use krill oil, a type of fish oil from shrimplike crustaceans.

• **Garlic**. Slice or dice a garlic clove, and a relatively inert compound called *allicin* undergoes an amazing cascade of chemical changes. Nearly all allicin-generated compounds function as antioxidants that prevent the types of cell mutations that give rise to cancer. Evidence suggests that garlic might help protect against cancers of the colon, prostate, esophagus, larynx, ovaries and kidneys.

Advice: Consume garlic regularly. Because chopping and cooking garlic seem to increase its biological activity, sauté or bake it rather than eating it whole or raw. There is no recommended serving size for garlic, but the more you consume, the better.

• **Spinach**. Spinach and other "greens," such as chard and collard greens, are rich in antioxidants that protect cells from the type of damage that can create cancerous mutations. One study published in *Journal of Agricultural and Food Chemistry* gave spinach the top "bioactivity index" ranking of vegetables for its ability to protect against cancer.

Advice: Eat spinach and other greens daily. You can make spinach salads or 50/50 lettuce and spinach salads, or gently sauté spinach. A single serving is equivalent to one cup of raw or one-half cup of cooked spinach or greens.

My top anticancer supplements

Research on the role of individual supplements in reducing cancer risk has been especially confusing. *Taking all evidence into account, I'm convinced that these five supplements have clear benefits…*

• **Vitamin D**. If you were to take just one immune-enhancing supplement to lower your long-term risk for cancer, vitamin D would be the one to choose. More than 60 studies have found that high levels of vitamin D offer broad protection against many types of cancer. A recent German study reported that people with low vitamin D levels were one-third more likely to die of any type of cancer.

Advice: Take at least 1,000 IU of vitamin D-3 daily. Vitamin D-3, with its slightly different molecular structure than D-2, is a more bioactive form of the vitamin, which means that the body can use it more readily. Take 2,000 IU if you don't get much sun or have a dark complexion. (Dark skin absorbs less of the rays necessary for conversion to vitamin D.)

Best: Have your blood tested to determine how much vitamin D you need.

• **Vitamin K**. Two recent studies have shown an unexpected benefit of vitamin K—that it reduces the odds of developing breast and liver cancers.

Possible mechanism: Vitamin K activates *osteocalcin*, a protein involved in making strong bones. Recent research found that osteocalcin also may function as an anticancer nutrient.

Advice: Take 300 mcg of either vitamin K-1 or vitamin K-2, the forms most often studied.

Caution: Vitamin K may increase blood clotting. Do not take vitamin K if you also are taking blood-thinning medication unless you are being monitored by a doctor.

• **Selenium**. This essential dietary mineral forms part of *glutathione peroxidase*, an antioxidant enzyme that helps the liver break down cancer-causing toxins. A study published in *The Journal of the American Medical Association* found that 200 mcg daily of selenium led to significant reductions in the risk for prostate, colon and lung cancers within just a few years.

Advice: Take 200 mcg daily. Don't take a higher dose (which could be toxic) without the supervision of a nutrition-oriented doctor.

• **Coenzyme Q10** (CoQ10). I believe that modest amounts of this vitamin-like nutrient may reduce an individual's general risk for cancer. Studies have shown that large amounts of CoQ10 can inhibit the spread of breast cancer and boost immunity… and may have benefits in other types of cancer as well. A recent study of women with breast cancer who were on the drug *tamoxifen* found that a combination of 100 mg of CoQ10 daily and vitamins B-2 (10 mg) and B-3 (50 mg) boosted the activity of enzymes that can repair genes.

Advice: Take 100 mg daily. If you already have been treated for cancer, you should take 300 mg daily.

• **Lycopene**. This antioxidant helps prevent cell damage. Several small studies have shown that lycopene supplements can reduce the size of prostate tumors and their tendency to spread. They also can lower levels of *prostate-specific antigen* (PSA), a common marker of prostate cancer risk.

Advice: For prostate cancer prevention and for men with elevated PSA levels, I recommend taking five mg to 10 mg of lycopene daily, even if you eat lycopene-rich foods. If you have been diagnosed with prostate cancer, discuss taking 30 mg daily with your physician. Use tomato-based (not synthetic) lycopene, which contains other beneficial antioxidants.

Note: Some multivitamins may contain these nutrients but not in the amounts recommended for cancer prevention. Check the label of your multivitamin, and add to it, based on the recommendations above.

Ultimate Cancer-Fighting Food... Now in Capsule Form, Too

"I do not like broccoli. I haven't liked it since I was a little kid and my mother made me eat it. I'm president of the United States, and I'm not going to eat any more broccoli!" George H.W. Bush spoke these words early in his tenure at the White House. Unfortunately, Mr. Bush is missing out on a potent cancer-fighting food.

If you share the former president's aversion to broccoli, you'll be happy to learn of convenient new alternatives that provide even more health benefits. *First, some background information...*

Deficient diets

Researchers have published some eye-opening studies on the compound *sulforaphane*, found in broccoli and similar vegetables. Sulforaphane helps prevent cancers of the breast, ovary, prostate, bone, brain, bladder, liver, lung and stomach and combats other conditions associated with aging and cell death.

It is no secret that the average American fails to consume the seven to nine daily servings of fruits and vegetables recommended to provide dietary protection against cancer and other diseases. And for many people, the produce they do eat seldom includes the recommended one to two daily servings of *cruciferous* vegetables (so called because the plants' flowers have four petals arranged like a crucifix), such as cauliflower, kale, bok choy, rutabagas, radishes, turnips, brussels sprouts and, of course, broccoli. An analysis published in the *Journal of Nutrition*, which looked at dietary data on 4,806 men and women ages 25 to 75, revealed that just 3 percent of the group consumed broccoli during either of two typical days. Consumption of dark green vegetables averaged just one-fifth of a serving per day.

Cruciferous vegetables are a rich source of healthful plant chemicals called *phytochemicals* or *phytonutrients*. These include cancer-fighting *thiols* (such as the sulfur-containing *glucosinolates*) and *indoles* (which bind chemical carcinogens and activate detoxifying enzymes). Yet even veggie lovers may find it difficult to ingest therapeutic amounts of cruciferous vegetables on a regular basis. This problem is compounded by the fact that cooking can destroy phytonutrients, so health benefits are diminished unless the vegetables are consumed raw or lightly steamed.

SGS discovered

Scientists at Johns Hopkins University School of Medicine identified the compound *sulforaphane glucosinolate* (SGS)—a naturally occurring precursor to sulforaphane—in 1992 and began to research its cancer-fighting potential. Leading this effort was Paul Talalay, MD, a professor of pharmacology and director of the university's Laboratory for Molecular Sciences.

His strategy: To support the body's natural detoxification capacity to fight cancer-causing chemicals and cell-damaging free radicals. It is well accepted that cell DNA controls replication of cells and that damage to cell DNA is an important factor in the development of cancer.

In 1994, Dr. Talalay looked at the impact of SGS on mammary (breast) tumors in rats exposed to a potent carcinogen. Results were astounding. The number of rats that developed tumors was reduced by as much as 60 percent... the number of tumors in each animal was reduced by 80 percent… and the size of the tumors that did develop was reduced by 75 percent. Subsequently, hundreds of other test-tube and animal studies have confirmed the anticancer properties of sulforaphane.

Toxins (natural and man-made) go through phases of breakdown in the cells of the body, particularly the liver. *Sulforaphane promotes detoxification by…*

• **Supporting enzymes** that destroy carcinogens.

• **Stimulating longer-lasting protective antioxidant effects** than other nutrients do.

• **Replenishing the cells' supplies of the amino acid glutathione**, strengthening the immune system.

• **Inhibiting COX-2**, an inflammatory enzyme that contributes to cancerous changes in cells.

• **Limiting DNA damage and abnormal cell growth.**

Super sprouts

Dr. Talalay discovered that various types of fresh and frozen broccoli differed significantly in the amounts of SGS they contained—and that the older the broccoli was, the lower its SGS. Painstaking research uncovered certain varieties of three-day-old broccoli sprouts—which look like a cross between alfalfa sprouts and bean sprouts—that contained up to 50 times more SGS than mature, cooked broccoli. One ounce of these sprouts could provide as much SGS as *three pounds* of cooked broccoli.

This set the stage for a fascinating study, published in *Cancer Epidemiology Biomarkers & Prevention*. The study was conducted in a rural area near Shanghai where liver cancer is common because local grain is contaminated with *aflatoxin*, a carcinogen produced by mold.

In the study, broccoli sprouts with known levels of SGS were grown at the site in China. Three days after the shoots emerged from the soil, the sprouts were picked and used to prepare a liquid extract to ensure standard dosages. One hundred local residents drank five ounces of diluted extract in tea form (equal to eating two ounces of sprouts) daily for two weeks. A control group drank a tea indistinguishable in taste and appearance but containing no SGS.

Great results: Analysis of the participants' urine showed that in people who drank the SGS extract, carcinogens were being removed from the body—providing the first direct evidence that broccoli sprouts can enhance the human body's detoxifying system, reducing the risk of cancer.

New ways to get greens

Broccoli sprouts and SGS are safe for everyone. (If you have thyroid problems, check with your doctor—there is a slight risk that broccoli sprouts may suppress thyroid function. There is no concern with the SGS supplement.) Because the SGS content of broccoli sprouts can vary greatly depending on seed type and growing methods, I recommend the sprouts developed by the Johns Hopkins team. These are now available under the brand name BroccoSprouts, from Brassica Protection Products (877-747-1277, www.broccosprouts.com). Offered in health-food and grocery stores nationwide, these broccoli sprouts contain standardized and therapeutic amounts of sulforaphane.

Alternatively, you can grow your own sprouts using seeds. Order from Caudill Seed Company, www.caudillseed.com.

For optimal health, have one-half cup (one ounce) of BroccoSprouts every other day. Each serving contains 73 mg of SGS. They are most beneficial when eaten raw, so sprinkle them on salads and sandwiches. The taste is similar to that of a radish, with a spicy flavor that results from the release of sulforaphane as you chew. Even people who hate broccoli usually enjoy the tangy taste of broccoli sprouts.

Cancer-prevention pill

Some people don't have the time—or taste buds—for a full day's worth of fruits and vegetables. That's when the capsule form of SGS comes in handy. I recommend it for people with a family history of cancer... as a complement to ongoing cancer treatments (with your doctor's approval)... for those who have been exposed to toxins... and for all who want to reduce their risk of cancer.

The supplement company Xymogen (www.xymogen.com) markets OncoPLEX, which contains SGS. Though it does not require a prescription, it is not sold in health-food stores and usually is purchased through holistic doctors.

In general, I advise taking one capsule daily. If you have had cancer or are undergoing cancer treatment, increase to two to four capsules daily, under the supervision of your doctor.

The Seafood Secret to Stopping Cancer and Halting Heart Disease in its Tracks

While mainstream medicine continues to stick its head in the sand, those of us with a clue *already* know that chronic inflammation is one of the main factors behind cancer and heart disease. It hardens your arteries and causes tumors to grow. So, naturally, the goal should be preventing the "sparks," the cause the "fire" of inflammation in the first place.

Head off inflammation with the power of omega 3s

We know that special compounds—found in foods like fish, nuts, and seeds—are powerful inflammation fighters. (More on those compounds in a moment.)

Now, new research shows us *why* they work.

It turns out these compounds have the power to reduce the amount of inflammatory proteins—known as *intercellular adhesion molecules* (ICAMs)—that your body produces. This is important because ICAMs help cells stick to each other and to their surroundings—which is not always a good thing.

ICAMs are found even in the healthiest people. But when blood tests show that they're elevated, it's a sure sign of trouble. It can mean an increase in white blood cells, blood platelet cells, and cells that make up the lining of blood vessels. This can cause a serious inflammation of your arteries. Plus, your body may react by producing too many immune cells, called monocytes, opening the door for cancer cells to develop.

Research proves "fats" keep your heart healthy and cancer free

Now let's get back to those powerful compounds I mentioned earlier. Nuts, seeds, and fish all contain omega-3 fatty acids. These fats, found in plant and marine oils, are nature's inflammation fighters.

At China's Jilin University, researchers looked at 18 randomized clinical trials on omega-3 supplements. They studied blood levels of a specific kind of adhesion molecule known as sICAM-1. They found that those who took omega-3s had lower blood levels of sICAM-1, even in people with unhealthy blood fat profiles. And remember, fewer ICAMs means fewer of those sticky cells setting the stage for disease.

But the benefits of omega-3s don't stop there. The researchers found they were able to essentially block the "on" switch for a type of white blood cell that rapidly reproduces when there's inflammation. And remember inflammation drives the build up of plaque in your arteries called atherosclerosis.[1]

Another study, out of Paris, looked at how omega-3s affect sICAM-1 levels and cancer risk. Researchers compared data from 408 people with cancer and 760 healthy people. They found that the higher a person's omega-3 level, the lower their sICAM-1 level was. And the more omega-3s they were taking, the lower their risk for four kinds of cancer, including breast and prostate.

On the other hand, people who ate fewer omega-3s had higher blood levels of sICAM-1 and, of course, a higher cancer to go with it. The researchers believe that the omega-3s decrease the number of adhesion molecules. Or perhaps they block a pro-cancer pathway that's normally set off by them.[2]

Fill up on fish packed with fatty acids

Clearly omega-3 fatty acids are good for both your heart health and for reducing your cancer risk. I tell my patients that the easiest way to up your omega-3s is to eat cold-water fish like wild salmon at least four times a week. Also take 1,000 to 2,000 mg of combined EPA and DHA daily. If you're a vegetarian… or just not a fan of fish… you can take one to two tablespoons daily of flaxseed or hempseed oil, or two scoops of chia seeds along with eight ounces of water a day.

Supercharge Your Immune System and Fight Cancer with the "Secret" Medicinal Mushroom Remedy from the East

Have you ever heard of turkey tail? No, I'm not talking about the tail feathers of our favorite thanksgiving bird. It's actually a mushroom with a rather colorful name and a surprising ability.

The turkey tail is a potent medicinal mushroom that has been found to boost your immune system. In fact, there are over 400 published studies showing just how powerful this mushroom is. Several human studies have even shown that it may be able to fight cancer. But don't feel bad if you haven't heard of turkey tail before, because even most cancer doctors are clueless about this "secret" wonder of nature.

The truth is, most mainstream <u>doctors</u> don't even know medicinal mushrooms like turkey tail exist. Not so surprising since drug companies sponsor both the medical schools they attend and the continuing education seminars they go to. And, of course, drug companies have no interest in cheap natural remedies that they can't patent. Individual doctors can, of course, venture a look outside of the box and do their own research, but the reality is most don't.

Even worse, doctors are often so brainwashed that they develop a bias against natural therapies. They're not willing to admit that some natural remedies work even if the science <u>proves</u> that they do. I've seen this happen countless times with my own patients who respond well to a complementary therapy I recommend. Their oncologists often ignore the positive results. Or, if they do acknowledge them, they refuse to learn more about the therapy that led to them.

Talking turkey tail mushrooms

Although here in the West few of us have ever heard of turkey tail, it's well known in East Asian medicine. In fact, in Japan and China there's a long history of using it in both traditional and modern medical practices. In Traditional Chinese medicine the mushroom is used to treat pulmonary infections, hepatitis, and cancer. And in Japan it's a folk remedy commonly used to treat cancer.

The scientific names for turkey tail mushrooms are *Coriolus versicolor* and *Trametes versicolor*. The Latin translation of Trametes is "one who is thin" and versicolor means "variously colored."

The fungus grows naturally on dead logs and on trees around the world. It has a fan-shaped, multicolored cap that some say resembles the tail feathers of a turkey. However, in Japan you would ask for *kawaratake* or "the mushroom by the river bank." And in China you'd look for *yun zhi* or the "cloud mushroom."

In the 1960s a Japanese scientist saw that a neighbor with late stage stomach cancer was treating himself with turkey tail. He became interested in the mushroom and he and his colleagues began to study it. Eventually the group developed an extract that they named PSK, an abbreviation for polysaccharide-K. Soon after, Chinese researchers developed their own version of the extract naming it PSP, an abbreviation for polysaccharide-peptide. Here in America, non-drug versions of turkey tail extract are available in the form of a nutritional supplement.

Building "super immunities" with glucans

The secret to the immune boosting power of many mushrooms are compounds called glucans. Turkey tail has its own unique "super" version of glucans. These glucans are pulled from the mushrooms using a special water extraction process. The result is a powerful immune enhancing extract.

Research shows that these special glucans pass right through the gut wall and into the bloodstream unchanged. (This means that when they go to work they're just as potent as when they were extracted.) Next, the extract switches on receptors on your immune cells, including neutrophils, monocytes/macrophages, natural killer cells, and T- and B-lymphocytes. So, in other words, the glucans essentially supercharge your entire immune system not only turning on your body's own cancer killers, but also the immune cells that fight off bacteria and viruses.

Turkey tail is obviously great for building up your immune system. But what I prescribe it for most often is as a complimentary therapy for treating cancer. Studies show it does the most good for: Esophageal, lung, colon, and stomach cancers.

Leaving lung cancer behind

One ten-year study looked at how good turkey tail extract (PSK) is at protecting your health when you're *already ill*. Researchers recruited 185 people with lung cancer who were getting radiation. Half of the group received a placebo and the other half received the PSK extract. And it turns out that the mushroom does an excellent job of protecting the immune system of lung cancer patients.

The researchers found that those receiving the turkey tail did much better overall than those on the placebo. The five-year survival rates of the patients who got the extract were 39 percent for those who had stage I or stage II cancers, and 22 percent for those who had stage III. And while those numbers may not seem huge at first glance, when you compare them to the placebo group's numbers of 16 percent and five percent it's instantly clear just how significant a difference the extract made.

Plus, those lung cancer patients who were 70 years old or older who got the PSK had a much better chance of surviving than those that only got radiation.

Conquering colon cancer

Another ten- year study showed just how good turkey tail is against colon cancer. The randomized double-blind trial divided a group of 111 volunteers with colon cancer into two. After surgery for colorectal cancer the first group of 56 patients took a turkey tail extract (PSK). The second group of 55 was given a placebo.

The results were pretty stunning. The rate of patients in remission (or disease-free) in the PSK group was more than double that of the placebo group! Researchers also found that the PSK patient's white blood cells showed, in their words, "remarkable enhancement in their activities." (White blood cells are the ones that fight disease by attacking things that don't belong in the body like germs, bacteria, and cancers. So anything that boosts their abilities is welcome in the fight against cancer.)

Striking back at stomach cancer

Turkey tail may be an important player in the fight against stomach cancer. One study, published in *The Lancet*, examined the effect of PSK in stomach cancer patients. All of the volunteers had stomach surgery and were starting chemotherapy. The two hundred sixty-two patients got either standard treatment alone or with PSK.

The survival rate of the group using both turkey tail extract and chemotherapy was 73 percent after five years. The group who got chemo-

---

One mushroom many uses

In Japan and China turkey tail extract is commonly used for immune enhancement for those who have had surgery, are undergoing chemotherapy, or are receiving radiation treatments.

therapy alone had a survival rate of only 60 percent. The researchers said that PSK had "a restorative effect in patients who had been immunosuppressed by both recent surgery and subsequent chemotherapy."

Slashing chemo and radiation side effects

One of the biggest sins in medicine today is that <u>proven</u> complementary therapies are being ignored and aren't being used on cancer patients The fact is, turkey tail can work wonders when it comes to beating the toxic side effects of cancer treatments.

Researchers at the University of Shanghai, wanted to find out if Coriolus polysaccharides (PSP) could reduce the side effects of chemotherapy or radiation. They recruited 650 people with cancer who were undergoing chemotherapy and radiation and gave them either PSP or a placebo. Then they measured how severe the side effects from the cancer treatments were in both groups. It turns out that those volunteers who received PSP had a lot fewer side effects than those that got the placebo.

And as anyone who has been through the nightmare of chemo or radiation can tell you, the cure can sometimes seem worse than the disease. So fewer side effects are a Godsend.

Talk to your doc about turkey tail

If you have esophageal, lung, stomach, or colon cancer I recommend you talk to your oncologist about turkey tail. Now don't be surprised if you meet some resistance at first. But remember, the science proves that the mushroom extract can reduce the side effects of conventional therapies, supercharge your cancer killing cells, and even reduce your chances of a cancer coming back. So if your doctor is willing to take an honest look at the evidence he should also be willing to give it a try.

And if after looking at all the studies he's still resisting it might be time for you to find a new doctor. Your life could *literally* depend on it.

I usually recommend 1,000 to 1,500 mg of a standard hot water extract twice a day (of course make sure to check with your *own* doctor before starting supplementation). As with any immune modulator you should not use turkey tail extract if you've had an organ transplant, or if you're taking immunosuppressive drugs. Side effects from turkey tail supplements are rare. Look for a standardized extract at your local health food store or from your holistic doctor.

Say Goodbye to Chemo and So Long to Those Harsh Drugs... Starve Cancer Cells to Death Instead!

Throughout military history a key strategy for defeating an enemy has been to cut off the food supply. The enemy surrenders or faces death from starvation. It turns out the same concept is true for cancer cells! Without their energy source, they die.

Cancer cells have a huge appetite for glucose—a simple sugar. Cancer cells require a byproduct of glucose metabolism for energy. Normal cells can use fats as fuel in addition to glucose. In 1924, German medical doctor, physiologist, and Nobel Laureate Otto Warburg discovered that cancer cells are fueled by the metabolism of sugar inside cells. He published several works on this concept, including *The Metabolism of Tumours*.

"Chicken or the egg" cancer debate

A debate has gone on for years about this. On the one side is the argument that this different metabolism is what fuels the cancer cells. On the other side is the argument that it's a *byproduct* of the changes that come from the cancer itself. Warburg felt strongly that this metabolic switch was the primary cause of cancer. But this was never accepted by the medical establishment as a primary cause of cancer. Sadly, I still hear from cancer patients today that their oncologists tell them that dietary improvements are of little benefit in the treatment of cancer. This is kind of like heart attack victims being served hamburgers during their hospital recovery. How foolish.

The latest research reveals that Warburg was right. A team of researchers from University of California, Los Angeles (UCLA) and collaborators from Memorial Sloan-Kettering Cancer Center and Weil-Cornell Medical College showed that depriving cancer cells of glucose does indeed cause them to die. When you take away the glucose your body responds by creating free radicals that destroy the cell.[1]

Remember the term *free radicals*? These molecules play a key role in the immune system's offensive maneuvers destroying infections and cancer cells. On the other hand, free radicals from pollution, poor diet, and stress can overwhelm the body and contribute to disease. The body must maintain a balance between the production of free radicals and the production of antioxidants (like vitamin C, E, selenium, polyphenols in green tea) that neutralize free radicals.

The simple sugar cancer connection

Holistic doctors such as myself have long recommended people with cancer, as well as those using nutrition to prevent cancer (which should be everyone), limit the amount of simple sugars in the diet. We know that when you eat too many your levels of the glucose-transporting hormone insulin spike. This in turn contributes to inflammation, which is pro-carcinogenic, or cancer causing.

With two-thirds of the population overweight, and an epidemic of diabetes on our hands, this means that there are a lot of people walking around with cancer-inducing levels of insulin. In addition, high levels of sugar in the bloodstream have been shown to suppress the immune system, feed fungus (another potential cancer-causer), and promote a favorable environment for cancer cells to thrive.

So how do you starve cancer cells so that they self-destruct? Obviously you should avoid high-sugar foods such as candy (if you can even call that a food), soda pop, fruit juice (minimize to a few ounces diluted in water), and processed grains such as white breads, cookies, crackers, chips, white rice, and sweets. And these foods are a problem for many Americans.

The Whole Wheat Wolf in sheep's clothing

There's one food your nutritionist actually *recommends* you consume to fight cancer, diabetes, and weight gain. But the harsh reality is that it's actually a wolf in sheep's clothing. I'm talking about whole wheat! I know what you are thinking: Whole wheat contains fiber and complex carbohydrates that should reduce the absorption of sugars and not lead to a spike in blood glucose and insulin levels.

And that *was* true about 50 years ago. But today's wheat has been so genetically modified that its carbohydrate content has changed and it's rapidly broken down into glucose.

Let me prove this by looking at the Glycemic Index (GI) score of whole wheat. The GI assigns foods a score based on how that food affects blood sugar and insulin. The lower the GI score the less it spikes blood sugar and insulin levels.

You also have to take into consideration how much of that food you are consuming (for example, one serving of a certain food will have a lesser effect than two servings of that same food). The highest and worst rating is glucose, which has a score of 100. Lentils at a weight of 150 g have a GI of 29, 250 mL of orange juice (unsweetened) has a score of 50, Coca-Cola at a volume of 250 mL has a score of 63, and 30 g (two slices) of whole wheat has a GI score of 71![2] And just in case you like your white bagels the GI is a whopping 95.[3]

The point is that you should not be duped into thinking that whole wheat is a super food. Wheat products are not only giving people "belly drop" as my mother calls it, but they're feeding those dreaded cancer cells.

Restricting carbs to restrict cancer

German doctors have been experimenting with a ketogenic diet. This is a severely carbohydrate-restricted diet already shown to have some success with controlling seizures. Alternative and nutrition-based approaches for cancer treatment are quite mainstream in Germany. And the early research *is* showing some benefit from this carbohydrate-restricted diet.[4] However, much more study is required before this type of diet can be recommended for all cancer patients. A ketogenic diet requires medical supervision.

So Dr. Warburg was right after all. His proposed theory of sugar metabolism in cancer cells may have been incomplete, but his premise was correct. I strongly urge you to limit the amount of wheat and simple sugars in your diet.

This is even more important if you have active cancer or a history of cancer. Focus your diet on vegetables; proteins such as beans, nuts, and seeds (not peanuts since they contain aflatoxin known to be a potent carcinogen); fish; and organic meat. Limit fruit.

Starve those cancer cells... don't feed them!

Fight Cancer Fatigue and Beat Exhaustion with This Native American Herbal Gem

If you… or someone you know… is fighting cancer, chances are you're *also* familiar with the debilitating fatigue that often goes hand in hand with the disease. In fact fatigue—the kind that makes it hard to even get out of bed sometimes—is one of the *most* common complaints that cancer sufferers have… and for good reason.

Not only is a cancer patient's body in a *literal* fight for its life, the chemotherapy and radiation treatments that they often must endure can lead to bone-wearying exhaustion. A common side effect of these harsh therapies is a drop in red blood cells (anemia), which causes other cells in the body to not receive enough oxygen and the nutrients they need, like iron or B12, for energy production.

In addition, chemo and radiation produce a number of toxic byproducts that must be detoxified. Not to mention the tremendous amount of harmful molecules known as free radicals that are created which the body must deal with as well.

To make matters even worse weight loss and tissue wasting, known medically as cachexia, is a common problem during cancer treatment and leaves cancer patients feeling spent and weak. And of course we can't overlook the sheer amount of physical and emotional energy that's expended when you're fighting cancer.

Recharge your energy stores naturally

In my practice I combat this fatigue in several different ways. I've had a lot of success with nutritional intravenous therapies. In addition, I've found that supporting the often-overlooked adrenal glands (the stress glands on top of your kidneys) can be tremendously effective. In fact, I think it's *so* important that I'm willing to say that it's an **essential** step in re-energizing those with cancer related fatigue as well as other energy sappers.

This support comes in the form of herbal extracts—known as *adaptogens*—that can help the body and the adrenal glands adapt and cope to physical and mental stress. They have helped thousands of my patients with cancer revitalize over the years. Common ones I use with patients include ashwagandha, rhodiola, and various ginsengs.

But there's one ginseng in particular that's a shining star when it comes to beating cancer fatigue. Researchers have confirmed that one of America's native plants—American ginseng—may be just what's needed for getting over that energy slump.

While many people have heard of the more common Asian ginseng… often referred to as Panax ginseng… few are familiar with the American variety. Also known as Panax quinquefolius, American ginseng is indig-

---

Supercharge your energy levels

If you don't have cancer, but are suffering from general fatigue supporting your adrenals can help you too! When a patient comes to me complaining of exhaustion I have found that adrenal supporting ashwagandha, rhodiola, and Siberian ginseng can make a huge difference in their energy levels.

enous to the forests of northern and central US. China imports American ginseng where it is highly revered in traditional Chinese medicine. It contains active constituents known as ginsenosides, which support adrenal gland function. These ginsenosides contain nerve relaxing, anti-inflammatory, anti-fatigue, pain relieving, and digestive tonic properties.[1]

American herb helps restore balance

Recently, mainstream researchers confirmed what holistic doctors like myself have already known about herbal adaptogens like American ginseng... and that is that they work! A recent study headed by Mayo clinic, and reported on at the 2012 Annual Meeting of the American Society of Clinical Oncology, found that American ginseng was effective in treating cancer related fatigue.

The study involved 340 patients with cancer who were receiving treatment at one of 40 community medical centers. Sixty percent of the patients had been diagnosed with breast cancer. Participants received 2000 mg of pure American ginseng in capsule form daily or a placebo.

During the first four weeks of the study those taking the ginseng had only a slight reduction in their fatigue. However, by week eight there was a significant improvement in fatigue when they were compared to those taking a placebo. In addition, there were zero side effects found in those taking the ginseng.[2]

When you add these new findings to previous studies using American ginseng that have demonstrated the herb inhibits cancer cell proliferation and tumor growth and this becomes a must-have therapy in my book.[3,4] If you're suffering from cancer related fatigue speak with your holistic doctor or oncologist about using an adaptogen such as American ginseng to help relieve your exhaustion naturally.

Miracle Mineral Could Reduce Your Risk of Prostate Cancer by 40 Percent or More!

Utter the words prostate cancer and most men are filled with dread. And for good reason, after all we've all heard the horror stories… impotence, incontinence, or worse. But I can usually get a guy to crack a smile when I explain that a very inexpensive mineral could significantly reduce his risk of ever getting aggressive prostate cancer in the first place.

Now holistic doctors like me have known for quite some time that people with higher levels of selenium in their blood have lower rates of death from cancer, including the prostate variety. But what has remained unclear however, is just how *much* selenium you need on board to avoid getting prostate cancer. With the goal of figuring out that level, researchers in the United Kingdom looked at a number of studies (a meta-analysis) that included reported measurements of selenium intake or status (plasma, serum, or toenail selenium), assessments of prostate cancer cases (number of events), and the relative risk (the risk of developing the disease relative to exposure) in the adult population.

Prostate cancer risk plummeted

Using sophisticated statistical analyses, the researchers determined that blood concentrations of selenium between 135 and 170 ng/mL reduced the risk of an aggressive form of prostate cancer by up to 40 percent![1] Your doctor can order your blood selenium level with any of the standard laboratories.

Selenium is a "trace mineral." But don't make the mistake of thinking that it's of limited importance. The truth is the human body requires small, or trace, amounts of the mineral to function. Selenium is actually essential for life. It's required for the proper functioning of a number of enzyme systems in the body which control cell metabolism. Some examples include the proper functioning of glutathione—your body's master antioxidant—as well as other antioxidant systems in the body. Selenium is also needed to produce the most powerful thyroid hormone in the body known as triiodothyronine (T3). And it's a key nutrient involved in ridding your body of toxins including carcinogens.

Low selenium levels linked to weakened immunities

Selenium deficiency contributes to a weakened immune system. According to the Linus Pauling Institute at Oregon State University, "There is a great deal of evidence indicating that selenium supplementation at high levels reduces the incidence of cancer in animals. More than two-thirds of over 100 published studies in 20 different animal models of spontaneous, viral, and chemically induced cancers found that selenium supplementation significantly reduces tumor incidence."[2]

Other studies have shown a link between low dietary selenium intake and prostate cancer risk. For example, a large prospective study published in the *Journal of the National Cancer Institute* involved over 30,000 male health professionals in the US. Toenail selenium samples were tested and researchers found *higher* selenium levels were associated with a significantly *reduced risk* of advanced prostate cancer.[3]

It's best to raise your selenium through diet

They also found that men with toenail selenium content consistent with an average daily dietary intake of 159 mcg/day of selenium had a 65 percent lower risk of advanced prostate cancer compared to those with toenail selenium content consistent with an average intake of 86 mcg/day.[4]

As with most nutrients, it's best to raise your selenium through diet. Good food sources of selenium include:

- **Brazil nuts**—Three nuts contains approximately 270 mcg

- **Sardines**—Three ounces contains approximately 50 mcg

- **Halibut**—Four ounces contains approximately 50 mcg

- **Eggs**—One egg contains approximately 15 mcg

- **Brown rice**—One cup contains approximately 19 mcg

- **Sunflower seeds**—A quarter cup contains approximately 19 mcg

A good daily intake of selenium for adults is 200 mcg. You can get this through diet and supplementation if needed. The upper limit for selenium intake is 400 mcg daily. Remember that more is **not** better when it comes to trace minerals like selenium. Excessive selenium intake can cause side effects; although research shows this requires significantly higher levels than 400 mcg. Talk with your doctor about measuring your own levels and determining how much you need.

Prostate cancer affects one in six men in the US. A diet that consistently includes selenium rich foods is one of the best ways for men to stave off this all too common disease.

PART III

Heart and Blood

Brush Teeth to Keep the Cardiologist Away

Now there is additional proof that dental problems don't end in your mouth. Researchers from University College London found that people who reported brushing their teeth less than twice daily, on average, had a 70 percent increased risk for heart disease compared with those who brushed at least twice daily. That's even more reason to get your toothbrush busy twice a day.

Pomegranate Juice and Your Heart

The pomegranate recently has been acclaimed for its numerous health benefits. Pomegranate juice, which is available at most health-food stores and most grocery stores, contains a blend of powerful, disease-fighting antioxidants, including *phenolic compounds, tannins* and *anthocyanins.*

Researchers in Norway found that pomegranates contain a higher concentration of antioxidants than 23 other fruits. This big red fruit has about 10 times more antioxidants than those with the next-highest levels, including grapes, oranges, plums, pineapples, lemons, dates, clementines and grapefruits.

Cleans your arteries

One of the major benefits of pomegranate juice is that it prevents the oxidation of "bad" *low-density lipoprotein* (or LDL) cholesterol—a major cause of artery damage and subsequent plaque buildup.

For several years, researchers in Israel have studied the protective antioxidant and cardiovascular effects of pomegranate juice. In one of their most recent studies, pomegranate juice was found to reduce oxidation of LDL cholesterol by 40 percent. In another study, they found that pomegranate juice reduced the buildup of plaque in the carotid (neck) arteries, which supply blood to the brain.

Protects diabetics' arteries

Researchers from Shaheed Beheshti University of Medical Sciences in Tehran, Iran, found pomegranate juice to be helpful for people with diabetes. In this study, participants who consumed 40 g (about 1.4 ounces) daily of concentrated pomegranate juice for eight weeks, saw significant reductions in their total cholesterol and LDL cholesterol levels. This definitely is good news for diabetics because elevated blood glucose and insulin levels raise the risk of *atherosclerosis*.

I recommend that those with *carotid stenosis* (narrowing of the carotid arteries) and/or diabetes drink at least two ounces and up to eight ounces of 100 percent pomegranate juice daily. (Those with diabetes should drink no more than two ounces at a time, and take it with meals to slow down blood sugar absorption.)

For people trying to lower their blood pressure and those with a strong family history of heart disease, I recommend eight ounces a day.

You can, of course, dilute it by half with water (as I do) or combine it with other juices, such as grape or cranberry, for better flavor. One widely available brand that I use regularly is R.W. Knudsen Just Pomegranate.

New to the market are pomegranate supplements, which may prove to be a good alternative for people who wish to avoid the calories in pomegranate juice.

Does Red Wine Protect the Heart?

You might have read the headlines in recent years—moderate consumption of alcohol, especially red wine, decreases the risk of cardiovascular disease. Before you assume that is reason enough to consume alcohol on a regular basis, let's look at this issue more closely.

It is true that alcohol consumption provides some cardiovascular protection. For example, when researchers combined data from 51 epidemiological studies, they found that the risk of heart disease decreased by about 20 percent when one to two alcoholic drinks were consumed per day. (One drink of alcohol is equivalent to 1.5 ounces of liquor, five ounces of wine or 12 oz of beer.) The people who seemed to benefit most from light drinking (about 1.2 drinks a day) to moderate drinking (2.2 drinks daily) were middle-aged men and women.

Red wine has additional benefits over other alcoholic beverages, studies suggest. That's because several chemicals in red wine may protect heart health, including *resveratrol*, a *polyphenol* (plant pigment) with antioxidant effects. (White wine has smaller amounts of resveratrol.)

The natural compounds in red wine seem to prevent buildup of plaque in the arteries by reducing inflammation and promoting good tone in blood vessel walls. The compounds also play a role in preventing blood clots, which can obstruct blood flow and cause a heart attack or stroke. Alcoholic beverages of any type increase HDL "good" cholesterol, which removes LDL "bad" cholesterol from circulation, thereby minimizing plaque formation.

Despite these positive effects, I don't recommend that people rely on wine or any alcoholic beverages for heart disease prevention. If you do not drink alcohol on a regular basis, don't start. One of the obvious risks of regular alcohol consumption is alcoholism, a very serious and common disease in our country. *Other reasons not to drink alcohol…*

• **Cancer risk**. According to the American Cancer Society, men who have two alcoholic drinks a day and women who have one alcoholic drink a day increase their risk of certain cancers—of the esophagus, pharynx, mouth, liver, breast and colon. If you enjoy drinking each day, limit consumption to half a drink for women and one drink for men so as not to increase cancer risk.

• **Heart risk**. Paradoxically, the same amount of alcohol that has been shown to have a heart-protective effect—two drinks daily for men and one for women—also has been shown to raise triglyceride levels. High levels of these fats increase heart disease risk. Excessive drinking also raises the risk of high blood pressure, heart failure and stroke.

• **Obesity risk**. Alcohol contains simple carbohydrates. Consuming large amounts of simple carbs increases the risk of obesity and diabetes.

• **Fetal risk**. Mothers who drink alcohol during pregnancy predispose their babies to birth defects.

You can dramatically reduce your risk of heart disease without negative effects by not smoking, avoiding secondhand smoke, exercising regularly and consuming a Mediterranean-style diet. This diet is rich in fruits and vegetables, whole grains, nuts, seeds, legumes and olive oil—and has low to moderate amounts of dairy, fish and poultry and little red meat. You also might take fish oil with a combined *EPA* and *DHA* total of 500 mg daily to get heart-healthy essential fatty acids.

Also drink purple grape juice. It makes arteries more flexible and reduces the susceptibility of LDL cholesterol to cause damage in patients with coronary artery disease. Purple grape juice has potent antioxidant activity and, like red wine, contains resveratrol. It is high in simple sugars, so drink only six ounces daily—with a meal to slow sugar absorption. If you have diabetes, have no more than four ounces daily with a meal.

Poor Circulation Help

If poor circulation in the legs is of concern to you, consider supplementing with ginkgo biloba. This herb dilates arteries in the limbs.

Dosage: 120 mg of a ginkgo extract (including 24 percent *flavone glycosides* and six percent *terpene lactones*) twice daily for eight weeks.

Also take *nattokinase*, the enzyme extracted from *natto* (the by-product of fermented boiled soybeans), which is a natural blood thinner.

Dosage: 2,000 *fibrin units* (FU) per day on an empty stomach for eight weeks. Both are sold at health-food stores and generally are safe, but they should not be taken if you use blood-thinning medication, such as aspirin or *warfarin* (Coumadin).

In addition, every day sprinkle one-half teaspoon of cinnamon onto toast or apple slices, or add it to a smoothie. Cinnamon improves circulation by dilating the arteries, can be used indefinitely, is safe for everyone—and is tasty, too.

Blood Pressure Breakthrough

B lood pressure regulation is a complex process, which is one reason why blood pressure problems are so common. Half of people over age 60 have high blood pressure, or hypertension—pressure of 140/90 or greater, measured in millimeters of mercury (mmHg)—and some develop it as early as their mid-30s.

Blood pressure is determined by the amount of blood your heart pumps and by the arteries' resistance to blood flow. Excess weight, a high-salt diet, stress and high cholesterol can contribute to hypertension. In such instances, dietary changes, exercise, relaxation techniques and/or cholesterol-lowering therapies can help.

In 95 percent of hypertension cases, however, the cause is unknown—and often the therapies above are not enough to keep blood pressure in check. Uncontrolled hypertension raises the risk for heart failure, heart attack, stroke, kidney damage and diabetes.

Reason: When blood pressure rises, arteries take a beating as blood pounds through them. The body responds by patching damaged arterial walls with plaque (a mix of fat and cholesterol)... but this makes arteries narrower, increasing blood pressure even more.

Often medication can lower blood pressure—but it may take considerable experimentation to find the most effective drug or drugs for an individual. Also, these drugs can have side effects, such as dizziness, chronic cough, muscle cramps, fatigue and erectile dysfunction.

That's why I am always exploring natural ways to reduce blood pressure—and why I am so enthusiastic about a device with the brand name Resperate, designed for use at home.

Encouraging evidence

So far, nine clinical trials published in medical journals confirm that Resperate successfully lowers blood pressure. The first, from the *Journal of Human Hypertension* in 2001, involved 61 men and women with blood pressure averaging 155/95. For 10 minutes daily, one group of participants used the Resperate device and the other listened to quiet music on a Walkman portable CD player. After eight weeks, Resperate users' average reduction was 15.2 points for systolic pressure (top number) and 10 points for diastolic pressure (bottom number)... compared with the CD player group's reduction of 11.3 points (systolic) and 5.6 points (diastolic). Six months after treatment stopped, the Resperate group's diastolic pressure remained lower than the CD player group's.

The principle behind Resperate—sustained deep breathing—is not new. Yet the way the device accomplishes this goal is quite innovative. Before I describe this, let me explain some important facts about breathing. Most people breathe shallowly, taking air only into the tops of the lungs... unconsciously hold their breath whenever they feel anxious or are concentrating on a task... and hold in their stomachs, a practice that slims the silhouette but prevents the long, deep "belly breaths" that carry oxygen all the way down into the lungs.

Breathing slowly and fully from the abdomen helps to reduce blood pressure, because it balances the messages from the nervous system that constrict or relax the arteries and helps control the "fight or flight" stress response. As the body relaxes and anxiety eases, constricted blood vessels dilate and blood flows more easily.

How resperate works

Resperate has three components—a small computer unit, a headphone set and a sensor belt. The first time you use the device, it detects your baseline (normal) breathing pattern. Using this information, the computer develops a personalized melody—with high tones indicating inhalation and low tones indicating exhalation—that gradually guides you into a slower breathing pattern. You can follow this tailor-made breathing pattern effortlessly and almost unconsciously, the same way your toes automatically tap out the rhythm as you listen to music.

Resperate is designed to slow your respiration rate from the average of 12 to 19 breaths per minute to the hypertension-lowering rate of 10 or fewer breaths per minute. You use it for at least 40 minutes per week, typically in three or four 15-minute sessions. After you complete a session, your breathing returns to its normal rate—but the decreased blood pressure achieved during your session usually remains throughout the day. The more you use Resperate, the greater its effects are likely to be.

A blood pressure reduction of 10 points systolic and five points diastolic yields measurable health benefits. After three to four weeks of use, Resperate reduces blood pressure, on average, by 14 points systolic and eight points diastolic. Some users have experienced decreases of as much as 36 points systolic and 20 points diastolic. Among my own patients, 15 have used Resperate in the last six months—and 13 have successfully lowered their blood pressure by 10 to 14 points systolic and five to 10 points diastolic.

This device is safe for everyone and has no side effects. It can be used in conjunction with blood pressure drugs. After 10 weeks of regular use of Resperate, many patients can reduce their hypertension drug dosage, under a doctor's supervision. Note: For sustained health benefits, you must use Resperate for the rest of your life—just as it is necessary to exercise regularly and eat healthfully for life.

To order: Resperate is available without a prescription from the manufacturer, InterCure (1-800-220-1925, www.resperate.com) and at some pharmacies. The cost is $299.95, plus tax and shipping. It is not covered by insurance, though it may be tax-deductible (ask your accountant) or reimbursible through a flexible spending account. I consider it money well spent.

Additional natural treatments

The following substances can lower blood pressure. Take them all for eight weeks. Then, if blood pressure readings show that you have improved, continue indefinitely. Supplements are sold in health-food stores and, unless noted, generally are safe for everyone.

Best: Use these natural therapies in conjunction with Resperate.

Note: Do not stop taking blood pressure drugs without your doctor's approval.

• **Calcium**—500 mg twice daily. This mineral aids transmission of nerve impulses that relax arteries and muscles, improving blood flow.

• **Coenzyme Q10 (CoQ10)**—300 mg daily. For unknown reasons, many people with hypertension have low levels of this vitamin-like substance. It is especially beneficial if you have type 2 diabetes.

• **Hawthorne extract**—250 mg three times daily. This herb has a blood-thinning effect, which improves blood flow. Ask your doctor before using if you take a pharmaceutical blood thinner, such as aspirin or warfarin (Coumadin).

• **Magnesium**—250 mg twice daily. This mineral promotes normal function of nerves and muscles that affect blood flow. Reduce dosage if stools become loose.

• **Vegetable juice** high in potassium and low in salt (such as Low Sodium V8)—four ounces twice daily. Potassium helps to normalize blood volume. If you have a history of kidney disease, ask your doctor before drinking high-potassium juice.

Fun fact: In a recent study, hypertensive patients who ate about one-quarter of an ounce (30 calories) of dark chocolate daily for 18 weeks reduced blood pressure by about three points systolic and two points diastolic. Try a daily morsel. Evidence isn't strong enough to recommend it is as a treatment for hypertension, but for most people it can't hurt and might help.

27 Percent Lower Blood Pressure Readings with "Hypertension Soup"

Hippocrates once said "Let food be thy medicine." Now a new study allows us to follow that sage's advice when it comes to high blood pressure. Recent research has uncovered a food so powerful that it actually competes with the strongest of pharmaceutical hypertension medications. It's the traditional Spanish cold vegetable soup called Gazpacho.

According to researchers, people who consume this soup on a regular basis have overall blood pressure readings that are 27 percent lower than people who eat little or no gazpacho.[1] The scientists believe the benefit comes from the nutrients found in the raw vegetables, namely carotenoids, vitamin C, and antioxidants that reduce the damage done by free radicals in other foods we eat and in the air we breathe.

I believe the soup is *also* effective because of the large amount of potassium it contains. Potassium is a proven blood pressure lowering nutrient. The researchers believe that the synergistic blend of the foods is more powerful than any one ingredient and I absolutely agree.

Elevated blood pressure is the leading risk factor for death worldwide. It affects one in four adults globally and is expected to increase by 60 percent between 2000 and 2025.[2] The statistics in America are even worse as this silent killer affects approximately one in three adults.[3]

Approximately 70 percent of Americans with high blood pressure take drugs to treat the condition.[4]

I see patients all the time who are taking those medications and suffering their notorious side effects including fatigue, dizziness, and dry coughs. My goal is always to reduce or eliminate their need for these drugs using natural therapies. I'm adding Gazpacho to my list of effective natural approaches.

Making gazpacho at home is easy. Just choose organic produce and use a light hand with the saltshaker. For a nutritional boost, you can garnish the soup with slices of ripe avocado.

Powerful Herb Beats High Blood Pressure Without Drug Side Effects

High blood pressure, also known as hypertension, is far too common in Americans. More than half of those over age 60, and about three-fourths of those 70 years of age and older, have elevated blood pressure.[1]

With so many people being diagnosed with hypertension the chances are good that you, or someone that you care about, is suffering with the condition. And if that's the case, you've probably already heard conventional medicine doctors give lip service to making lifestyle changes to reduce blood pressure including keeping a healthy weight, exercising daily, eating healthy, cutting down on salt, managing stress, and giving up smoking.

It all sounds good. But, the reality is that, most people with hypertension walk out of their doctor's office clutching a prescription or two for treatment. (So much for those lifestyle changes huh doc?) And, of course, those prescriptions are far from harmless. They come along with a slew of potential side effects including dizziness, fatigue, memory loss, diabetes, impotence, and muscle cramps.

As a holistic doctor I certainly work with patients on diet and lifestyle issues that can be the cause of their hypertension. A number of factors can influence your blood pressure including:

- Viscous (thick) blood

- Sleep apnea

- Kidney abnormalities such as blockage of the renal artery or chronic kidney disease

- Low potassium and magnesium intake

- Use of alcohol or caffeine and other stimulants

- Cancer

- Hyperthyroid

- Heavy metal toxicity such as lead or cadmium

- Side effect from some drugs including NSAID's—ibuprofen or naproxen; cough and cold medicines; migraine medications; weight loss drugs, and steroids

But, by far, the two most common reasons I see for high blood pressure are being overweight or living with too much stress.

Some of my patients are able to quickly get their blood pressure back

Understanding your blood pressure reading[2]

	Systolic	Diastolic
Normal Blood Pressure	Less than 120	Less than 80
Prehypertension	Between 120–139	Between 80–89
High Blood Pressure	140 or more	90 or more

Note: A diagnosis of high blood pressure should be made only after several readings on different days are elevated. Keep a diary at home of your blood pressure since many people have elevated blood pressure only at the doctors office. This is known as white coat hypertension.

under control by dropping a few pounds or following a stress management program. Others, I find, do well with chelation therapy, acupuncture, or supplements such as magnesium and fish oil. However, many of my patients do require more support to bring those blood pressure numbers back into the normal range. Prescription blood pressure medications are an option, but they're never my first choice. I look to nature first.

Herb lowers blood pressure naturally

When lifestyle changes and some standard natural therapies haven't done the trick for one of my patients I often turn to a little know, but powerful herbal wonder called Rauwolfia or African Snake Root. And while my patients *do* get a kick out of reading a supplement label that lists Snake Root on it, the truth is this herb is the opposite of useless "snake oil."

African Snake Root is a potent blood pressure lowering herb that's regularly used by herbalists in other parts of the world. It can be found growing naturally in the tropical forests of Asia and South America. Rauwolfia *serpentine* is traditionally the most commonly used form of the herb; however, it's now considered endangered so the serpentine variety is being replaced with Rauwolfia *vomitoria*.

Reserpine relaxes blood vessels

Rauwolfia contains several medicinal compounds known as alkaloids. The best researched in terms of blood pressure lowering is reserpine. Reserpine calms the nervous system and directly lowers blood pressure by relaxing blood vessels. It also is believed to block the effect of the stress hormone adrenaline on blood vessels, which would help prevent their constriction.[3]

Reserpine already has a history of being used in medications to lower blood pressure. But isolating a single isolated substance like reserpine from an herb and concentrating it comes with a price. Without the synergistic and balancing properties of the other medicinal substances in the herb you often end up with severe side effects. In fact, this method of isolating one substance from a plant is what changes a promising *medicinal plant* into a potentially dangerous *drug*.

American drug companies aren't using reserpine anymore because of the concern over side effects. However, when taken as one of the many ingredients found in the whole plant, reserpine's side effect potential plummets! In this way it reminds me of green tea which contains caffeine. Since green tea also contains the amino acid L-theanine, which has a calming effect, any potential over-stimulating effects of the caffeine are greatly minimized.

An analysis of four studies involving 237 people found reserpine to be as effective as normal first line drug agents in the treatment of hypertension. None of the four trials had any participants withdraw due to adverse side effects.[4]

Target stress-induced hypertension with Rauwolfia

Millions of people suffer from high blood pressure as a result of anxiety, depression, or just an inability to handle stress. Since Rauwolfia has a calming and possibly anti-depressant action I find it can be very helpful for patients whose hypertension that's caused by any of these factors. For example, one of my patients relied on several glasses of wine each evening to unwind and help keep his blood pressure under control. Rauwolfia was a much healthier choice for him and has worked well to control his hypertension. However, do keep in mind that if you suffer with fatigue Rauwolfia could be too sedating for you and may potentially aggravate your fatigue.

I like to use Snake Root as part of a formula that contains other blood pressure lowering herbs. Additional natural remedies that can help reduce blood pressure include:

- Hawthorn- 250 mg three times daily

- Magnesium- 400-500 mg daily

- Garlic extract- 600 mg twice daily

- Fish oil- 3,000 mg daily

- Hibiscus- Tea or capsule form three times daily

Talk with your own doctor about giving Rauwolfia a try. This powerful herb could be just what you need to keep you off of the harsh blood pressure drugs for good. And although Snake Root isn't commonly available over the counter, it should be readily available through your local holistic doctor.

"Full-Body" CT Scans

It was not so long ago that a CAT scan—a computerized X-ray technique, also called a CT (for "computed tomography") scan—seemed very exotic. In fact, if you are age 35 or older, there were no CT scanners in clinical use when you were born. Today, of course, CT scans are commonplace.

Now there's an even more advanced, and highly touted, version— *electron beam computed tomography* (EBCT), often (erroneously) referred to as a full-body scan. EBCT scans examine the abdominal cavity and chest (including coronary arteries and lungs). These scans are available in cities nationwide and are being promoted as a way to detect coronary artery disease and other abnormalities, including tumors and aneurysms in the chest, abdomen and pelvic area. In many states, a prescription is not required to get a scan. Even if you're healthy, you can just contact an imaging center and ask—and pay—for the test. The idea is to find trouble before any symptoms appear.

EBCT scans use very rapidly processed X-rays that capture images in a fraction of a second. This allows for clear, freeze-frame pictures of the heart and arteries while the heart is beating. Images are captured from many angles, allowing a three-dimensional view of the heart as well as other organs and systems.

The test is painless. While the patient lies on a table, an overhead scan machine takes images in an open environment—not in an enclosed space as with some other CT and magnetic resonance imaging (MRI) scans. Testing usually takes 10 to 15 minutes. Typically, a center's radiologist or cardiologist determines if there are any visible abnormalities and reviews the results with the patient within minutes. Upon your request, a copy of the report and images can be sent to your primary care doctor.

One purpose of an EBCT scan is to determine the amount of calcium buildup in the lining of the arteries, including the coronary arteries. Several studies, including one conducted at the respected Cooper Institute in Dallas and published in the *American Journal of Epidemiology*, have shown a correlation between the degree of calcification and the severity of hardening of the arteries, known as atherosclerosis. A low level of calcium buildup in the arteries means that your risk for coronary artery disease is low. A high level means that you are at higher risk for cardiovascular problems in the future.

There are a few downsides to EBCT scans. One is the radiation exposure from the X-rays—which can be two to 10 times more than that of a standard X-ray. Radiation is a known risk factor for cancer (although the risk appears small with occasional scans). The EBCT scan also may result in "false positives"—meaning that doctors may spot a suspected lesion that requires follow-up tests, possibly even an invasive biopsy and it may turn out to be nothing serious. Lastly, many insurance companies don't cover EBCT preventive screening. A scan costs $850 to $1,500.

Despite the financial cost, I do recommend that people age 40 and older get a preventive EBCT screening. If the results are normal, then follow up with another in five to 10 years. The test is even more important for those with a strong family history of heart disease or cancer. While EBCT scanning is not foolproof, it can help detect life-threatening diseases that are best treated with early intervention.

The Overlooked Artery Enemy: Knowing Your Levels of This "Hidden Heart Menace" Could Save Your Life!

It's hiding in your body right now. You can't see it but it's lurking in your bloodstream threatening your health as it silently packs plaque onto the interior walls of your arteries. The tests your doctor normally orders are essentially useless for revealing it. Total cholesterol, LDL, HDL, triglycerides, and C-reactive protein measurements don't provide any useful information about it. And chances are you've never even heard of the stuff before.

This silent killer is called oxycholesterol, or oxidized LDL cholesterol (OxLDL), and its sinister role in cardiovascular disease has been well documented. And knowing how to lower OxLDL levels, and keep them low, is critical to preventing or reducing the plaque buildup in your arteries known as atherosclerosis.

The LDL cholesterol story

LDL cholesterol plays many important roles in the body including transporting antioxidants, building muscle, and fighting infection. It also carries cholesterol to your arteries, which, despite what you may have heard before, is a good thing because all cell membranes, including those of your arteries, <u>require</u> cholesterol for both their structure and function.

The problem arises when LDL cholesterol becomes *oxidized*; in other words, when the LDL molecule becomes damaged by oxygen molecules. The easiest way to picture this oxidizing process is to think about rust, which is *also* caused by oxidation. If you leave a shiny new metal shovel out for months on end, exposing it to rain and snow, it will start to change color as it becomes rusty or "oxidizes." Eventually, over a long period of time, the metal will weaken because of the oxidation. This same sort of thing occurs with cholesterol, but this oxidation happens in your bloodstream or in your artery walls. And if it stopped here you would *already* have a problem but things get worse when inflammation then kicks in.

The "hidden" heart menace

You see, once the LDL cholesterol oxidizes and transforms into Ox-LDL it becomes like a magnet for a type of inflammatory immune cells called macrophages. The macrophages, a kind of white blood cell, seek out the OxLDL particles in your blood vessel walls. And then, like a game of Pac-Man gone horribly wrong, they start gobbling up the OxLDL.

What happens next, frankly, isn't pretty. The bloated macrophages transform into fat-laden foam cells causing even more inflammation in your artery walls. And to make matters worse there are a host of *other* immune cells that find the OxLDL irresistible too, and they also rush to your artery walls leading to... yes, you guessed it... yet *more* inflammation.

And that's not even the worst of it. While all that plaque formation is going on, OxLDL is also reducing the elasticity of your arteries. It literally blocks your body from making enough of the nitric oxide that it needs to keep your arteries dilated so your blood can flow easily.

The OxLDL's health-destroying rampage doesn't even stop there. The sinister lipid also increases blood clot formation in your arteries leading to atherosclerosis and sending your stroke risk skyrocketing.

Not surprisingly, when blood vessels get all inflamed and gunked up with plaque they just don't work well anymore. When this happens we docs call it *endothelial dysfunction*. I know it's a mouthful, but you don't need to know the term, just what it means for your heart.

The endothelium is a thin layer of cells that lines the inner walls of blood vessels. These cells control your blood vessels' ability to flex. (Inflexible arteries are bad news because they raise your risk for arterial ruptures and clots.) In fact, this cell layer is *so* important that many physiologists consider the endothelium to be an organ, just like your heart or brain.

Mainstream medicine misses the point

The mainstream medicine answer to preventing or reversing heart disease is... shall we say... predictable. Press the play button on almost any conventional doc and he'll tell you the same things. You start by running tests. Then you work on lowering your total and LDL cholesterol levels while you increase your good HDL cholesterol levels. And, finally, you focus on lowering the amount of fats, known as triglycerides, in your bloodstream.

That's all well and good, and *overall* not totally terrible advice. But, you may be wondering just *how* that doctor expects you to accomplish these things. Simple, by prescribing cholesterol-lowering statins of course! And this is where we run into trouble. Because, as I've explained to you before, the statin approach is so full of holes you could practically drive a Mack truck through it.

Want an example? A huge meta-analysis of 65,000 people published in *Evidence Based Medicine* found no link between using a statin drug and living longer. That's right, nada.

In fact, the researchers didn't even find any relationship at all between cholesterol levels and survival rates. And, don't forget, statins *also* come with a laundry list of potential side effects including increased cancer risk, muscle damage, liver damage, kidney damage, and memory loss.

Taking advantage of the test NOW

Clearly the tired old mainstream medicine approach is missing the mark. And a big part of what's sending them so far from that target is that the OxLDL levels… that they essentially ignore… must be addressed. Fortunately, the technology to measure OxLDL levels is available. In fact, I'm *already* using it myself with patients, and you can have your doctor use it too.

I believe in the next three to five years this type of testing will become much more mainstream. But why wait? Knowing your OxLDL levels and working on lowering them, and keeping them low, can mean the difference between no plaque buildup and *severe* plaque buildup in your arteries!

This blood test is already available through Shiel Medical Laboratory (www.shiel.com) and will soon be available through a national diagnostic laboratory as well. And the good news is that insurance coverage *is* available for the test. I suggest you seriously consider getting one done if you have any family or personal history of heart disease. But even with no history it's a great preventative tool if you're concerned about keeping your heart healthy.

The often overlooked warning sign

Research clearly shows us that OxLDL levels are linked to heart disease and that they serve as a good warning sign for future heart attacks and strokes. For example, in a study published in *Circulation* the plasma OxLDL level in patients who had had heart attacks skyrocketed about 3.5-fold over control subjects.[4] That's a HUGE leap!

Another study, published in the *American Journal of Cardiology*, looked at a variety of heart disease risk factors, including the old mainstream medicine favorite *traditional lipid levels*. The study included 431 healthy men and women who didn't have any signs of coronary artery disease who were matched with 490 men and women of about the same age who *did* have heart disease.

It turned out that the number-one marker for discriminating between the people with and without coronary artery disease was the ratio of OxLDL to HDL cholesterol.[5] In fact, as that ratio was by far a better predictor of heart disease than the standard total cholesterol or LDL cholesterol measurements!

Pursuing the cause of the cause

Knowing if the amount of oxidative damage to your LDL cholesterol is elevated or not is critically important. That's why testing is essential. But equally as important is to know *why* the oxidative damage is occurring in the first place so you can do something about it.

Our Creator designed special defense systems in our bodies to remove OxLDL. These weapons include special scavenger receptors in blood vessel walls that clean up the OxLDL, as well liver cells that hunt down and remove the stuff.[6] While the experts aren't positive yet what triggers the oxidation of LDL molecules, I believe the research will eventually show that much of it is related to diet, stress, and environmental toxin exposure.

Dining to drive those levels down

The good news is that there are things that you can do to start bringing down, and controlling, your OxLDL levels starting with your diet. In fact, several studies have already shown that a Mediterranean-style diet, high in monounsaturated fats, reduces LDL oxidation. For example, a study of 372 adults at high risk for heart disease found that diets rich in olive oil or nuts caused OxLDL to take a welcome nosedive. In contrast, people following a traditional… *supposedly* "heart healthy"… low fat diet had <u>no</u> change in their OxLDL levels.[7]

On the other hand, it appears that a diet high in polyunsaturated fats—like the ones you'll find in fast foods, junk food, and baked goods—increases OxLDL. In fact, corn oil, sunflower oil, safflower oil, cottonseed oil, and soy oil *all* seem to raise OxLDL levels more than mainstream medicine's favorite boogeyman… saturated fat.

Avoid these bad-news oils by saying no to fast foods and avoiding packaged and processed foods. Eating fresh is tastier. Besides I'm a big fan of the antioxidant-rich Mediterranean-style diet anyway. Knowing that it will *also* reduce LDL oxidation is like icing on the cake.

Besides the Mediterranean diet there are a couple more dieting "secrets" that can drive down LDL oxidation. For example, both vegan and gluten-free diets have been shown to reduce levels of OxLDL.[8] (It's likely that this is why so many of my patients feel better when following a gluten-free or gluten-limited diet.) And the flavonoids in pomegranate juice have been shown to ward off LDL oxidation.[9] Fresh vegetable juice, which is rich in antioxidants, is also a good addition to your diet. And don't forget, green tea—which is already known for protecting against heart disease—fights LDL oxidation as well.[10]

Choose cholesterol-fighting nutrients

Vitamin E is a powerful antioxidant that gobbles up free radicals and prevents oxidation damage in the body. And that's what makes it such a potent player against the oxidation of LDL molecules.[11] Good food sources of vitamin E include seeds, nuts, and brown rice.

However that's not the only OxLDL fighting nutrient on the block. You've probably heard of the heart supplement superstar Coenzyme Q10 before. But what you might *not* know is that CoQ10 goes well beyond general heart support by targeting and reducing the oxidation of LDL cholesterol molecules.[12] CoQ10 is found in peanuts, seafood, and meat. I also recommend 60 mg to 200 mg daily as a supplement for all adults.

Other natural solutions for fighting oxidation include garlic, Resveratrol, and grape seed extract. In addition taking a daily full-complex multivitamin and mineral formula will provide a base of antioxidants to protect against LDL oxidation.[13]

Other cholesterol elevators

Hormone balance can affect OxLDL levels as well. Research has shown that either a low functioning or an over-functioning thyroid gland can drive up your OxLDL levels.[14] There's also emerging research that hints that estrogen may fight LDL oxidation. Just one more reason to have your hormone levels checked and balanced!

There's evidence that chronic infections can increase levels of OxLDL and I'm willing to bet that future research will confirm that toxins in our environment can have an effect on them also.

Be sure to get your OxLDL level tested and work with a holistic doctor to treat the root reasons if your level is elevated.

Stop the Silent "Thick Blood" Killer That's Putting Your Heart and Health at Risk—Before it's Too Late!

"I don't understand it. My cardiologist has tried all the different drugs for my high blood pressure and we can't get it under control!" As I looked across my desk at Frank, a 65-year-old executive, it was clear that he was frustrated. And for good reason... he felt like he was fighting a losing battle.

I guided Frank through his lab results, "You have too many red blood cells, which is making your blood too thick. This not only increases your blood pressure, but puts you at direct risk for a heart attack or stroke," I explained.

Now you may never have heard of "thick blood" before, but that doesn't mean it isn't a serious threat to your *own* health. At this very moment it could be putting you at high risk for cardiovascular disease just like Frank. But also, like Frank, my stunningly simple two-step approach could help you turn the tables fast.

When Frank put my plan into action his blood pressure dropped like a rock in water. I'll tell you more about this natural approach a bit later, but first let's talk about one recipe you're never going to want to follow.

Thick and sticky blood is a recipe for heart disease

Everyone knows about the common risk factors for heart disease: Poor diet, diabetes, genetics, high blood pressure, smoking, inflammation, elevated lipid levels, and stress. But, as a *Health Revelations* reader, *you* know that there's much more to the story. Over the years I've given you the inside scoop on deficiencies of magnesium, coenzyme Q10, vitamin D, and omega-3 fatty acids that put you at risk. And I've explained how LDL particle size, the oxidation of LDL cholesterol, and endothelial (inside lining of the artery walls) dysfunction are all major risk factors for heart disease. Now I want to take it a step further and look at the role of thick, viscous (sticky) blood.

The stickier your blood becomes the bigger your risk for cardiovascular disease. When blood is too thick and gooey it can't flow easily through your blood vessels and your poor heart ends up having to work extra hard to keep it moving. This means less oxygen is being delivered to your body tissues (an under-diagnosed reason for fatigue). And the increased friction from trying to force this thick blood through thin blood vessels creates a shearing force on the walls of the vessels (picture trying to trying to pump molasses syrup through a straw and you'll have the right idea) can leading to inflammation, plaque formation, and blood clots.

Understanding your BP numbers

The viscosity of blood changes with each heartbeat. When blood is being pumped out of your heart—the period known as systole (first number in a blood pressure reading)—your blood is less sticky. When blood is moving more rapidly it disperses the components of blood, which decreases the stickiness. During diastole when your heart is at rest (the second and lower number in your blood pressure reading) blood viscosity greatly increases. The viscosity can be up to 20 times more than the same blood at systole. The good news is that during both phases of the heart pumping cycle one can take natural measures to reduce the stickiness.

Studies highlight link between thick blood and heart issues

There is a lot of data linking thick blood to a host of cardiovascular problems. In fact, Dr. Gregory Sloop from Louisiana State University School of Medicine at New Orleans has proposed that *all* the major risk factors for atherosclerosis ultimately do their damage because they increase blood thickness.[1]

One commonly cited study is the Edinburgh Artery study. It involved 4,860 men between the ages of 45 and 59 years and women aged 55 to 74 years. The researchers found that the 20 percent of study participants with the thickest and stickiest blood had the majority (55 percent) of the major cardiovascular events over a five year period. Researchers found that the link between blood viscosity and cardiovascular events was at *least* as strong as that of diastolic blood pressure and LDL cholesterol, and stronger than that of smoking.[2]

When you combine high blood pressure and thicker blood you have a deadly combination on your hands. A study published in the *European Journal of Clinical Investigation found those men in a group with the highest blood viscosity had more than a three-fold risk of cardiovascular events compared with those in a group with the lowest blood viscosity.*[3]

Where the pressure is greatest so is the plaque

Heart disease experts have been pondering a question for some time now. The fact is, most plaque formations occur in arteries close to the heart. But, if accepted cardiovascular risk factors such as elevated cholesterol are *really* the culprit behind plaque buildup in the arteries, why don't these blockages occur uniformly throughout the blood vessels of the body?

The answer has to do with pressure. The blood vessels that experience the strongest and most turbulent blood force are the most prone to inflammation, injury, and plaque (a sticky mix of cholesterol, fat, and calcium) formation. Thick blood, of course, increases this pressure on the blood vessels.

For example, as your heart pumps blood the large exit area known as the left ventricle is under a lot of pressure and the thicker your blood is the more intense that pressure becomes and the more likely it is for plaques to form in this spot. The carotid arteries of the neck and the large arteries of the legs are other areas that are prone to atherosclerotic plaques. These arteries split into different branches creating more turbulent blood flow and pressure. This increases blood viscosity as well as plaque formation.

Oncologists (cancer doctors) are well aware of the health problems associated with high-viscosity blood. There are a number of cancers, including leukemia, multiple myeloma, and Waldenström macroglobulinemia, which affect the bone marrow production of cells. Oncologists monitor the stickiness of the blood in patients with these cancers because it can lead to confusion and changes in mental status; hemorrhage of the retina; bleeding; various cardiovascular and lung problems, including heart and respiratory failure; and even death if not treated promptly.[4] It stands to reason that people without these cancers but who have increased blood viscosity can experience similar symptoms and risks.

Five risk factors for "fat and sticky" blood

There are five known risk factors that affect blood viscosity. These are hematocrit, erythrocyte deformability, plasma viscosity, erythrocyte aggregation, and temperature.[5] I know they're a mouthful, but don't worry you don't need to remember their actual names. All you really need to know is a little bit about what they are and that, fortunately, there are natural ways to improve abnormalities in each of them.

1   **Hematocrit** is the proportion of your blood that is made up of red blood cells. The higher your hematocrit is the thicker your blood is. A normal adult male range is 42 percent to 54 percent hematocrit and for an adult woman it is 38 percent to 46 percent hematocrit. It's best to be on the lower end of the hematocrit range.

The proportion of hematocrit in blood can be lowered by donating blood (therapeutic phlebotomy is a treatment where a doctor prescribes regular blood draws). When my patients have an elevated hematocrit I recommend 450 cc blood draws every few weeks until an optimal level is reached. This relatively painless process only takes about 15 minutes.

Testosterone replacement can increase your hematocrit, so I monitor this blood marker in patients who are receiving testosterone replacement therapy. An even simpler way to decrease hematocrit is to be well hydrated by drinking enough water.

2 **Erythrocyte deformability** is the ability of your red blood cells to change shape when force is applied. An example of this is blood cells bending and folding to move through capillaries. The more flexible your red blood cells are, the less viscous your blood is.

Red blood cells are kind of like us as we age, the older they get the less flexible they become. Blood donations and therapeutic phlebotomy can improve erythrocyte deformability because older red blood cells are removed, causing the formation of new red blood cells. Taking omega-3 supplements and improving your blood-sugar control can also help.

3 **Plasma viscosity** refers to the thickness of the fluid portion of your blood. This is the part of your blood that doesn't contain red blood cells, white blood cells, or platelets. Drinking enough water will improve plasma viscosity.

4 **Erythrocyte aggregation** refers to the tendency of your blood cells to clump together under pressure. Our blood needs to be able to clump, for example to stop the bleeding from a cut or bruise. But ideally, this clumping doesn't happen so aggressively that artery-blocking blood clots appear. Controlling factors like plasma viscosity and the ability of blood cells to change shape

(the erythrocyte deformability described above) can help you reach the right clumping balance.

5 **Temperature** is the last factor. Blood flows better at higher temperatures. More research is required, but it appears that keeping your thyroid… which regulates body temperature… in top shape can help improve the stickiness of your blood. Also, regular exercise improves body temperature regulation and circulation. The use of saunas and hydrotherapy (alternating hot and cold applications) can be beneficial as well.

Step One:
Blood pressure dips with blood donation

As I mentioned, blood donation is a great, natural way to reduce blood viscosity. It sure worked with Frank!

Research shows that blood donation can reduce systolic (21 percent) and diastolic (32 percent) blood viscosity values.[6] A study published in the *American Journal of Epidemiology* found an 88 percent reduced risk of sudden heart attack in those who donate blood regularly when compared with non-donors.[7] So donating blood can not only save the lives of others, but your own life as well!

Step Two:
Test blood thickness and then treat naturally

Everyone should find out his or her blood viscosity. This is particularly important if you have heart disease already or a strong family history of this common disease. If you're a smoker you have a much higher risk for thick blood and should be tested. I recommend testing for anyone with a history of stroke, blood clots, high blood pressure, elevated lipid levels, diabetes, chronic fatigue, migraine headaches, autoimmune disease, decreased cognition, or glaucoma. If you are an athlete, don't drink enough water, receive hormone therapy (especially testosterone and birth control pills), take diuretics, or have certain cancers (especially when the bone marrow is affected) I also typically recommend getting your levels checked as well.

Hematocrit level is a common test that is part of a routine blood panel known as a complete blood count. However, more direct testing, using an automated device that measures systolic and diastolic viscosity, can be done. Your doctor can get this test through Meridian Valley Lab (www.meridianvalleylab.com).

Should you be diagnosed with increased blood viscosity it is important to work with a holistic doctor to treat the *underlying* problem. Aspirin is *not* a good solution. Aspirin use is one of the leading reasons people end up in the hospital with bleeding ulcers. It's also a cause of tinnitus. And a recent study found regular aspirin use can nearly triple the risk of a serious, irreversible, and potentially blinding condition called wet age-related macular degeneration![8]

Drinking enough water is critical to keeping your blood from getting too thick. Depending on your activity level during the day, and the temperature you're in, most people need 50 to 80 oz daily.

One of the reasons that fish oil supplements (as well as eating fish) decreases your cardiovascular risk is that it reduces blood viscosity. Supplement 1,000 to 1,500 mg of EPA and DHA combined daily.

The best overall natural blood thinner is nattokinase. I regularly use nattokinase with my own patients. The dose for most brands is one to two capsules taken on an empty stomach. Check with your holistic doctor for the proper dose for your situation.

And the most effective means to lower your blood viscosity is therapeutic phlebotomy or blood donation that I've already mentioned. Regular monitoring with blood testing will let you, and your doctor, know when your blood has reached the right viscosity level.

The Up-and-Coming Heart Health Superstar That Everyone Will Be Talking About: Put the MEGA into Your OMEGA

It's the biggest success story in natural health: Heart-friendly omega-3 fatty acids are now so widely used that they've become one of the best-selling supplements in the entire nation.

For once this isn't the power of marketing at work. It's a triumph of science—and a triumph for natural health, as the millions of people who take these essential fatty acids see the results for themselves.

But what if I told you there was "another omega" out there... one that's showing so much promise in early research that it might actually turn out to be _**even better**_ than the omega-3s for cardiovascular health you've come to depend on?

I know—that's a little hard to believe. And I wouldn't blame you for a minute for being skeptical. I was a doubter myself... at first. Then I saw the research that made me a true believer—research that could greatly impact the way we approach heart health in the very near future.

And it started in the most unlikely place...

A fried chicken restaurant!

OK, now I know you think I'm pulling your leg… along with your wing, thigh, and drumstick. After all, fried chicken might be delicious—but it's the farthest thing in the world from anything that could ever possibly be healthy.

It's not the chicken itself that's so bad for you. It's the fats in the deep-fryer—fats that are absorbed by the breading, skin, and even the chicken meat itself.

And you should see what they do to deep fryers. Anyone who's ever worked in a restaurant will tell you that cleaning those things at the end of the night is the worst job in the kitchen.

Well, one restaurant owner who was famous for his fried chicken was tired of the mess. So he asked a friend for help—a biochemist with 30 years of experience who knew a thing or two about how fats and oils work on a molecular level.

And after dumping just about everything he could think of into the deep fryer, he was stumped. Nothing could eat through that greasy buildup.

Then, almost as a last resort, the biochemist tried a completely natural oil he had read about.

Did it work? Did it ever! And if the story ended there, it would be great news for the fast food industry… but I wouldn't be writing to you about it today.

So of course, the story doesn't end there. The biochemist began to wonder what a natural oil that can clean kitchen machines might do if it was used in another "machine."

That "machine" is YOU…

The human "machine"

The biochemist recruited some of his fellow scientists to look into this—and not just any old scientists. He hired some of the best on the planet to perform this study: The crack research team at the world-famous Cleveland Clinic who are leading researchers in medicine, specifically cardiovascular health.

Now, you know how it is with science. You don't go right from the deep fryer to experiments on humans. You have to start with something else—something with a similar system to humans, but something that wouldn't be missed if you had to chop them up at the end of the study.

And—sorry, rodent lovers—you start with mice.

More specifically, you start with mice that have been specially bred for cardiovascular research. And after 12 weeks, the same natural oil that cleaned the deep fryer clearly helped support cardiovascular health in these mice.

I saw the study at the time. It came with photos of the arteries, which you can see for yourself online—and believe me, you don't need to be a doctor or a scientist to see the results.

Now this was a mouse study, so I'm waiting to see the results from future human studies to know this natural oil's *full* potential. But trust me when I tell you that what I've seen so far is quite impressive.

So what was this "magical" oil? It was the *other* omega, of course. Specifically…

Omega-7

If you're like most people, you've heard plenty about omega-3 and absolutely nothing about omega-7. But while this might be the first time you've ever heard of omega-7, it certainly won't be the last.

As I write this, nearly all the major supplement makers are rushing to create their own omega-7 formulas. You'll read about them in magazines and see doctors talking about them on television.

In fact, I wouldn't be surprised if "omega-7" quickly becomes the next big buzzword in natural health. And with *Health Revelations* I typically give you breakthroughs years ahead of any other source.

But there's one thing you won't hear about anywhere else—one thing all the high-priced marketing teams and even some of the TV doctors won't talk about… but I will.

Not all omega-7s are created equal!

The omega-7 used in the study showed such promise in supporting heart health—but it came at a price: The form they used in the mouse study, which came from macadamia nuts, also contained higher levels of palmitic acid, an unhealthy saturated fat.

And, when all is said and done, macadamia nut oil isn't even the best source of actual omega-7 anyway.

That got my own wheels turning, and I set out to find a better source of omega-7—one that's low in unhealthy palmitic acid and high in the actual omega-7 everyone is trying to get.

And it's in a form of fish oil that the other guys were throwing away.

It's called Provinal™, and its levels of palmitic acid are seven times lower than what you'll find in macadamia nut oils. More importantly, it's got 22 percent more omega-7 content than the next highest source on the market today.

I'm not just a believer in this stuff. I'm a big believer—which is why Dr. Stengler's Health Products made an exclusive deal with the creators of Provinal™ to make this available to my customers at the lowest cost possible, and I put it at the heart of my new formula, Provicor.

Because of this exclusive relationship, you won't find this top source of omega-7 in any other doctor's formula—so when you see omega-7 somewhere else, you know you might be getting something less.

Now, I could have just stopped there and called it a day—and it would be a pretty good day, too, since I truly believe omega-7 alone will change the face of natural health.

But that's just not how I operate.

I know many people are tired of swallowing pill after pill after pill—even essential all-natural supplements—and the last thing I want to do is add yet another one to the list. Also, I recognize that there are many factors that contribute to cardiovascular health.

So I've combined the power of omega-7 with some of the biggest superstars in natural cardiovascular support.

Provicor isn't one more pill to take—it's an easy-to-swallow gel capsule that could actually reduce the number of pills you take by combining the great all-natural supplements you *already* depend on with the next big thing in heart health.

That's why I think of this formula as a one stop shop for natural cardiovascular support. And just like a one-stop shop for cars would contain plenty of sparkplugs, Provicor contains plenty of coenzyme Q10.

After all, this essential enzyme is literally…

The sparkplug that powers your heart

That might sound like a wild exaggeration, but coenzyme Q10 kicks off the reaction that allows the body to convert nutrients into energy. This process is so critical to cardiovascular support that one major study on 2,359 patients found that volunteers who took CoQ10 saw improved heart function in just three months.

In addition, research has shown that, once converted into its antioxidant form in the body, CoQ10 can fight free radicals in the bloodstream.

It's like having a team of trained Navy SEALS on your side.

Some people pay big money just for a quality CoQ10 supplement on its own. It's worth every penny, too, in my opinion—but you don't have to pay extra for it here. You'll find 100 mg of this essential in every daily dose of Provicor.

And I didn't stop there, either.

One of the things my patients ask me about most is a natural way to support healthy cholesterol levels. They've seen the commercials and read the newspaper reports and know they should be doing something… but what?

Well, there's the usual approach of diet and exercise. And as you know I am not a fan of the conventional approach that only targets cholesterol. But if you're like my patients, you're already doing that—and you want to do more. And if that's your story, I've got just the thing for you:

The ancient secret backed by modern science!

It's called Indian gooseberry, also known as amla. But it's not the name that matters here—it's what it does.

Let's start with triglycerides. If you've been in to see your own doctor lately, he's probably mentioned these blood fats, and with good reason: Triglyceride levels are an important heart health marker.

Clearly, you want to support healthy triglyceride levels naturally— and one recent small study found that AmlaMax may help do just that. In three months, this ancient secret from the Near East cut triglyceride levels by 21 percent in comparison to their starting values.

Think that's good? This gets even better—because over six months, triglyceride levels plunged by 34 percent compared to their starting values.

Along with triglycerides, your doctor has probably also mentioned HDL cholesterol. And again, he's right on the money if he does. HDL is known as the "good" cholesterol because it's like a street cleaner for the arteries, sweeping LDL ("bad") cholesterol out into the gutter.

Or, more specifically, out into your liver.

Clearly, it's essential to get healthy HDL support—and in one study, volunteers who took AmlaMax saw a 16 percent increase in HDL levels in just 12 weeks.

As a doctor, I can't tell you enough how big that is. HDL can be as stubborn as a cranky old mule. No matter how much you push, sometimes it seems like you just can't get those levels to budge.

Now, if you're a regular *Health Revelations* reader, you know HDL, LDL, and triglycerides are just three pieces of the cholesterol puzzle. They're important—but there's so much more to heart health than just tracking those levels on a chart and watching them rise or fall.

The other pieces of that puzzle involves a few things your own doctor probably isn't talking about—yet—including oxidation and particle size. And in my opinion, one of the most important pieces of all is…

INFLAMMATION

If I could pick just one thing to measure—total cholesterol or inflammation—I'd go with inflammation every time, because those levels tell me so much more than all the cholesterol tests in the world combined.

A critical marker of inflammation is CRP, or C-reactive protein—and once again, AmlaMax is showing great promise here. In one of the studies mentioned above, volunteers who took this extract saw a 35 percent plunge in CRP levels in three months.

Some of the most promising studies on AmlaMax, including the ones I just mentioned, used levels of 500 mg a day—and that's exactly what you'll find in each daily dose of my Provicor.

But I'm not a believer in putting all my eggs in one basket, especially when it comes to supporting heart health. So as great as AmlaMax is, I also included some backup—and it's the healthy plant sterols many people already swear by.

Plant sterols inhibit the body's ability to absorb cholesterol in the intestines, which may be why one major analysis of 84 clinical trials confirmed that they can help support healthy LDL levels.

And believe it or not, I still didn't stop there.

You've heard a lot in recent years about the healthy polyphenols in grapes and especially wine. What you don't hear as much is that wine itself is actually a lousy source of those great polyphenols.

In fact, you'd have to drink hundreds of bottles a day to get some of the amounts used in top studies.

That's not just impossible—it would be deadly to even try.

Well, thanks to Provicor, you can now get healthy levels of grape seed polyphenols without swallowing a drop of alcohol—because I've included some of the best of the best in the form of MegaNatural-BP.

MegaNatural-BP is a blockbuster blood-pressure supporting compound made from the polyphenols found in grape seed extract—and in one double-blind clinical trial, volunteers with normal blood pressure levels who took it enjoyed a significant dip in both systolic and diastolic blood pressure.

Patients who took a placebo, on the other hand, saw no real changes at all.

All-in-one heart support

Provicor—featuring the groundbreaking heart-support of omega-7s—is an all-in-one exclusive formula you won't find anywhere else. It can help support healthy LDL cholesterol, HDL cholesterol, triglycerides, blood pressure, CRP levels, and supercharge your heart's energy all at the same time.

Normally, I'm not one to brag. But I can't help but be proud of Provicor—and I'm so confident that it can help you that I want you to try it risk-free. So here's the deal: Set your expectations as high as you want… and if Provicor doesn't meet or even exceed those expectations, send it back to me.

Even if you're down to the very last capsule—send it back, and I'll refund every penny.

You won't find an offer like that anywhere else. If you're ready to take me up on it—if you're ready to see what Provicor can do for you—visit www.besthealthnutritionals.com or give us a call at 1-800-539-1447 and be sure to use your special promo code G653PC04 to make sure to get your exclusive *Health Revelations* subscriber discount of 20 percent off the regular price of $69.95.

Part IV
Energy and Fatigue

Tired? Moody?
Adrenal Fatigue May Be to Blame

The epidemic of exhaustion affecting so many Americans today may have at its root one condition that is common and easy to correct—yet that condition often goes unrecognized by medical doctors. The culprit is *adrenal fatigue* (AF).

Adrenal glands produce stress hormones in response to stressful situations. With AF, the hormone response mechanism is so overwhelmed that it becomes ineffective. AF is usually triggered by long periods of mental, emotional or physical stress, and it is worsened by poor nutrition and unhealthful lifestyle choices.

In my estimation, 20 percent of Americans suffer from some degree of AF. And I find that this disorder often triggers—or contributes to—the development of numerous other illnesses, particularly chronic fatigue syndrome and diabetes. When AF is correctly diagnosed and treated, the other conditions often are relieved as well.

Stress hormone factory

Located on top of each kidney is a crescent-shaped adrenal gland. Hormones that these glands secrete affect blood pressure, heart rate, metabolism, liver function, immunity and the body's response to stress. Although the adrenal glands produce many hormones, two in particular become depleted in cases of AF—*dehydroepiandrosterone* (DHEA) and *cortisol*.

• **DHEA**. The body converts DHEA into *estrogen* and *testosterone*. Abnormally low DHEA levels may contribute to cardiovascular disease, autoimmune disorders, poor resistance to infection, diabetes, weight gain, osteoporosis, sexual dysfunction, menopausal symptoms and mood disorders. DHEA also plays a role in aging. On average, the citizens of the Japanese Island of Okinawa (one of the world's longest-living people) have much higher DHEA levels at age 70 than Americans do—30 percent higher for men and 172 percent higher for women.

• **Cortisol** plays an important role in fighting infection... stabilizing blood sugar... controlling the body's use of proteins, carbohydrates and fats... and regulating the sleep cycle. Cortisol is secreted at higher levels during the fight-or-flight response to stress, providing a burst of energy, heightened alertness and decreased pain sensitivity. But when cortisol levels are elevated for long periods, production by the adrenal glands drops. Insufficient cortisol can make you more prone to fatigue, infection, allergies, diabetes and thyroid dysfunction.

Depletion of DHEA and cortisol adversely affects the way your body handles stress, inflammation, regulation of blood sugar, energy production, immune response and cognitive function. That's why AF can be a contributing factor in a surprising number of ailments. A weakened immune response plays a part in cancer as well as in recurring infections, particularly of the respiratory tract. And poor regulation of blood sugar can contribute to both diabetes and alcoholism (alcoholics often crave simple sugars, which are found in alcohol, so improving blood sugar balance can help reduce alcohol cravings).

Making the diagnosis

Conventional medical doctors often do not recognize AF—even though the condition was described in medical literature in the early 20th century. It was known then as *hypoadrenia*, which means low- or under-functioning adrenal glands.

If you show signs of AF your best bet for diagnosis and treatment is to see a holistic doctor. For a referral, consult the American College for Advancement in Medicine (949-309-3520 or www.acamnet.org). *In addition to assessing your symptoms, the doctor may perform...*

• **Saliva testing to measure cortisol levels.** This test is more accurate than a blood test. A pattern of low cortisol levels throughout the day indicates AF. I ask patients to collect saliva samples in test tubes upon waking... before lunch... in the late afternoon... and before bed. Cortisol levels are normally highest in the morning and decrease throughout the day. People with severe AF usually have below-normal cortisol readings during at least two of the four time periods. I also use a saliva test that measures the DHEA level in the morning, when it is normally highest.

Saliva testing of cortisol levels is used by many research institutions, particularly to assess the effects of stress. Several commercial labs offer saliva hormone testing—including Quest Diagnostics, the nation's largest conventional medical lab, which is used by medical and naturopathic doctors. To use Quest, you must have a prescription for the test from a doctor. A lab I have used for years that usually doesn't require a doctor's request is ZRT in Beaverton, Oregon (866-600-1636 or www.zrtlab.com).

• **Blood pressure measurements**, taken three times—first while you lie on your back, then when you sit upright and again when you stand up. Normally, *systolic* (top number) and *diastolic* (bottom number) blood pressure will increase between five mmHg and 10 mmHg from the first reading to the third. If blood pressure *drops*, it may indicate AF—the adrenal glands may not be producing the stress hormones required to maintain blood pressure.

• **Pupil testing**, performed in a darkened room. A practitioner shines a flashlight from the side across one eye, and the pupil should continue to get smaller. With AF, the pupil first contracts and then dilates again.

Healing strategies

Lifestyle changes and treatment reduce symptoms in most patients with AF in four to six weeks. In severe cases, full recovery may take several months. *My advice…*

• **Curb stress**. A hectic lifestyle sets the stage for AF. Are you working too hard? Is your job emotionally draining? Are your relationships unsatisfying? Try to alleviate stress and seek out emotional support.

• **Get enough rest**. Get to bed by 10 pm, and aim for eight to nine hours of sleep nightly. Whenever possible, take a 15- to 30-minute nap after lunch, even if you're getting the required amount of sleep. On weekends, nap for an hour or two.

If you have insomnia, it's vital that your sleep problems be resolved. Take a walk in the early evening or listen to relaxing music. One hour before bedtime, take 100 mg to 200 mg of *5-hydroxytryptophan* (5-HTP), an amino acid that increases brain serotonin levels and promotes relaxation… or take 0.5 milligrams to three milligrams of melatonin, a hormone that induces sleep. Both are available at health-food stores.

• **Eat right**. People with AF are prone to blood sugar swings that sap energy, so it is imperative to eat breakfast. I also recommend between-meal snacks, such as whole-grain toast or whey protein drinks. My favorite is Jay Robb's Whey Protein, which is naturally sweetened. It is available at major health-food stores and at www.jayrobb.com (877-529-7622). Almonds, walnuts and macadamia nuts are good snack foods, since they provide protein for blood sugar stabilization. Avoid simple sugars, such as those found in fruit juice and soda, as well as processed grains, such as white breads and pastas. These trigger a quick spike and subsequent drop in blood sugar levels.

Don't severely restrict salt intake unless you have high blood pressure. People with AF often benefit from salt because it helps maintain blood volume and proper circulation. Aim for 2,400 mg of sodium daily. Limit caffeinated beverages, such as coffee, tea and cola, to one cup daily because caffeine stimulates the already overtaxed adrenal glands. Avoid alcohol, which contains simple sugars.

• **Exercise in moderation**. Too little exercise is harmful, since exercise helps balance stress hormones. But overexercising worsens fatigue.

General guideline: If you're exhausted after your workout or feel more worn out than usual the next day, you're doing too much. Start by walking 15 minutes daily. As your adrenal glands recover, you can gradually increase to 45 minutes of moderately intense exercise daily.

• **Avoid lung irritants**. Cigarette smoke, air pollution and allergens can worsen AF by stimulating cortisol release. If you smoke, please quit. Avoid secondhand smoke, and reduce exposure to allergy triggers with a *high-efficiency particulate air (HEPA) filter*.

• **Clear up infections**. Acute and chronic respiratory infections as well as other types of infections can exacerbate AF symptoms. To quicken recovery, work with a holistic doctor, who can recommend natural immune boosters, such as the herb *astralgalus*.

Helpful supplements

The following nutritional supplements are invaluable in promoting adrenal function. Take them until you recover. All are available from health-food stores. (Do not use if you are pregnant or breast-feeding.)

• **Adrenal glandular extract (AGE)** is made from cow or sheep adrenal tissue. It contains growth factors (substances that promote cell healing and regeneration) and nutrients that support gland function and adrenal repair. Take one to two tablets, two to three times daily, on an empty stomach. If you get a headache, have insomnia or feel jittery, lower the dosage.

• **Ashwagandha** is an herb that's used traditionally in Ayurvedic medicine for normalizing adrenal gland function. Jarrow's Sensoril Ashwagandha uses a form of the herb that has been well studied and standardized. Take one to two capsules of this product daily on an empty stomach. Side effects are rare.

• **Rhodiola rosea**, an herb that has been extensively researched, supports normal adrenal function. I recommend using a product such as Paradise Herbs' Dual Action Rhodiola, which is standardized to three percent to five percent *rosavins* (the active ingredient). Take 500 mg twice daily, on an empty stomach. If you feel jittery, try a lower dose.

• **B vitamins** are involved in the production of stress hormones. Particularly important is *pantothenic acid* (vitamin B-5), which is best taken at a dosage of 500 mg, three times daily. Side effects are uncommon. The rest of the B vitamins can be taken as part of a multivitamin formula.

• **Vitamin C** is needed for the adrenal glands to synthesize hormones. I advise 1,000 mg to 2,000 mg twice daily. Reduce the dosage if you develop loose stools.

For severe cases of AF, hormone support with DHEA and cortisol may be required. This therapy should be administered by a knowledgeable doctor. The goal is to reduce the workload of the adrenal glands so they can heal. Over time, the hormone replacement can be reduced, then discontinued once the adrenals are functioning optimally.

For more information on AF, I recommend the book *Adrenal Fatigue: The 21st Century Stress Syndrome* by James Wilson, ND (Smart Publications).

Adrenal Fatigue symptoms

Patients with AF typically experience low energy or exhaustion (even after a good night's sleep), plus one or more of the following...

• **Light-headedness upon standing up**.

• **Mood swings, especially irritability**.

• **Decreased ability to cope with stress**.

• **Low libido**.

• **Poor concentration**.

• **Impaired memory**.

• **Slow recovery from illness**.

• **Low back pain**.

• **Salt and/or sugar cravings**.

• **Inability to lose or gain weight**, despite calorie reduction or increase.

Conditions associated with Adrenal Fatigue

Although AF is not the direct cause of all the conditions below, it can be a contributing factor in…

• **Alcoholism**.

• **Arthritis**.

• **Asthma**.

• **Exercise burnout** (becoming ill after intense workouts).

• **Autoimmune disorders**, like lupus and multiple sclerosis.

• **Cardiovascular disease**.

• **Chronic fatigue syndrome**.

• **Depression and/or anxiety**.

• **Diabetes or hypoglycemia** (low blood sugar).

• **Insomnia**.

• **Menopausal symptoms**.

• **Osteoporosis**.

• **Recurring infections**.

Fixing Fatigue After a Quadruple Bypass

Many who have been through a bypass surgery experience uncomfortable aftereffects, such as shortness of breath and fatigue. Some patients have reported that taking hawthorn improves these symptoms, but there are other supplements to be considered as well.

Coenzyme Q10 (300 mg daily) and *L-carnitine* (2,000 mg) are nutrients that help the heart contract with better force. Studies have shown that they can improve congestive heart failure. One other supplement I frequently recommend is *ribose* at a dosage of five grams twice daily. This nutrient helps heart cells produce energy more effectively. A European study found that *ribose* supplementation significantly improved heart function in cardiac patients.

Magnesium also is important to proper heart function. A good dosage is 250 mg to 400 mg twice daily. In addition, I have written about the mushroom *cordyceps* in the past and how it supports heart function. The recommended dosage is 1,500 mg to 1,600 mg twice daily of the Cs-4 extract. Be sure to talk with your cardiologist before taking any supplements. You also may want to consult with your cardiologist about *enhanced external counterpulsation* (EECP). This involves the use of pressure cuffs on the legs that are inflated by a machine in sequences. The blood vessels in the legs are gently compressed, which improves the rate at which blood returns to the heart.

Cordyceps—The Champion's Choice for Fatigue, Kidney Health and More

The use of medicinal mushroom extracts has gained tremendous popularity in North America and Europe over the past decade. Centuries of use by Asian herbalists and doctors, solid scientific research and publicity about the unique health benefits of medicinal mushrooms have created interest by doctors and consumers.

Much of this excitement has been generated by research that shows mushroom extracts restoring immune function and improving the condition of people with a variety of serious illnesses. I have been using a variety of mushroom extracts with patients for over a decade and am very impressed by their clinical effectiveness.

One of my favorites and an emerging superstar is *Cordyceps sinensis*. What I find fascinating is that *Cordyceps* is also called "caterpillar fungus," as it grows on and acquires nutrients from several species of caterpillars. It is also referred to by traditional Chinese herbalists as "winter worm" or "summer grass." This fungus is found at high altitude such as on the mountaintops of China, Nepal and Tibet.

Cordyceps attracted the attention of the general public and the health profession in 1993 when a group of Chinese runners broke nine world records in the World Outdoor Track and Field Championships in Germany. Their coach attributed those results from the regular use of a *Cordyceps*-based tonic. However, we do have reason to think that performance-enhancing steroids were rampant at those events as well.

Cordyceps subsequently became a sought- after nutritional supplement, and it does have reputable science behind it. *Cordyceps* helps increase stamina, energy levels and endurance. It has become one of the top-selling sports supplements among elite competitive athletes and has caught the attention of health-food consumers.

In traditional Chinese medicine *Cordyceps sinensis* is considered to benefit the lung and kidney channels. It is commonly used with the elderly in China as a type of "superginseng" for rejuvenation and stamina.

Since it is difficult to cultivate enough *Cordyceps* from the wild, commercial fermentation methods have been developed in China. These methods are now used here in the West. Cs-4 is an isolated strain of wild *Cordyceps* that has been the focus of much study and is used by clinics throughout China and recently in the US, including my own clinic. What do the studies show?

Improves Fatigue

One of the most popular uses of *Cordyceps* is to improve energy levels. More than two thousand patients with a variety of medical problems have been involved in clinical trials of Cs-4. Placebo-controlled studies have found *Cordyceps* to benefit elderly patients with fatigue. Subjective improvements included improvement of fatigue, cold intolerance, dizziness, frequent nighttime urination, tinnitus (ringing in the ears), low libido and loss of memory. Animal studies suggest that *Cordyceps* improves the ability of cells to use oxygen more efficiently to produce energy.

Sexual revitalizer and adrenal booster

The adrenal glands are one of the most important glands (in addition to your thyroid) for energy production and to produce sex hormones such as testosterone. Studies have shown *Cordyceps* to have a homeostatic or balancing effect on adrenal hormones and to protect against adrenal atrophy. Many holistic doctors prescribe *Cordyceps* for supporting and regenerating the adrenal gland. I have found it to be one of the best supplements for this purpose.

Human studies have demonstrated benefit in patients reporting low libido.

For example, in a double-blind, placebo-controlled clinical trial, patients who reported decreased sex drives were treated with *Cordyceps*. Participants who took *Cordyceps* had a subjective improvement rate that was significantly higher than those receiving a placebo. In addition, the group who received *Cordyceps* had a much higher increase in sex-hormone production as compared to those who received a placebo. *Cordyceps* has been used in traditional Chinese medicine for the treatment of sexual dysfunction and male impotence.

Respiratory support

Cordyceps also has a long history of use in the natural treatment of chronic respiratory disorders such as asthma, chronic bronchitis and other diseases. Various studies have demonstrated positive effects to improve respiratory function. In Chinese medicine there is a strong link between kidney/adrenal gland function and lung performance. One of the ways that I and other holistic doctors help patients with chronic asthma and other lung problems is to improve adrenal gland function. *A note about patience:* It takes up to six weeks to notice improvement with chronic lung conditions. *Cordyceps* can be safely taken in conjunction with asthma medications.

Kidney health

This remarkable fungus has been relied upon by physicians in China for benefit in the treatment of chronic kidney diseases such as chronic nephritis, kidney failure, chronic pyelonephritis, and others. Studies also show that it has a protective effect against chemicals that are toxic to the kidneys.

One study of thirty patients with chronic renal failure found that treatment with *Cordyceps* resulted in an overall significant improvement in kidney function.

A significant increase in creatinine clearance and reduction in BUN were noted (signifying the kidney's ability to filter the blood). In addition, there were significant improvements in anemia with increases in hemoglobin and red blood cell counts. It appears that *Cordyceps* stimulates the kidney's production of erythropoietin (EPO), a hormone that stimulates the bone marrow's production of red blood cells.

Cardiovascular benefits

Human and animal studies have demonstrated diverse benefits for the cardiovascular system. These include positive studies in regards to arrhythmias, ischemic heart disease, and chronic heart failure. Animal and human studies have shown *Cordyceps* to lower total cholesterol, triglycerides, LDL cholesterol, and VLDL cholesterol. Conversely, it improves the healthy HDL cholesterol.

In a double-blind, randomized placebocontrolled study, researchers looked at the effects of *Cordyceps* on elevated cholesterol levels. More than half of the patients on *Cordyceps* therapy had a greater than 10 percent decrease in total cholesterol and a more than 20 percent decrease in triglycerides, while 76 percent of patients had a greater than 10 percent increase in HDL cholesterol.

Interestingly, animal studies have demonstrated that *Cordyceps* can dilate the coronary arteries and increase blood flow to the heart. This circulatory effect has been shown to also occur with the smaller arteries that supply blood flow to the brain.

Potential new uses: Preliminary studies have shown *Cordyceps* to have value in the treatment of Hepatitis B and diabetes. *Cordyceps* also has a diverse effect on the immune system. It has been studied in combination with chemotherapy and radiation treatment for lung cancer. Patients showed improved tolerance of these therapies with the supplementation of *Cordyceps*.

What makes it work?

Scientists have not completely determined why *Cordyceps* offers so many benefits to the human body. *Cordyceps* has several active constituents—Cordycepin, d-mannitol, adenosine, and various polysaccharides—that may contribute to improved cellular energy production and immune system enhancement.

Dosage: I recommend a dosage of 800 to 1,600 mg of a standardized water/ethanol extract from fermented mycelia of *Cordyceps sinensis* strain Cs-4. There are several brands available in health-food stores, online sellers and pharmacies that carry this Cs-4 extract. Brands include Mushroom Science, Pharmanex and Planetary Formulas.

Safety profile: *Cordyceps* is an extremely safe supplement to use. The key is to use a Cs-4 extract from a reputable manufacturer. One word of caution. As an immune modulator it should be avoided in organ-transplant patients using immunosuppressive agents.

Uses of Cordyceps include…

- Athletic performance
- Cancer
- Adrenal fatigue
- Hepatitis B
- Asthma
- Emphysema
- Hypercholesterolemia

- Chronic fatigue
- Decreased libido
- Chronic renal failure
- Diabetes
- Chronic bronchitis
- Heart disease
- Tinnitus

Supercharge Your Metabolism... Supercharge Your Energy

Imagine a simple nutritional protocol that not only boosts your metabolism but also your energy levels! It is one I prescribe in my clinic daily—and I want to share it with you.

Even if you are in good shape and in relatively good health, you probably don't have the vitality that came so naturally when you were younger. Many of my patients also complain about putting on weight even when they still eat and exercise much as they did when they were younger. You already know that carrying excess weight contributes to or complicates a multitude of serious conditions—among them diabetes, arthritis, heart disease, and even several types of cancer. Carrying even a few extra pounds makes us feel slower... less ready to live with energy and zest... older.

Many people are resigned to these changes, assuming that slowing down and fattening up are inevitable parts of aging. Not so! You can't turn back the clock, but you can rev up your metabolism so it is closer to where it was when you were younger. In recent years, I have had great success prescribing "metabolism superchargers"—critical nutrients that revitalize the body's energy production. My patients tell me that these substances give them more energy, and I have seen many patients of all ages lose excess pounds.

The energy thieves

Your basal metabolic rate is the speed at which your body burns calories while at rest. When it slows, as it usually does with age, you burn fewer calories.

Result: Your energy level begins to flag... you gain weight.

But what is "energy" to our bodies? Here's a brief (I promise!) biology refresher to help you understand. Our physical strength, stamina and vigor originate within cell structures called mitochondria. Mitochondria generate *adenosine triphosphate* (ATP), a chemical that affects our metabolism and produces energy—both the fuel that cells need to do their work and the vitality we feel in our bodies. As we age, mitochondrial function gradually declines... as does the actual number of mitochondria.

One reason: The numerous toxins to which the body is exposed over the years, including environmental metals and other pollutants, radiation, alcohol, infections... hormone imbalances, such as hypothyroidism... inherited mitochondria mutations... some medications... and, in elite athletes, the stress caused by chronically overexercising—ultimately damage some mitochondria and interfere with replication of new mitochondria cells.

The natural way to boost your energy

Considerable research demonstrates that certain natural nutrients, taken as supplements, can increase energy by directly increasing mitochondrial functioning and ATP production. In other words, they can supercharge your metabolism. Healthful foods do boost metabolism, but not enough to make a real difference in energy or weight to people who need help in those areas.

My suggestion: For three months, take all of the following nutrients daily (there is no one energy supplement that combines these nutrients in the amounts I recommend) (All are available at many drug stores and most health-food stores.) Then assess whether your energy has increased and whether it feels as if your weight has become easier to control with appropriate food choices and exercise. I find that most people experience an energy boost (if you don't experience this, stop taking the supplements), and about 75 percent of patients find that this regimen helps with weight control. If you are pleased with your increased energy, you can continue to take these supplements indefinitely—as I do.

• **Coenzyme Q10 (CoQ10).** This nutrient is found in every cell in the body and is required for ATP production. It is a potent antioxidant, helping to protect mitochondria from damage. Researchers at the Southeastern Institute of Biomedical Research in Bradenton, Florida, examined 20 women with chronic fatigue syndrome who became so exhausted after even mild exercise that they required bed rest. Testing revealed that 80 percent of them were deficient in CoQ10. After three months of taking 100 mg of CoQ10 daily, they were able to exercise for twice as long, and 90 percent of them showed fewer symptoms of fatigue—or none at all. The generally recommended dosage is 100 mg once daily with a meal. For people with severe fatigue—those who have trouble carrying out daily activities—I advise taking 100 mg two or three times each day with meals. Continue the higher dosage for a few months. When your energy level improves, try to cut back to 100 mg daily. CoQ10 is a mild blood thinner so if you are on blood-thinning medication it is particularly important to consult your doctor before taking this supplement.

• **L-Carnitine.** This chemical derived from the amino acids *lysine* and *methionine* exists in most cells and serves a dual purpose—it transports long-chain fatty acids into the mitochondria to be used as fuel… and removes waste products such as lactic acid and ammonia. I was particularly impressed by the results of a study at the University of Catania, Italy, on the beneficial effects of L-carnitine. For the study, 66 centenarians were divided into two groups. For six months, one group took two grams of L-carnitine once a day and the other took a placebo. The study authors concluded that the L-carnitine helped to reduce body fat… increase muscle mass… increase the capacity for physical activity… minimize fatigue… and improve cognitive functions, such as arithmetic, memory and orientation (an awareness of one's environment with reference to time, place, and people). My recommended dosage is 1,500 mg (1.5 grams) twice daily. Side effects are uncommon, but can include digestive upset—in which case, take it with food or reduce your dosage slightly.

• **Resveratrol**. Recently publicized as the "healthful" component of red wine in animal studies, this potent antioxidant has been shown to help increase the number of mitochondria in muscles and other tissues and to reduce fat deposits in the body. Resveratrol activates the SIRT1 gene, which promotes longevity, and also contributes to better glucose and insulin control in men with type 2 diabetes (which leads to better energy and weight control). In my practice, I am also finding that resveratrol helps with metabolism in general. My colleague, Carrie Louise Daenell, ND, in Denver, works extensively with fatigue and weight issues. She has her patients take all the nutrients discussed here and says that 75 percent of her patients improve in energy and weight—but, she adds, it is resveratrol that seems to give the greatest benefits for weight control.

My recommended resveratrol dosage for adults to improve metabolism and weight control: 125 mg daily. It is generally well tolerated, though occasionally people experience nausea or loose stool—in which case take with food or start with a lower dose and build up over time.

• **D-ribose**. This is a type of sugar found in all the body's cells. It helps to restore energy by prompting the mitochondria to recycle ATP that has broken down… and it acts as another fuel source besides glucose, especially in the muscles and in particular the heart. In a study at The Fibromyalgia and Fatigue Centers in Dallas, patients with either fibromyalgia or chronic fatigue syndrome were given five grams of d-ribose three times daily for between 15 and 35 days. Patients had few side effects, and 66 percent showed significant improvement in energy, sleep, mental clarity, pain intensity and overall well-being. My recommended dosage of d-ribose for the average person is five grams twice daily. If you feel light-headed after taking d-ribose, take it with meals. Although d-ribose is a type of sugar, it can be safely taken by people with type 2 diabetes.

You aren't likely to hear much talk about mitochondrial dysfunction from practicing physicians in the conventional Western medical community. That's because researchers are just beginning to demonstrate that it is very common and plays an important role in our metabolism, energy levels and weight. Furthermore, new research is on the horizon. The recommendations you read here are well ahead of the curve, but you can adapt them into your life now. These plus a healthful diet and regular exercise should enable you to enjoy vibrant energy, a greater zest for life—more happiness!

The Antidote to Your Exhaustion: Regain Your Lost Energy with the Doctor-Recommended Method for "Superhuman Power" in 30 Days—Guaranteed

Let me clear one thing up right from the start. There's no doubt in my mind that CoQ10 is every bit of the wonder everyone says it is...

When I first saw Frank, he was a shell of his former self. He was tired, lacked the vitality of his younger years and was unable to work at his beloved nursery. He was also skeptical of natural supplements.

But I was able to convince Frank to give Co-Enzyme Q10 (CoQ10) a try, and what happened next was nothing short of a miracle.CoQ10 revitalized Frank so effectively he had a new lease on life. He even looked and felt like a new man!

Frank's story, which happened about 17 years ago, shows you the power of CoQ10. But that was then. Now, modern medical advances mean you can enjoy even greater health miracles!

It's now possible for you to boost your heart health… keep healthy blood pressure… revitalize your energy… and regain your youthfulness in even more powerful ways!

For years, my patients have been enjoying the full age-defying, health-boosting benefits of this special CoQ10 blend—and now, it's your turn.

If you're already taking some kind of CoQ10, you're off to a good start.

After all, CoQ10 plays a major role in…

- Converting carbs and fat into ATP energy, which is the raw form of energy desperately needed by your…

  - Heart

  - Brain

  - And ALL of your cells!

- Effectively suppressing age-robbing free radicals—which are known to damage cells and cause the tell-tale signs of aging…

In fact…

Studies show the power of CoQ10 for promoting…

A strong heart: In an international, three month, study of 2,359 people, up to 80 percent of those taking CoQ10 saw improvements in various markers of heart health when compared to their starting values.

Healthy cholesterol: The medical journal *Bio Factors* reports that CoQ10 has been shown in vitro to inhibit the oxidation of LDL "bad" cholesterol.

Healthy blood pressure: In a review of 12 clinical trials involving 362 people, taking regular CoQ10 was shown to promote healthy blood pressure levels.

Increased energy performance: In a double-blind study reported in *Molecular Aspects of Medicine*, top-level cross-country skiers took 90 mg of regular CoQ10 or a placebo—and 94 percent of those taking CoQ10 reported that it boosted their performance versus 33 percent of skiers given a placebo.

That's why everyone over the age of 40 would be crazy not to take CoQ10! No wonder sales of CoQ10 have soared. Yet, shockingly, the way most people take CoQ10 falls way short!

This is a travesty because I've seen first-hand how this breakthrough in natural medicine can do wonders for your health, vitality and youthfulness.

That's why I'm excited to tell you that now you can take the same special, bioactive forms of CoQ10 I give my patients in my exclusive formula RevitalizeQ Plus. Now, as one of my readers, you're invited to try it risk-free.

In a moment, I'll tell you how my exclusive formula, RevitalizeQ Plus can help you feel years younger and more revitalized in just 30 days—guaranteed... or your money back, less shipping.

First of all, ubiquinone is the most widely studied form of CoQ10 and stacks of papers, studies and reports all show that it supports energy production inside of your cells, and is especially important for strong and healthy blood flow—which not only helps your heart, but your entire circulatory system. So I'd never skimp on this powerful ingredient.

And the fact that ubiquinone supports energy production INSIDE your cells is the most important benefit.

With the power of ubiquinone, I believe you'll get the very best results—so you can keep your heart pumping strong, your blood flowing smooth, and your whole body energized so you feel young and vibrant.

Even better... For the very first time that I know of, a powerful form of CoQ10 is now combined with a unique and concentrated form of resveratrol.

Resveratrol first made headline news in the early 1990s as the secret behind "The French Paradox." You see, the French typically eat a lot of rich foods and drink wine daily. Yet their overall cardiovascular health is superior to many Americans. And resveratrol—a natural substance first found in grapes and red wine—may be the key to these unique anti-aging benefits.

Interest in resveratrol exploded in 2003 when Dr. David Sinclair of Harvard Medical School reported that resveratrol can activate the "longevity gene."

Newsweek reported in 2006, "A compound found in red wine may extend human life span."

Fortune headlined in 2007: "Drink wine and live longer."

And you've likely heard about resveratrol on Oprah, Dr. Oz and other national TV shows.

As you can imagine, sales of red wine and resveratrol rocketed. Even though these longevity claims haven't been proven in humans yet, more recent studies suggest resveratrol helps promote heart health, brain function and circulation

Recently scientific research suggests resveratrol does more than trigger the longevity gene. It also helps...

Promote proper inflammatory response: Controlling inflammation is an important part of maintaining your overall health and well-being. In a study published in the *Journal of Clinical Endocrinology and Metabolism*, individuals taking 40 mg of trans-resveratrol had a significant reduction in two major factors causing inflammation.

Promote circulation to the brain: To help maintain brain health as we age, it is important to keep the blood flowing. In a study reported by the *American Journal of Clinical Nutrition*, patients taking large doses of resveratrol experienced an increase in blood flow to the brain as quickly as 45 minutes after taking it.

Support cardiovascular health: Promoting increased circulation is also part of maintaining heart health. Great news! In another study published in *Nutrition, Metabolism & Cardiovascular Diseases*, overweight subjects taking resveratrol enjoyed healthy blood flow and improved dilation of blood vessels—all of which help cardiovascular health.

So, should you drink lots more red wine or take more resveratrol? Not so fast!

Yes, resveratrol is found in grapes and red wine. But those aren't your best sources. The truth is you have to drink cases of red wine to get enough resveratrol you'd need each day. The Linus Pauling Institute reports that a whole liter of red wine (a little more than a quart) gives you less than two milligrams of resveratrol—that's all!

To put it another way, to get the 100 mg of resveratrol you're getting from RevitalizeQ Plus, you'd have to drink 20 bottles of red wine!

Resveratrol supplements? You'd better carefully read the label to make sure you're getting the proper dosage and a concentrated source of resveratrol—that's not from red wine or grapes.

You see, most news sources will tell you how resveratrol comes from red wine—and how the French are healthy because they drink so much of the stuff... But the only resveratrol I recommend to my patients doesn't come from wine—or even grapes.

I prefer the resveratrol from a little-known plant called Japanese Knotweed. It might not be as exciting as a glass of wine—but Japanese Knotweed contains one of the highest concentrations of resveratrol you can find in nature.

That's why it's the same source of resveratrol you'll be able to get in my exclusive, RevitalizeQ Plus formula. Not to mention, getting your resveratrol from wine wouldn't be easy or safe considering you'd have to drink about 20 bottles to get the same dose you'll find in RevitalizeQ Plus.

Yet to feel younger and healthier, you need to fight premature aging at all levels—especially as it relates to free-radical damage. So I didn't stop with CoQ10 and Resveratrol. RevitalizeQ Plus also includes one of the most powerful of all age-fighting antioxidants: Grape seed extract.

It's a fact: To slow down premature aging and feel younger and stronger, you must stop free radicals. Nothing could age you faster than these destructive molecules which cause oxidative damage to your cells.

The good news is, special compounds in grape seeds known as OPCs (oligomeric proanthocyanidins) are one of the most powerful of all antioxidants to quell age-robbing free radicals.

In fact, OPCs in grape seeds have antioxidant power that's 20 times greater than vitamin E and 50 times greater than vitamin C. In addition, grape seed extract can help promote healthy blood vessels, vascular function and circulation.

And that's why grape seed extract is the third key ingredient in my exclusive, RevitalizeQ Plus formula.

To make RevitalizeQ Plus even better, Dr. Stengler added another secret weapon to help your body use CoQ10.

It's a patented botanical extract called BioPerine®.

BioPerine's entire job is to help you absorb CoQ10. In fact, one study done by the manufacturers found that people who took BioPerine with CoQ10 had up to 32% **more CoQ10** in their bloodstream than those who took CoQ10 alone.

And it took less than a month to get those results!

Until you turn 40, your body probably has plenty of CoQ10...but then a funny thing happens. Research shows that with each passing year, it gets harder for you to make CoQ10 and even harder to use it, too.

And that could be why your muscles tire more easily...because you just don't have all the CoQ10 you need to make as much cellular energy as you used to. But that's not all. This breakthrough formula also includes a proprietary blend of nutrients to help you feel young again.

RevitalizeQ Plus goes far beyond typical formulas with a special blend of the age-fighting nutrients I recommend to my patients. Together, this blend works synergistically to "power up" the other ingredients to give you nature's powerful age-defying nutrients in one capsule. These include…

Açai fruit extract: The tiny fruit from this Brazilian palm tree is hailed as a strong antioxidant to help you better fight aging.

Alpha-lipoic acid: A remarkable antioxidant that's both water and fat soluble—to help keep the inside and outside of your cells young and healthy.

Pomegranate fruit extract: The juice of this fruit, known since Biblical times, has been shown to have antioxidant activity three times that of red wine or green tea.

Quercetin dihydrate: A flavonoid found in onions and apple skins, it's a robust antioxidant that helps prevent oxidation of LDL "bad" cholesterol.

Curcuma longa root: This root, also known as turmeric, is a powerful antioxidant that may help promote a healthy inflammatory response throughout the body.

Bottom line: My exclusive RevitalizeQ Plus is uniquely formulated to help slow the aging process to a snail's pace and you could feel younger and revitalized in 30 days—GUARANTEED or your money back.

As you age, there is no reason why you cannot keep abundant energy, a strong heart, a healthy brain, a robust immune system and youthful vitality.

How do I know? Because I see the results every day with my patients who are using some of the most powerful natural supplements on earth, like CoQ10. Plus, resveratrol from Japanese knotweed… and the other unique nutrients in my RevitalizeQ Plus formula.

This formula gives you the very same nutrients I give my patients, and is the one that unleashes the full age-fighting, health revitalizing power of these discoveries.

What can taking my RevitalizeQ Plus formula mean to you? The nutrients you need to support...

- A healthy, strong heart—that performs at peak cardiac energy

- Flexible arteries and less oxidation of LDL "bad" cholesterol

- Healthy blood pressure levels

- A sharp mind and memory

- Youthful natural energy

- Support for your immune system

- Younger-looking skin

- Feeling rejuvenated and revitalized again

You could buy all the individual ingredients found in my RevitalizeQ Plus formula. But chances are good you won't be getting the active and concentrated forms of these natural health breakthroughs. And you'd have to buy two, three or even more supplements to get everything you get in one capsule of RevitalizeQ Plus.

To order RevitalizeQ Plus, visit www.besthealthnutritionals.com or call 1-800-539-1447 and mention code G653PC01 to receive an exclusive 20 percent discount. As a loyal *Health Revelations* reader, you are always covered by Dr. Stengler's "Anytime Guarantee." If you're not completely satisfied for ANY reason at all—at ANY time—return the unused portion for a FULL refund, less shipping, even if you're on the last capsule in the bottle! No questions asked, and no explanations needed.

The FALLACY of FATIGUE

Over the past 18 years, I've helped over 3,598 patients beat "hopeless" cases of fatigue... Including folks who were literally crying with exhaustion and sheer frustration...

Because they tried everything! Coffee, teas, juices, energy bars, energy drinks, exercise, diets...

And supplements like yerba mate, guarana, kola nut, bitter orange...

Sound familiar? But I'm going to let you in on a shocking little secret...

Everything on that long list is actually DRAINING YOUR ENERGY as systematically as a thief who siphons gas from your tank. In a moment, I'll explain why each of these "energy boosters" won't (and can't!) work, but first let me get to the great news. You see...

I've proven 3,598 times over that "hopeless" fatigue can be beaten and replaced with a "go get 'em" feeling that you may not have felt since you were a teenager.

Remember that feeling? Remember the joy of all that energy surging through your young body, as you'd bounce out of bed and tear through the day! Get ready to feel that great again...

THE SECRET: It's all about your adrenal glands.

How? Because your adrenal glands are practically ignored by most doctors, but they practically control the health of your entire body!

Perched atop your kidneys like tiny beanbags, your adrenal glands may not look important, but ignore them at your peril.

Your adrenal glands are your key to boundless energy, a sharp mind, sunny moods, flexible joints and so much more.

In fact, these overlooked little critters sit atop each of your kidneys, where they quietly control the health of your entire body. In fact, your adrenal glands are almost a "second brain," because...

- They make your bones and muscles strong by producing DHEA, the precursor to anabolic hormones like testosterone...

- They regulate your blood pressure in several different ways (for example, they can make your blood pressure soar and your heart pound like a drum, by secreting adrenaline)...

- They control your blood sugar by stimulating your liver to convert glycogen (to glucose) when your blood sugar gets too low...

Plus, they provide your body with the powerful stress hormone *cortisol*. Too much cortisol production for too long can be a bad thing, but, in small amounts it can:

- Sharpen your mind...

- Heighten your mood...

- Give you extra energy...

- Influence your sleep cycle...

When you get stressed, your adrenals respond by pumping out cortisol to help you cope. But when they run out of "juice," you're running on empty. You get anxious and forgetful, your blood sugar may rise, you may gain weight, you can't sleep, everyday aches and pains seem to be the rule, and you feel totally, utterly exhausted

But the great news is that, if you support your adrenals, your whole life can turn around...

Not just your health—your career, your marriage, your ability to *enjoy* every precious moment of your life. My patients have told me this so often and it makes great sense, because it's physically impossible to excel on the job, have great sex or simply feel good without healthy adrenal glands.

This is so important that 50 percent of my patients who come in with *other* health issues turn out to have adrenal imbalance...

And once we solve *that* problem, everything else usually falls into place. Your stiff joints, aching muscles, moodiness, jittery nerves, poor sleep patterns, senior moments, inability to concentrate—all these concerns can fade like the mist on a sunny morning, once your adrenal glands perform at their peak.

Better still, now it's never been easier to beat adrenal fatigue.

Whether you're just starting out your career or enjoying a well-earned retirement, healthy adrenal glands give you the gusto you need to *enjoy* every year of a long, fulfilled life. You'll feel sharper, calmer, happier and stronger than ever before...

So now it's *your* turn to reclaim your life...

To order Adrenal Performance Plus, visit www.besthealthnutritionals.com or call 1-800-539-1447 and mention code G653PC03 to receive an exclusive 20 percent discount. As a loyal *Health Revelations* reader, you are always covered by Dr. Stengler's "Anytime Guarantee." If you're not completely satisfied for ANY reason at all—at ANY time—return the unused portion for a FULL refund, less shipping, even if you're on the last capsule in the bottle! No questions asked, and no explanations needed.

PART V

Weight Loss

Why I Love Lasers to Zap Fat

How can I get rid of this belly fat?" That is the question countless patients ask when they come to my clinic. My answer to that question is a healthful diet, an exercise program and some hormone balancing. But as I have observed from countless patients, losing weight in these ways is not easy. *So before you sign up with some gimmicky program that promises to take inches off your abdomen and waist, find out about a new alternative…*

It is a low-level laser treatment (LLLT) called Zerona that is currently awaiting FDA approval for body contouring, although it has been used by physicians since 2008. (There are other LLLT devices made by other companies. Zerona is the one I am most familiar with.) The procedure is performed by holistic physicians, plastic surgeons and some dermatologists.

Are you wondering why I recommend a laser therapy for fat reduction? Because aside from diet and exercise, it is one of the most noninvasive therapies for eliminating fat cells—and I believe that there's nothing wrong with using technology to help make things easier. Zerona does not involve surgery or anesthesia—and there are no wounds and no pain. I recommend it for people who are five pounds to 25 lbs overweight, who really want to lose that fat and who haven't been able to do it.

What is a low-level laser?

One of the reasons I like LLLT is that the energy output of the laser is extremely low, only about 1/1,000 as intense as the lasers used to perform other procedures, such as those to eliminate age spots and skin blemishes. Known as cold laser technology (because it isn't hot and doesn't burn the skin), Zerona involves a focused light that penetrates below the skin, stimulating receptors inside individual cells. In the case of fat cells, the laser emulsifies some of the fat that they contain. The liquefied fat is then released as fatty acids into the bloodstream, where it is eliminated as waste. Unlike liposuction, the cosmetic surgical procedure that removes excess fat from the body, LLLT doesn't eliminate fat cells. LLLT patients retain all the fat cells that they started with—the cells simply contain less fat. And the body uses its own detoxification process to rid itself of the contents of the fat cells.

In a study conducted by Erchonia Medical, the manufacturer of the Zerona laser, and published in the peer-reviewed journal *Lasers in Surgery and Medicine*, researchers found that volunteers treated for two weeks with the laser lost about 0.7 inches from each thigh… 0.98 inches across the waist… and 1.05 inches across the hips. The weight loss can be long term if patients continue to maintain a healthful diet and exercise program. If they don't, of course, the weight loss is not permanent.

Thomas Barnes, MD, a cosmetic surgeon in Newport Beach, California, who uses the Zerona technique and serves as a consultant to Santa Barbara Medical Innovators (SBMI), the company that distributes the Zerona laser, explained how the technique works.

Losing inches of fat in weeks

During each treatment, the lasers are beamed from the waistline down to the middle of the thighs, first on the front of the body for 20 minutes and then on the back of the body for 20 minutes. Because the energy level is low, patients don't feel anything.

Patients undergo a 40-minute session every other day for 14 days. This sequence is necessary because pores in fat cells (which are opened by the laser) begin to close after 72 hours. The treatment works best for those who want to lose areas of fat and for those who need motivation to spur on their weight-loss efforts. It is not for obese patients, who usually need to lose several inches of waist circumference.

Dr. Barnes advises patients to drink eight glasses of water and walk for 30 to 60 minutes every day from the start to the end of treatment to help metabolize the released fat.

One of Dr. Barnes' patients, a 50-year-old woman who had been unable to lose fat in her midsection despite ongoing dieting, lost an average of 1.875 inches from her hips, waist, thighs and knees. Another patient, a woman of 35, lost an average of one inch from these areas.

SBMI reports that more than 15,000 patients have been treated with the laser over the last year. The cost for a full treatment regimen of six sessions is about $2,500. It is not covered by insurance.

Additional health benefits

Liposuction carries significant risk for complications (such as bruising, swelling and tissue damage), but LLLT has never been associated with any adverse effects. There also appear to be benefits associated with emptying fatty acids from the fat cells. The study published in *Lasers in Surgery and Medicine* found that those who had LLLT had significant reductions in total cholesterol and triglycerides.

LLLT is available around the country. To find a physician or other health-care provider in your area who offers Zerona treatments, visit www.find zerona.com.

Caralluma for Weight Loss

Legend has it that the hunting tribes of Western India chewed on the edible Caralluma cactus to suppress hunger and thirst when on long hunts. Today, Caralluma extract is being marketed as a weight-loss product that suppresses appetite and enhances metabolism.

For centuries, Caralluma fimbriata, the most common form, which grows in Africa, the Canary Islands, Arabia, southern Europe, Sri Lanka, Afghanistan and India, has been a normal part of the daily diet in India. It is commonly found growing wild in urban centers, as roadside shrubs and as boundary markers in gardens. It can be eaten in several forms—raw, cooked as a regular vegetable or used in preserves, such as chutney. There have been no reports of adverse side effects over centuries of use.

Two recent studies investigated a concentrated extract of Caralluma known as *Slimaluma*. In the first—a randomized, double-blind, placebo-controlled study—25 overweight or obese participants received 500 mg of Caralluma twice a day (a dosage that is equivalent to the traditional Indian intake of 100 g of raw cactus) and another 25 participants received a placebo for eight weeks. No other changes were made in the study participants' diets, and all were advised to walk 30 minutes every morning and 30 minutes every evening.

There was slightly greater average weight loss in the Caralluma group

(1.94 pounds) than in the placebo group (1.12 pounds). More impressive was the decrease in waist circumference—an average loss of 2.75 inches in the participants taking Caralluma, versus 1.29 inches in those taking the placebo.

Also, researchers found that there was a statistically significant decrease in body fat, blood pressure and hunger in members of the Caralluma group but not in the placebo group.

The second study consisted of 19 overweight participants who were given 500 mg capsules of Slimaluma twice per day—once before breakfast and once before dinner—and seven patients taking a placebo for one month. More than 60 percent of those taking the cactus extract lost six pounds or more in the month. Three of the seven participants in the placebo group lost an average of one pound... the other four gained weight or stayed the same.

I talked with Ronald Lawrence, MD, PhD, a former assistant clinical professor at UCLA School of Medicine, who reviewed the research on Slimaluma and has recommended the extract to many patients. He told me that most patients lose two pounds per week for the first one to two months of use, with no side effects, and most report an increase in energy.

We do not know exactly how Caralluma suppresses appetite and stimulates weight loss. Researchers theorize that substances in Caralluma known as *pregnane glycosides* prevent fat accumulation by blocking *citrate lyase*, an enzyme involved in fat formation. Pregnane glycosides also may inhibit the hunger mechanisms in the brain.

I believe that Caralluma fimbriata will become popular in the US because it is one of the few weight-loss supplements that has sound clinical data demonstrating its effectiveness.

Several companies offer the Slimaluma extract. Check Country Life (800-645-5768, www.countrylifevitamins.com), which provides a product known as Genaslim.

Cost: $25 to $30 for one month's supply. The recommended dosage of Slimaluma is 500 mg twice a day—30 to 45 minutes before breakfast and 30 to 60 minutes before dinner.

As with all supplements, pregnant or nursing mothers and children should use this only under a doctor's supervision.

Hormones May Be Your Allies in the Weight Wars

Are you fighting a weight-loss battle? By eating a healthful diet and exercising regularly, you can shed some weight—but then it's common to "get stuck." No matter how you modify your diet and exercise regimen, the pounds just stop coming off. What's going on?

Your hormones may be the key. They influence appetite (when and to what degree you desire food)... *metabolism* (how you convert food to energy)... and *insulin sensitivity* (the degree to which your cells respond to insulin, which allows your body to use glucose).

If you have hit a plateau—or even have had a reversal—in your weight-loss efforts, it may be time for you to look more closely at your hormone levels.

To start, have them tested by a physician. Hormone levels can be detected from samples of blood, saliva and urine. A knowledgeable holistic doctor will help you interpret the results and choose supplements or other natural solutions that will allow you to lose those additional pounds.

Important factors to consider...

How active is your thyroid?

Your body depends on thyroid hormones to regulate your metabolism. These hormones are produced in the butterfly-shaped gland just below your voice box. If thyroid hormones are in short supply, you can expect to gain weight. Assuming that your physician has ruled out any serious thyroid disease that must be treated in its own right, you can start to beat your weight problem by optimizing your thyroid function.

Natural solutions: For mild deficiencies—perhaps your levels are just a little off or are normal but you still have classic low thyroid symptoms, such as weight gain, fatigue, cold hands and feet, poor memory—look into one of these daily supplements or, even better, a formula that combines several of them. Take them until symptoms are better, and then taper off. If symptoms return, start taking them again—or have a doctor monitor you. If there is no improvement within four weeks, stop taking the supplements.

• **Bladderwrack** (a type of algae) contains iodine, which the thyroid requires for optimal functioning.

Typical dose: Two or three 500 mg capsules, in divided doses, for a total of 1,000 to 1,500 mg per day.

• **L-tyrosine** (an *amino acid*) helps the thyroid to manufacture hormones.

Typical dose: 500 mg twice daily on an empty stomach.

• **Homeopathic thyroid** (a minute dose of thyroid hormone or animal thyroid gland) stimulates your thyroid gland to produce hormones. Follow label directions.

• **Thyroid glandular** (an extract derived from animal thyroid tissue, typically that of a sheep) contains amino acids, vitamins and minerals that stimulate hormone production.

Typical dose: One to two capsules or tablets twice daily on an empty stomach.

Best formulas: I recommend Thyroid Support Liquid Phyto-Caps containing Bladderwrack and L-tyrosine from Gaia Herbs (800-831-7780, www.gaiaherbs.com) or Solaray's Thyroid Caps, which has L-tyrosine, iodine and thyroid glandular (800-669-8877, www.nutraceutical.com).

If your lab tests reveal a severe deficiency, you will be prescribed a thyroid hormone replacement program. Ask your doctor about natural thyroid replacement treatments, such as Armour Thyroid, Westhroid, Nature-Throid and compounded thyroid tablets.

The power of DHEA

Dehydroepiandrosterone (DHEA) is an adrenal hormone that enhances metabolism. DHEA levels naturally decrease with age. A study of 56 men and women at Washington University School of Medicine found that those who took 50 mg of DHEA daily for six months experienced a reduction in belly fat and visceral fat—the fat that builds up around internal organs—both of which are associated with heart disease, diabetes and other serious illnesses. Insulin levels also dropped significantly, indicating better blood sugar control and insulin sensitivity.

Natural solutions: If testing indicates that your DHEA level is low—less than 100 mcg/dL—take DHEA. If not, take one of the other supplements described below. Get your levels checked every six months.

• **DHEA supplements** increase DHEA levels.

Typical dose: Up to 50 mg once per day. DHEA is available over the counter, but its use should be monitored by a physician. Potential side effects include facial hair growth in women and prostate enlargement in men.

• **Sterols and sterolins** are plant fats that are chemically similar to animal fats but have different biological functions. Sterols and sterolins support DHEA production by the adrenal glands. Moducare Capsules (877-297-7332, www.moducare.com) contain both nutrients.

Typical dose: Two capsules in the morning and one before bedtime on an empty stomach.

• **Cordyceps sinensis** (a medicinal mushroom) also helps support DHEA production.

Typical dose: 2,400 mg of a standardized water and ethanol extract of Cordyceps sinensis strain Cs-4.

The cortisol factor

Prolonged elevation of the stress hormone cortisol can contribute to weight gain. High cortisol levels can interfere with normal thyroid function and decrease insulin sensitivity, both of which lead to weight gain.

Natural solutions: Stress-minimizing techniques curb your production of stress hormones. My favorite stress relievers include regular exercise, positive mental imagery and prayer.

Your doctor can order a saliva test to measure your cortisol level. *If yours is elevated, consider...*

• **Ashwagandha** (an herb) reduces cortisol levels when taken daily. Look for products containing the patented ingredient Sensoril, which offers optimal concentrations of ashwagandha. Widely available products are Liquid Anti-Stress Plus Adrenal Support from Life Solutions Natural Products (a company in which I have a financial interest, 800-914-8771, www.lifesolutionsnp.com) and Tribulus Complex with Ashwagandha by Jarrow Formulas (310-204-6936, www.jarrow.com).

If cortisol levels have not come down after two months of taking ashwagandha, try...

• **DHEA**, described above, which also can reduce cortisol levels.

Typical dose: Up to 50 mg daily, taken under a doctor's supervision.

Estrogen dominance

Most women understand the importance of *estrogen*, but they might not realize that excessive amounts of this hormone can increase body fat and promote fluid retention. Estrogen in women needs to be "balanced out" with *progesterone*, which has a *diuretic* (water-excreting) effect. Perimenopause, menopause and any health condition that interferes with ovulation (such as polycystic ovarian syndrome) will reduce levels of progesterone and give fat-building estrogen the upper hand. This is one reason why some women gain weight for no apparent reason.

Natural solutions: The nutrient *indole-3-carbinol* helps the liver metabolize estrogen. It is found in cruciferous vegetables—broccoli, cauliflower, cabbage and kale. I recommend eating at least one plentiful helping of any of these foods each day.

If a saliva, blood or urine test shows that your estrogen level is elevated even after you adopt an indole-3-carbinol–rich diet or if you just don't like to eat the above foods, try these daily supplements…

•**Indole-3-carbinol** helps the body metabolize estrogen.

Typical dose: 300 mg to 400 mg a day.

•*Vitex* (also called *chasteberry*, derived from the berries grown on the *Vitex agnus castus* tree) has been shown to improve the regularity of ovulation and raise progesterone levels.

Typical dose: 120 mg of a product standardized to 0.6 percent *aucubine* or 0.5 percent *agnuside* twice daily… or 800 mg of a nonstandardized supplement. Vitex is available from Nature's Way (to find a retailer, call 800-962-8873 or go to www.naturesway.com) and Enzymatic Therapy (800-783-2286, www.enzymatictherapy.com).

•**Natural progesterone cream** should be used as directed by your doctor for extreme progesterone deficiencies.

Typical dose: One-quarter teaspoon (20 mg) applied to the skin one or two times daily for two weeks before menstruation (stop when menses begin) or, if menopausal or postmenopausal, applied once per day. Consider Emerita ProGest (to find a retailer, call 800-888-6041 or go to www.emerita.com), a good brand that is commonly available in health-food stores.

The testosterone factor

Testosterone, a powerful hormone found in women and men, affects the body's ability to maintain lean muscle mass. It is primarily produced by the ovaries in women and the testes in men. A low level makes it more difficult to tone muscles and lose weight.

Natural solutions…

• **DHEA** is converted by women's bodies into testosterone. If a woman has low DHEA and low testosterone levels, then doctor-supervised supplementation of DHEA, as described previously, may improve both levels.

• **Panax ginseng** may help boost slightly low levels of testosterone in men and women.

Typical dose: 200 mg daily of a product standardized to five percent *ginsenosides*.

• **Tribulus terrestris** is a plant whose extract may increase testosterone amounts in men and women. So far, research has been done mainly with animals, but this herb appears to be safe. Tribulus by Source Naturals (for a retailer, call 800-815-2333 or log on to www.sourcenaturals.com) is a good choice, as is Life Solutions Natural Products' Liquid Natural Libido Enhancer (800-914-8771, www.lifesolutionsnp.com), which contains ginseng and, for a calming effect, the herb passionflower.

• **Natural testosterone** is available by prescription only and should be used when there is a moderate to severe deficiency. I prefer the transdermal gel or cream form, which is applied to the skin, because it requires less metabolism by the liver than pills.

Is insulin on your team?

Blood sugar (*glucose*) is terrific fuel for an active person, but you need the right level of insulin to transport the sugar from your bloodstream into tissue. A condition known as insulin resistance occurs when cells become less accepting of glucose and insulin levels spike. It is one factor that sets the stage for weight gain.

Natural solutions…

• **High-fiber diet** that includes seven to nine daily servings of fresh vegetables as well as three servings of whole-grain breads and cereals. Nuts, seeds and raw vegetables are especially good to help balance insulin levels. Stay away from simple-sugar food products, such as white breads, pasta, soft drinks, cookies and other sweets. For protein, avoid fatty red meats and favor quality sources, such as legumes, nuts, eggs, fish and poultry.

• **Help yourself to some cinnamon!** Studies show that it helps balance blood sugar levels.

• **Eat smaller servings** throughout the day rather than three big meals, so your body metabolizes food more effectively.

• **High-potency multivitamin/mineral supplement**. Everyone should take one daily for general health—it provides nutrients that, among other things, balance insulin levels.

If tests for fasting blood glucose and insulin indicate that you have insulin resistance, try taking all three of these additional supplements daily…

• **Chromium** (a mineral) is particularly important to balance blood sugar levels.

Typical dose: 400 mcg.

• **Alpha lipoic acid** (an enzyme that acts as a powerful antioxidant) reduces levels of insulin and blood sugar.

Typical dose: Up to 200 mg.

•**Fish oil** (an essential fatty acid supplement) improves insulin sensitivity.

Typical dose: One teaspoon daily or a one gram capsule, three times a day. Nordic Naturals fish oil supplements are widely available and free of mercury and other toxins (to locate a retailer, call 800-662-2544 or go to www.nordicnaturals.com).

Caution: If you are taking a blood-thinning medication, such as warfarin (Coumadin), check with your doctor before taking fish oil.

Root causes of weight gain

• Poor diet.

• Lack of exercise.

• Genetic predisposition.

• Hormone imbalance.

• Neurotransmitter imbalance, such as serotonin deficiency.

• Side effects of drugs.

• Toxins, such as chemicals (pesticides).

• Psychological reasons, such as stress, anxiety and depression.

Lose Weight by Changing Your Plate Size

Researchers at Cornell University observed three groups of dieters who either changed their environment, eating behavior or food choices. Those in the environment group—who used small plates and rearranged shelves so that high-calorie foods were harder to get—were able to stick with these changes longer than those in the other two groups. Make these changes in your own home, and see if they help you lose weight.

Melt Away Abdominal Fat

The size of your waist is believed to be a better indicator of health problems than the number on the scale or your body mass index (BMI), a measure of weight relative to height.

It is far more healthful to have a "pear" body shape (fat stored around the hips, buttocks and thighs) than an "apple" shape (fat stored around the middle). Both men and women with apple shapes (men with waists of 40 inches or more and women with waists of 35 inches or more) are more likely to be insulin resistant—a condition in which the cells do not receive insulin properly and which often leads to diabetes—than those with smaller waists. In fact, research shows that having just an extra four inches around your waist increases your risk for heart failure by 15 percent. Belly fat is associated with a greater risk for stroke, and every additional two inches around the waist in men increases the risk for deep-vein thrombosis and pulmonary embolism (blockage of the main artery of the lungs) by 18 percent.

Why abdominal fat is so bad: This fat, also known as visceral fat, produces hormones that work against you in the following ways...

• **Releasing free fatty acids** (the breakdown product of fat cells that circulate in the bloodstream)

• **Decreasing insulin sensitivity** (the degree to which your cells recognize insulin and use it properly)

• **Increasing cytokines**, compounds that contribute to inflammation and insulin resistance, including *resistin*, another chemical that reduces insulin sensitivity.

• **Decreasing hormones** such as *leptin* that help regulate metabolism and appetite.

Help is on the way

Abdominal fat often is associated with hormonal imbalances, such as high insulin (yes, even insulin is a hormone)… high cortisol… and high estrogen. Once the vicious cycle of abdominal weight gain and hormonal imbalance begins, it is hard to stop—especially because each one causes the other.

I put those who are caught in this cycle on a hormone-balancing protocol that they follow for at least two months and up to six months. The results are impressive.

The protocols

If you are a man with a waist measurement of 40 inches or more or a woman with a waist of 35 inches or more, ask your doctor to test your levels of cortisol, insulin and estrogen.

Note: Excess estrogen is not just a female problem. While high levels most often occur in women younger than 45 and in postmenopausal women, they can appear in men as well, especially when made worse by the presence of environmental estrogens, compounds found in many plastic household products.

If you have excess estrogen…

High levels of estrogen, particularly combined with low levels of progesterone, can cause abdominal fat. When either a male or female patient has excess estrogen, especially in conjunction with low levels of progesterone (a condition called estrogen dominance), I recommend an estrogen detox program. This includes eating two to three daily servings of cruciferous vegetables (such as broccoli, cabbage, brussels sprouts, cauliflower and kale), which contain plant compounds called *indoles* that help regulate estrogen metabolism and can make estrogen less toxic. Supplements that help include *indole-3-carbinol* and *diindolymethane* (DIM). These phytochemicals in supplement form are similar to those found in cruciferous vegetables. Patients take 300 mg to 400 mg daily of indole-3-carbinol and 200 mg to 400 mg of DIM daily. (I recommend both the food, for the fiber, and the supplements because it's difficult to get enough of these phytochemicals through food.) For women who are perimenopausal or menopausal (and some men with prostate problems) with this type of hormonal imbalance, I also may prescribe a bioidentical progesterone cream.

If you have insulin resistance…

Abdominal fat and insulin resistance often go together like the proverbial chicken and egg, and it isn't always easy to know which one was there first. Insulin resistance increases the chances of developing type 2 diabetes and cardiovascular disease. It can be effectively treated by eating a diet with high-fiber foods, including vegetables, legumes and grains. Regular exercise also helps keep insulin resistance under control. For my insulin-resistant patients, I also recommend PGX, a form of glucomannan fiber.

Brand to try: Natural Factors PGX Daily (800-322-8704, www.naturalfactors.com for a store locator).

Also helpful: Chromium picolinate, a trace mineral (start with 500 mcg daily and increase to 1,000 mcg daily, if needed), which can help balance blood sugar levels… and resveratrol (50 mg to 100 mg daily), which improves insulin resistance.

If you have high levels of cortisol…

Cortisol, the major stress hormone produced by the adrenal glands, can signal the body to store fat around the middle. For my patients whose blood tests reveal high cortisol levels, I prescribe a basic program of aerobic exercise (30 minutes daily of swimming, jogging, bicycling or walking)… strength training… stress reduction… and deep breathing, all of which have been found to lower cortisol levels. The herb *ashwagandha* also can help normalize blood cortisol levels.

Brand to try: Sensoril Ashwagandha made by Jarrow Formulas (310-204-6936, www.jarrow.com for a store locator). Take one 225 mg capsule daily. Women who are pregnant or breast-feeding should not take this herb.

Lose Weight with Apple Cider Vinegar

Patients often tell me that apple cider vinegar has helped them with a variety of ailments. Until just recently, there was little research to back up these claims.

Cure-all?

Apple cider vinegar has been singled out as beneficial for a variety of conditions, including leg cramps, stomach distress, sore throat, sinus problems, high blood pressure, obesity, osteoporosis and arthritis. It also has been used to help rid the body of toxins, improve concentration, slow aging, reduce cholesterol and fight infection.

It is used topically to remedy acne, sunburn, shingles and insect bites... as a skin toner... and to prevent dandruff. Many women add it to bathwater to treat vaginitis. Two of its most common uses are for weight loss and arthritis.

The scientific evidence

Recent studies have found that consuming apple cider vinegar can improve insulin resistance, a condition in which muscle, fat and liver cells have become resistant to the uptake of the hormone *insulin* and the blood sugar *glucose* needed to provide fuel for energy.

This is common among people who have diabetes as well as in some people we consider prediabetic—that is, their blood glucose and insulin levels are approaching the numbers that define diabetes. People with insulin resistance are more likely to be overweight and have increased cholesterol and triglyceride levels as well as high blood pressure.

A study at the University of Arizona examined the effects of apple cider vinegar on 29 participants (10 had type 2 diabetes, 11 had signs that they could become diabetic and eight were healthy and "insulin sensitive"). All participants fasted and were randomly asked to drink either a vinegar solution (two tablespoons or 20 g of apple cider vinegar, some water and a bit of saccharin for flavor) or a placebo drink. The drinks were followed by a high-carbohydrate meal of one white bagel, butter and orange juice.

Researchers found that postmeal spikes of insulin and glucose in the vinegar group were significantly lower in those who had insulin resistance and slightly lower in those who had diabetes, compared with those in the placebo group. Other research has shown that apple cider vinegar helps control insulin and glucose spikes in healthy people.

How it works

Researchers theorize that the *acetic acid* in any vinegar, including apple cider vinegar, interferes with the enzymes that digest carbohydrates, so carbs pass through the digestive tract without being absorbed. Acetic acid also has been shown to affect enzymes that alter glucose metabolism in liver and muscle cells, reducing insulin spikes.

Because high levels of insulin promote inflammation, taking vinegar to maintain insulin levels will control any inflammation in the body. This may explain why vinegar eases arthritis pain.

Dosage: People can try apple cider vinegar for weight loss, blood sugar balance and other traditional uses, including arthritis relief. Dilute one to two tablespoons (some people use as little as two teaspoons to start with) in an equal amount of water, and drink it at the beginning of a meal.

Sometimes it is more convenient to take it in supplement form. A good product is Apple Cider Vinegar Plus, which is made by Indiana Botanic Gardens (800-644-8327, www.botanicchoice.com). Take three capsules a day (one with each meal).

Apple cider vinegar can cause digestive upset in some people. If you have active ulcers, use caution when taking apple cider vinegar.

The Hormone That May Help You Decrease Belly Fat

Researchers say an over-the-counter hormone supplement, *dehydro-epiandrosterone* (DHEA), might help seniors to shed hard to lose belly fat. Preliminary evidence also suggests that increased levels of this natural hormone secreted by the adrenal gland might help older people avoid diabetes.

The study

Belly fat tends to accumulate with aging, just as DHEA levels begin to fall. "DHEA declines progressively with age," explains Dennis T. Villareal, MD, associate professor of geriatrics and nutritional science at Washington University School of Medicine in St. Louis. "When we're 70 years old, we only have about 20 percent of the DHEA we had when we were young." From animal studies conducted in their lab, he and co-researcher Dr. John O. Holloszy suspected that falling DHEA levels might encourage weight gain. So in a double-blind trial, they had 56 non-exercising, elderly individuals take either a daily 50 mg DHEA supplement or a placebo for six months.

Results

"The replacement of DHEA, at doses of 50 mg per day, brought back

DHEA levels in older persons to the range seen in youth. This resulted in a reduction in abdominal fat that was accompanied by an improvement in insulin action," says Dr. Villareal.

Participants taking the hormone supplements lost an average of six percent in visceral abdominal fat—fat deposits lying deep within the abdomen. "It averaged about one kilogram (2.2 pounds) of weight loss per person," Dr. Villareal says. Those on the placebo experienced no significant weight loss.

Patients taking these supplements also made significant improvements in insulin activity, lowering their risk for developing diabetes. That is not surprising, according to Dr. Villareal, since fatty acids released from abdominal fat cells are known to have a negative affect on insulin action. In terms of health, "what's important is that we saw a specific reduction in abdominal fat, instead of just overall weight loss," he says.

Implications

Dr. Villareal notes that it's still much too early to recommend DHEA as a weight-loss supplement. "This is only a preliminary study, and we should wait for the results of large-scale, longer studies," he says. "The risks of DHEA haven't been fully defined in this short-term, relatively small study." A larger, five-year trial, involving 176 subjects, is currently under way, he says.

Roberta Anding, a clinical dietitian at Texas Children's Hospital in Houston and a spokeswoman for the American Dietetic Association, calls the findings "exciting," adding that they "open up another avenue for the management of obesity."

However, she says the supplements industry remains largely unregulated. "For the consumer, it's 'buyer beware' out there. I don't know that you can necessarily get high-quality DHEA in every health-food store, that they are all created equal."

She adds that DHEA supplements might be harmful for people with a history of hormone-sensitive cancers, such as tumors of the breast or prostate. Anding says participants in a St. Louis study who took DHEA supplements experienced a "significant" spike in blood levels of *estradiol* (an estrogen-like hormone) and testosterone, hormones commonly connected to breast and prostate cancers, respectively.

Bottom line

Long-term safety data holds the answer to the widespread use of DHEA. "There are going to be some people—individuals with estrogen-sensitive breast cancer or individuals who may have prostate cancer—who really should not take DHEA," Anding says.

How to Safely and Easily Shed 20 to 30 Pounds in Just Three to Four Weeks Flat

I'm a skeptic by nature. I want hard facts before I'm convinced that something is real. This is especially true if that something sounds "too good to be true." For example, I believe any quick fix weight loss program should be approached with a healthy dash of skepticism. Marketers will use one gimmick after another to separate you from your money but, if you're not careful, in the end you're likely to be disappointed with the results. Even worse than throwing your money away you can, all too easily, leave yourself with a health problem brought on by dangerous stimulants and wacky diets.

Years ago when patients started asking me to prescribe hormone human chorionic gonadotrophin (HCG) and a low calorie diet I resisted. After all, I need to be sure that what I prescribe for my patients is safe and effective. I needed more information. So I started my research to find out what the HCG protocol was all about. I sought out credible doctors and nutritionists and asked them what kinds of results they were seeing with the protocol. The feedback was positive.

Next, I read the book *Pounds and Inches* (available on the Internet) which was written by British endocrinologist A.T.W. Simeons the original developer of the HCG method. I also reviewed the available studies on these types of programs. In the case of *Simeons* HCG weight loss program the results were mixed with some positive results and some less than impressive findings. But the positive ones were enough to keep me intrigued.

Real life results

Only then—with all the facts in, and convinced of its safety—did I decide it was okay to try the program with patients. The first was a 50-year-old patient I had seen for several years for general health issues including hormone balancing protocols. She was very health conscious. Even though she exercised for an hour five to five days a week and consumed a 1,300 calorie diet she could not lose a stubborn extra 20 lbs.

I started her on daily HCG injections and a 500 calorie diet. She returned to the clinic once a week to follow up with me. Every visit when I asked her if she was hungry she always assured me that she wasn't. She reported that her energy levels were fine. Yet, she was losing, on average, a half-pound to a pound a day. At the end of her 30 day program she had lost 20 lbs and two inches off her waistline. And, needless to say, she was thrilled! She went back to her original diet and exercise program and now, several years later, has kept the weight off… even during a diet-sabotaging cruise.

Seeking out the truth

HCG is a hormone that's produced naturally by the placenta in pregnant women. Doctor A.T.M. Simeons is credited with being the first person to realize the hormones potential for use in weight loss. While some in the weight management arena want to treat Dr. Simeons as a heretic—and his HCG protocol as fringe medicine—the truth is he was no academic slouch.

Simeons was born in London, and like many of his American and British peers pursuing a career in medicine he chose to attend a German university. He graduated from the University of Heidelberg and completed his post-graduate studies in Germany and Switzerland. Simeon then worked at a surgical hospital near Dresden, Germany. Eventually he became interested in tropical diseases and joined the School of Tropical Medicine in Hamburg. After completing two years of work in Africa, Dr. Simeons headed to India where he continued to practice medicine for the next 18 years... from 1931 to 1949.

Simeons was a medical pioneer and even critics can't dismiss his credibility as a researcher and clinician. During his years in India he developed a drug treatment for life threatening malaria. Malaria, which is transmitted to people through mosquito bites, affects over 200 million people a year and hundreds of thousands die from the infection yearly. Simeons also pioneered a blood staining test to better identify the malaria parasite. For his work on medical advances for malaria he was awarded the prestigious "Order of Merit" by the Red Cross. In addition, he did extensive research on the bubonic plague and developed a model leper center for the treatment of leprosy. Later he maintained a private practice in Bombay India and was regularly consulted by the Government of India. In 1949 he moved to Rome and worked at the Salvador Mundi International Hospital until he passed away in 1970.

Simeons describes his first uses of HCG with young male patients in India who had large abdomens, buttocks, hips, and thighs along with undescended testicles. He referred to them as "fat boys." He discovered that daily injections of the bio-identical hormone HCG, along with a restricted diet of 500 calories (high protein diet with little fat and lots of water) a day, resulted in a loss of fat around the midsection and a normalization of their appearance. Amazingly his patients were able to follow the extremely low-calorie without suffering from hunger. He comments:

"I found that as long as such patients were given small daily doses of HCG they could comfortably go about their usual occupations on a diet of only 500 calories daily and lose an average of about one pound per day. It was also perfectly evident that only abnormal fat was being consumed, as there were no signs of any depletion of normal fat. Their skin remained fresh and turgid, and gradually their figures became entirely normal. The daily administration of HCG appeared to have no side-effects other than beneficial ones."[1]

In essence, Simeon discovered that HCG mobilizes fat away from undesired areas such as the waist, buttocks, and hips. My own experience using HCG with patients confirms Simeons' findings. My patients lose fat around the midsection, yet their faces don't become skinny or withdrawn. Simeons hypothesized that HCG and a very low calorie diet may somehow have a revitalizing effect on a metabolic center of the brain. However, the exact mechanisms of how HCG affects metabolism and fat distribution are still not completely understood.

The elephant in the room

If you're like most people I talk to about HCG you're likely wondering if it's the very low calorie diet and *not* HGC that accounts for the weight loss seen in patients on this protocol. The answer is actually yes *and* no. Let me explain.

When people first hear the diet is 500 calories they often gasp and say that it is no wonder people lose weight. They also comment that it would be a difficult diet to follow. The reality is that a 500 calorie diet in conventional medicine *is* an accepted medically supervised diet. Plenty of large, well known conventional medical institutions have patients follow a 500 calorie liquid diet. In those programs patients typically drink calorie-controlled shakes throughout the treatment and never eat any solid foods.

So it's important to understand that the 500 calories advocated by the Simeon diet is not particularly unusual and is regularly prescribed by *conventional* weight loss specialists. However, with the HCG program, unlike the liquid diets promoted by conventional weight loss programs, patients do eat real food. This alone makes HCG more attractive to many patients.

In addition, while it's true that many people can lose a similar amount of weight on a very low calorie diet without HCG some... like my patient I spoke of earlier… are unable to lose weight by lowering calories alone. Their metabolism is unbalanced and weight loss is difficult no matter how many calories they consume. The HCG component is often what's needed in these cases to finally kick-start the loss.

The fact is HCG makes it easier for almost anyone to lose weight for several reasons. First, HCG is a surprisingly powerful appetite suppressant. It's a great safe alternative to the common conventional appetite suppressant known as phentermine which can cause serious side effects including: Increased blood pressure, heart palpitations, restlessness, dizziness, tremor, insomnia, shortness of breath, chest pain, dizziness, swelling of the legs and ankles, and difficulty doing exercise.[2] HCG is not a stimulant and typically has none of the troubling side effects that you can expect to see with a *stimulant* appetite suppressant. Frankly, I'm still amazed when patients tell me they're not overly hungry on my HCG program. But the proof is in the results.

Another advantage for the use of HCG along *with* a lower calorie diet is that the hormone appears to target fat in the typical problem areas including the abdomen, hips, thighs, and buttocks. A double blind study with adults confirmed this unique ability when researchers found that HCG, plus a low calorie diet, significantly decreased waist and abdominal circumference compared to a low calorie diet alone.[3] I can clearly see this occurring with my own patients as we measure the inches they have lost.

HCG also has one other major benefit. The hormone combats the fatigue, mood swings, and irritability that often affect those on a very low calorie diet. In fact, there's data suggesting that HCG acts like an endorphin (a mood benefiting and pain reducing chemical) in the brain. One study, done by Argentinian researchers, found those on a 500 calorie diet plus pharmaceutical grade sublingual HCG "improved their attitude towards their environment, in the sense of an enhanced well-being, less irritability and lack of fatigue."[4] A side benefit of HCG's endorphin-like action is that patients with arthritis or other types of chronic pain often find a dramatic reduction in their pain levels.

Dr. Mark's HCG Modifications

Simeon's program was ingenious. However, I found it necessary to modernize his program for today's patient. Keep in mind he developed it over 50 years ago and we have learned a lot more about the body and nutrition since then. I have modified the HCG program to make it easier for people to follow, while still producing substantial weight loss.

The Simeon diet is a high protein diet consisting of 500 calories. I have found patients often do just as well starting at 660 calories. If you are prone to fatigue or low blood sugar 160 calories can make a big difference. If a patient still has any low blood sugar or fatigue issues I will increase their calorie intake. A small percentage of patients require 800 to 900 calories a day to feel good. Yet, even on this higher calorie protocol, they still lose weight and inches effectively.

The original diet includes only tea or coffee without sugar for breakfast. I have replaced this with a high protein, low sugar, meal replacement. Patients tend to feel better with this modification and it prevents mid-morning blood-sugar swings and the risk of burning muscle for energy. I prefer a protein meal replacement with added soluble fiber like glucomannan or chia seeds.

The original program calls for patients to fat load for the first two days. Simeon felt it was important to increase "fat reserves" before starting a very low calorie diet. On the original program patients would typically gain four to five pounds after eating the unhealthy fats for two days and then spend the next three days of the program losing the weight they just gained. This is psychologically unhealthy for people who already have a weight issue. Besides, I have found this step is unnecessary to safely lose the weight so I have patients skip the "fat loading" phase altogether.

Simeons' original program doesn't allow any fat in the menu. This means no fish or eggs (he did make an exception for an *occasional* boiled egg). However, during Simeons' era they simply didn't know the difference between good and bad fats. We now know how important good fats can be for our health. Totally avoiding good fats, like omega-3s, is not only *not* necessary to see results, it can leave your skin dry.

In my adapted program I allow lean fish such as salmon or trout, but I tell patients to avoid shellfish. I also encourage them to use egg whites instead of whole eggs while on my adapted program. Simeons' program didn't allow different vegetables to be mixed together. Since they are so low in calories (except for root vegetables) I have found this restriction is unnecessary. Instead I encourage patients to feel free to mix different vegetables and eat as much of them as they want, especially greens. This allows for more flexibility in meal planning.

My general HCG diet consists of a high protein meal replacement (preferably with added soluble fiber for additional blood sugar stabilization, appetite suppression, and binding of fat in the blood) for breakfast. A snack such as an apple with the skin is eaten mid-morning and again in the mid-afternoon. Lunch and dinner consist of a protein such as egg whites, poultry, or fish, along with a large salad and small portion of carbohydrate such as a gluten free piece of toast or brown rice.

Like on Simeons' original program, I encourage patient's to drink plenty of water throughout the day. Most patients drink 50 to 80 oz daily. This helps maintain hydration, suppress appetite, and allows for detoxification as fat stores are being broken down and metabolized. Remember that many toxins are stored in fat tissue.

Making HCG more effective

Although Simeon's program has a strict policy against any topical agents including makeup and lotions being used while on his program my adapted version does not. My own informal studies on this restriction haven't found that it makes any difference.

Simeon discouraged the internal use of medications such as hormones. I don't recommend stopping meds while on my adapted version of the program. If a patient *is* to stop a medication before starting a HCG cycle I have them do this with medical supervision before starting the program to sidestep any potential withdrawal side effects.

Simeon advised against using vitamin supplements during his HCG program. I feel this is a mistake. A restricted calorie diet can put you at risk for nutrient deficiencies. Since nutrients have no caloric value they don't block weight loss. Actually the opposite is true. Taking nutrients during a HCG cycle helps to optimize energy, promote detoxification, and helps with the metabolism of fat. I have patients take a multivitamin and a mineral supplement along with a calcium, magnesium, and vitamin D supplement. Many of my patients also receive a B12 shot once a week to maintain better energy levels.

I find that some of my patients require additional supplementation. For example, if you are prone to blood-sugar swings... such as patients who are hypoglycemic, prediabetic, or diabetic... you will benefit from blood-sugar balancing nutrients including, vanadium, soluble fiber, , and berberine. If you struggle with insomnia melatonin, passionflower, GABA, or other relaxing nutrients can help. For additional appetite suppression I use the non-stimulant supplement Caralluma Fimbriata. And, for stronger fat-burning support, green tea extract without caffeine and L-carnitine can both help burn fat as energy.

The role of exercise

Only light exercise should be done during an HCG program. A light walk for 20 minutes is fine. Weight loss is achieved through the very low calorie diet and moderate to heavy exercise is not required. In fact, too much exercise while on the program can lead to fatigue and the loss of muscle mass since the body would need to burn muscle tissue in addition to fat. Too much exercise can also backfire by causing your metabolism to slow down.

I once had a patient on the program that ignored my exercise restriction. On a hot summer day in California she went on a four hour long fundraising walk. She called me the next day complaining of fatigue and a black tongue... a sign of severe dehydration! When I asked her what she had been doing for the last 24-hours the reason for her problem was immediately clear. Fortunately quick rehydration solved her problem.

Exploring your options

I use a prescription form of HCG with my patients. Since it's an off label use there's no insurance coverage.

There are three ways to administer the HCG. Since it's done daily the patient is responsible for taking the HCG on their own. The first method is the traditional Simeon method of injection into the buttocks or thigh. We show patients how to do this at our clinic before starting the program. The second option is sublingual liquid or tablet HCG taken under the tongue. The last method is a nasal spray.

The traditional dosage is an injection of 125 IU of HCG daily. But no matter if it's an injection, sublingual, or a nasal spray I have found a higher dosage of 250 IU works better. If a patient is following the diet closely and they start to plateau I will have them increase the dosage of HCG to help with weight loss.

Going from start to finish

Before starting the program I give patients a physical exam and do blood work. For some patients I also have an EKG done to check on heart function. Balanced hormones helps with metabolism so it's important to get them balanced before or during the program. Thyroid hormone balance is particularly important, but I test all the major hormones to make sure they are where they should be.

Patients follow up at the clinic once a week to get their vital signs and measurements checked to be sure they're doing well on the program. Most patients follow the program for 30 days. I have found that after that period the weight loss plateaus and patients become sensitized to the HCG. If a repeat cycle is needed I will have you follow a healthy, higher calorie diet with exercise for at least 30 days first. Women who are fertile and sexually active are notified their fertility may be enhanced and birth control measures are implemented.

The truth about side effects

I have never seen any major side effects on this program. Some patients can feel tired. This is normally fixed by increasing the amount of calories they're eating or by giving nutrient support such as B vitamins. With the decrease in calories constipation can occur. This can usually be overcome simply by drinking more water and taking extra fiber. More stubborn cases may require the temporary use of laxative herbs such as cascara. Women who have a menstrual cycle may notice a temporary change in their cycle length.

Patients often ask me if taking HCG is a cancer risk. Human data doesn't show that it's a risk and actually there's some preliminary evidence that it may have a *protective* effect against breast cancer. A study published in *Cancer, Epidemiology, Biomarkers and Prevention* found that women 40 years and younger who had used HCG injections for weight loss or fertility had significantly less breast cancer than a control group who did not use HCG.[5]

A report published in *Molecular and Cellular Endocrinology* found HCG therapy had an inhibitory effect on breast cancer for postmenopausal women who were newly diagnosed. Researchers found that HCG reduced the growth of breast cancer cells that were stimulated by estrogen and progesterone.[6] I recommend anyone with a history of cancer consult with their physician before starting treatment with prescription HCG.

Making the most of HCG

Ninety percent of people who try HCG will lose at least 15 lbs per cycle. Heavier patients... those with 60 or more pounds to lose... will often drop 30 lbs in the first cycle. The HCG program is a kick start to dropping the pounds and inches, improving insulin resistance, and boosting overall metabolism.

However HCG is *not* a magic bullet. After losing weight with the program you will still need to maintain a healthy diet and exercise program. Your goal should be to keep the weight off long term, otherwise there's no point to doing the program. I do have some patients that repeat a round every couple of years to lose the extra pounds they have put back on due to things like "holiday weight gain."

Regardless of HCG, a comprehensive analysis of your hormones and natural hormone balancing can do wonders for increasing your metabolism. In addition, I've found that food and environmental sensitivities can be a barrier to weight loss so I typically test patients for these and have them avoid any trigger sensitivities. Lastly, many patients benefit from occasional detoxification programs that cleanse out toxins and keep the bowels regular which prevents weight gain.

Success stories show HCG is the REAL thing

I have hundreds of success stories I could share with you, but for now let me tell you about just two more recent ones. The first is Bernice who is in her late 60s. When I first saw Bernice she was walking very slowly with the aid of a cane. She weighed 300 lbs and her hip had no cartilage left in it. Her surgeon refused to do surgery to help relieve the pain until she lost 100 lbs. So we started Bernice on my adapted HCG program. After four cycles she had lost 95 lbs and her surgeon was very pleased with her results. I recently just got word that her hip surgery went very well, mission accomplished.

The next success story is also a woman in her 60s. Joan had just been diagnosed with type 2 diabetes when she came to see me. She wanted to avoid having to take diabetes drugs. After losing 65 lbs on the HCG program Joan now has no sign of diabetes at all. She doesn't take any diabetic medications. She has had a complete reversal of her disease!

Most patients that come to see me need to lose a little less weight than Bernice and Joan did. Typically they're struggling with losing 20 to 40 lbs and HCG allows them to do that. When they follow up that loss with a good diet and exercise program and I get their hormones balanced and their digestion and detoxification systems working properly—they have long term success.

For proper medical supervision of a HCG program you can find a physician through the American College for the Advancement of Medicine (949-309-3520, www.acam.org) or the American Association of Naturopathic Physicians (866-538-2267, www.naturopathic.org). Or, if you're in the California area, you can schedule a visit at the Stengler Center for Integrative Medicine.

PART VI

Diabetes

Say Goodbye to Your Diabetes Medication

Some of my patients with type 2 diabetes are able to keep the disease under control with diet, exercise and supplements. Lucky them! But for other diabetes patients, that's not enough and they must take pharmaceutical medications.

I'm happy to report that there is another natural treatment option for diabetes patients who currently take pharmaceutical medications. Research has found that the plant extract called *berberine* can control diabetes as well as, or better than, common medications such as *metformin* (Glucophage) and *rosiglitazone* (Avandia). And it does this with no side effects—and without damaging the liver, as some medications do. Here's how berberine can help people with diabetes…

A naturally occurring chemical compound, berberine is found in the roots and stems of several plants, including *Hydrastis canadensis* (goldenseal), *Coptis chinensis* (coptis or goldenthread) and *Berberis aquifolium* (Oregon grape). Long used as a remedy in Chinese and Ayurvedic medicines, berberine is known for its anti-microbial properties and as a treatment for bacterial and fungal infections. Several decades ago, berberine was used to treat diarrhea in patients in China. That was when doctors noticed that the blood sugar levels of diabetes patients were lower after taking the herbal extract—and berberine began to be investigated for this purpose.

Over the past 20 years, there has been much research on berberine and its effectiveness in treating diabetes. In 2008, Chinese researchers published a study in *Metabolism* in which adults with newly diagnosed type 2 diabetes were given 500 mg of either berberine or the drug metformin three times a day for three months. Researchers found that berberine did as good a job as metformin at regulating glucose metabolism, as indicated by *hemoglobin A1C* (a measure of blood glucose over several weeks)... Fasting blood glucose... blood sugar after eating... and level of insulin after eating. Berberine even reduced the amount of insulin needed to turn glucose into energy by 45 percent! In addition those taking berberine had noticeably lower triglyceride and total cholesterol levels than those taking metformin.

In another 2008 study published in the *Journal of Clinical Endocrinology and Metabolism*, researchers found that type 2 diabetes patients who were given berberine had significant reductions in fasting and postmeal blood glucose, hemoglobin A1C, triglycerides, total cholesterol and LDL (bad) cholesterol—and also lost an average of five pounds, to boot, during the three-month study.

In a 2010 study in *Metabolism*, Chinese researchers compared people with type 2 diabetes who take either 1,000 mg daily of berberine or daily doses of metformin or rosiglitazone. After two months, berberine had lowered subjects' fasting blood glucose levels by an average of about 30 percent, an improvement over the rosiglitazone group and almost as much as people in the metformin group. Berberine also reduced subjects' hemoglobin A1C by 18 percent—equal to rosiglitazone and, again, almost as good as metformin. In addition, berberine lowered serum insulin levels by 28.2 percent (indicating increased insulin sensitivity)... lowered triglycerides by 17.5 percent... and actually improved liver enzyme levels. Pharmaceutical medications, on the other hand, have the potential to harm the liver.

These were remarkable findings. Here was a botanical that was holding up to scientific scrutiny—and performing as well as, or better than, some drugs patients had been taking for diabetes for years.

How berberine works in the body

Berberine helps to lower blood glucose in several ways. One of its primary mechanisms involve stimulating the activity of the genes responsible for manufacturing and activating insulin receptors, which are critical for controlling blood glucose.

Berberine also has an effect on blood sugar regulation through activation of incretins, gastrointestinal hormones that affect the amount of insulin released by the body after eating.

How berberine can help

I recommend berberine to my patients with newly diagnosed type 2 diabetes to reduce their blood sugar and prevent them from needing pharmaceutical drugs. When a diet, exercise and supplement program (including supplements such as chromium) is already helping a diabetes patient, I don't recommend that he/she switch to berberine.

Some patients are able to take berberine—and make dietary changes—and stop taking diabetes drugs altogether. People with severe diabetes can use berberine in conjunction with medication–and this combination treatment allows for fewer side effects and better blood sugar control. I don't recommend berberine for prediabetes unless diet and exercise are not effective. Berberine is sold in health-food stores and online in tablet and capsule form. The dosage I typically recommend for all diabetes patients is 500 mg twice daily.

For patients with diabetes who once used berberine, I recommend talking to your doctor about taking this supplement. It's also important for every patient with diabetes to participate in a comprehensive diet and exercise program.

Note that berberine helps patients with type 2 diabetes, not type I diabetes (in which the body does not produce enough insulin).

The Dangers of Diabetes

More Americans than ever before have *diabetes mellitus*, a disorder characterized by elevated levels of blood sugar (*glucose*). About 21 million Americans (approximately seven percent of the US population) are afflicted with the disease, according to the National Institutes of Health. More than six million of these people don't even realize that they have it.

But that is not all. A staggering 41 million Americans show early signs of diabetes (*prediabetes*) but do not know that they are at risk of developing the full-blown disease. This alarming trend is due, in part, to the ever-increasing number of Americans who are overweight, which sharply increases diabetes risk.

If you have been gaining weight, eating a lot of high-fat and high-sugar foods and/or not getting much exercise, I'm afraid that you're already in danger of getting diabetes.

Even though this is a frightening scenario, there is some good news. If you identify the warning signs early enough, you can help stop diabetes from developing. If you already have diabetes, proper monitoring and healthful eating can help you control your glucose levels and avoid many of the disease's serious complications, such as heart failure, stroke, kidney failure, eye disease, nerve damage and/or amputation, due to poor circulation caused by plaque buildup.

What is diabetes?

Whenever we eat or drink, the food or liquid we ingest is broken down into nutrients that our bodies need to function. Glucose (a simple sugar that acts as the main energy source for our bodies) is one of the key nutrients. When glucose is absorbed into the bloodstream, it stimulates the pancreas to produce *insulin*. This hormone transports glucose into our body's cells, where it is then converted to energy for immediate or later use.

There are two main types of diabetes...

• **Type 1** (formerly known as *juvenile-onset*) diabetes affects only about 10 percent of people with diabetes. Although the disorder usually develops in childhood or early adulthood (before age 30), an increasing number of adults are now being affected.

Researchers theorize that the increasing incidence of obesity in adults may accelerate the autoimmune destruction that characterizes type 1 diabetes—specifically, the body's immune system attacks and destroys the insulin-producing cells of the pancreas.

People with type 1 diabetes need frequent doses of insulin, which is typically delivered by injection with thin needles, a pen that contains an insulin-filled cartridge or a special pump that delivers a continuous dose of insulin.

• **Type 2** (once known as *adult-onset*) diabetes affects 90 percent of people who suffer from the disease. Most cases occur during adulthood, and risk increases with age. Over recent years, many overweight children and teenagers have been diagnosed with type 2 diabetes.

In type 2 diabetes, the pancreas produces insulin (often more than the usual amounts), but fat and tissue cells are "resistant," preventing the hormone from doing what it's supposed to do—which is to "unlock" cells so that blood glucose can enter.

Your risk of type 2 diabetes increases significantly if you eat a lot of foods that are high in simple carbohydrates (which are rapidly transformed into sugar) and foods that are low in dietary fiber (needed to slow the absorption of sugars from the food we eat and digest). Also, people who don't get much exercise are more likely to develop type 2 diabetes because of the insulin resistance that results from weight gain and an imbalance of stress hormones.

In addition to obesity, risk factors for type 2 diabetes include a family history of the disease (especially in parents or siblings)… apple-shaped body type… high blood pressure… high cholesterol… or, among women, a history of diabetes during pregnancy ("gestational diabetes," which usually disappears after delivery). People with type 2 diabetes who have difficulty controlling their glucose levels may require oral medication, such as *glucophage (Metformin)*, and/or insulin injections.

Heading off diabetes

Prediabetes affects 40 percent of Americans between the ages of 40 and 74. In these people, blood glucose levels are elevated but not enough to be considered type 2 diabetes. Detecting the telltale signs of prediabetes—which show up in blood tests—helps you prevent the full-blown disease. Without these measures, there's a good chance that a person diagnosed with prediabetes will develop type 2 diabetes within 10 years.

I advise my patients (and readers) to get yearly blood tests to help identify many early-stage diseases, including diabetes. *Diabetes-related tests should include…*

• **Fasting blood glucose to determine signs of prediabetes**. Before you go to your doctor's office for the test, you will need to fast for at least eight hours. Then blood is drawn and sent to a lab for a measurement of the glucose concentration, which is expressed in milligrams of glucose per deciliter (mg/dL). A fasting level of 100 mg/dL to 125 mg/dL is considered prediabetes.

Too often, patients who have glucose levels of 100 mg/dL to 115 mg/

dL are told by their doctors that they don't have a problem. In my view, a fasting blood glucose level in this range indicates prediabetes. I consider my patients to be free of any immediate risk only if their glucose levels are in the range of 70 mg/dL to 86 mg/dL. If a patient's glucose level is 87 mg/dL to 100 mg/dL, I recommend some of the same strategies that I prescribe for people with prediabetes.

• **Oral glucose tolerance test can be used to check for prediabetes**. After fasting for eight to 12 hours, a blood sample is taken to determine your fasting blood glucose level. Then your doctor will ask you to drink a solution with a high sugar content. After one, two and three hours, your doctor draws a blood sample and checks your glucose reading. A level of 140 mg/dL to 199 mg/dL for any of the readings indicates prediabetes. A reading of 200 mg/dL or above indicates diabetes.

I recommend that doctors also check insulin levels with the blood sample used for the glucose tolerance test. If insulin levels are abnormally high (15 to 20 microunits per milliliter or higher), it's a sign that you are developing insulin resistance—a hallmark of early diabetes.

Better diabetes monitoring

If you have diabetes, proper monitoring of your condition literally can save your life. Blood sugar levels can change dramatically within a matter of minutes, causing confusion, dizziness, fatigue and, in serious cases, a life-threatening coma. People with diabetes can easily measure their blood sugar levels with a small portable device that analyzes a drop of blood obtained by pricking a fingertip with a lancet. I recommend self-monitoring at least twice daily (upon awakening and 30 to 60 minutes after dinner). In addition, people with diabetes should make regular visits to their primary care doctors, have annual physicals and get yearly eye exams from their ophthalmologists.

Other tests for people with diabetes…

• **Hemoglobin A1C.** This test measures the amount of glucose sticking to the hemoglobin in red blood cells. It can be used as a marker of average blood glucose level over the past two to three months. Studies indicate that for every percentage point drop in A1C blood levels, risks for circulatory disorders as well as eye, kidney and nerve diseases drop by 40 percent. Most doctors say that a hemoglobin A1C reading below sevenpercent is acceptable. However, I believe that a reading below sixpercent is more desirable, because it shows better blood glucose control. People with an A1C reading of seven percent or less should have this test twice a year. If your reading is above eight percent, you should have it every three months.

• **Oxidative stress analysis**. This test measures the amount of tissue damage, or *oxidative stress*, caused from *free radicals* (harmful, negatively charged molecules). So few medical doctors know about oxidative stress testing, but I recommend it for patients with diabetes because they have high levels of oxidative stress, which accelerates the disease's progression. The markers of free radical activity can be measured by blood or urine tests. Elevated levels mean that the antioxidants that are normally produced in the body and ingested from foods and supplements are not effectively neutralizing the overabundance of free radicals. Your doctor can use Genova Diagnostics (800-522-4762, www.gdx.net) or Metametrix (800-221-4640, www.metametrix.com) for the test. It costs about $100, but most health insurers will cover it. People with diabetes should receive this test every six months until their values are normal.

• **Cardiovascular markers**. Individuals with diabetes are more susceptible to heart disease. That's because elevated glucose levels accelerate the buildup of plaque in the arteries. For this reason, I recommend blood tests for *homocysteine, C-reactive protein, fibrinogen, lipoprotein a, apolipoprotein a* and *b* and iron. Abnormal levels of these markers are linked to the development of heart disease. I recommend a baseline test and yearly follow-up testing for people who have abnormal readings for any of these markers. Most health insurers will cover the costs of these tests.

The sugar connection

Everyone knows that people who have diabetes or who are at risk for it should pay close attention to their diet. However, I'm convinced that few people realize just how damaging certain foods can be.

For example, about 20 percent of the average American's energy intake comes from foods such as burgers, pizza, chips, pastries and soft drinks. A 2004 study in the *American Journal of Clinical Nutrition* found that between 1980 and 1997, the average American's daily calorie consumption increased by 500 calories. Eighty percent of this increase was due to increases in carbohydrates, which include almost all sweet and starchy foods. During the same period, the prevalence of type 2 diabetes increased by 47 percent and the prevalence of obesity increased by 80 percent.

One of the worst culprits in the war on diabetes is the simple sugar *fructose*, which is naturally found in fruit and honey. Table sugar is half fructose (the other half is glucose, which is chemically the same as blood glucose). A type of fructose known as *high-fructose corn syrup* (HFCS) is especially harmful because it worsens insulin resistance. It has become the sweetener of choice for many soft drinks, ice creams, baked goods, candies/sweets, jams, yogurts and other sweetened products.

My recommendation is to put a strict limit on your consumption of foods that contain HFCS. This can be done by decreasing your intake of packaged, processed foods, avoiding drinks that are high in fructose and eating as many fresh foods as possible. (Natural sources of fructose, such as fruit and honey, can be safely consumed in moderation.)

There is one exception—some liquid nutritional supplements, such as the liquid vitamin formulas, contain *crystalline fructose*, a natural sweetener that is far less processed than HFCS and is not believed to cause dramatic increases in insulin levels.

Symptoms of diabetes

• **Increased thirst**.

• **Frequent urination** (especially at night).

- Unexplained increase in appetite.

- Fatigue.

- Erection problems.

- Blurred vision.

- Tingling or numbness in the hands and/or feet.

Test for Diabetes

You have diabetes if any one of the following test results occurs on at least two different days…

- **A fasting blood glucose level** of 126 mg/dL or higher.

- **A two-hour oral glucose tolerance test result** of 200 mg/dL or higher.

- **Symptoms of diabetes combined with a random (nonfasting) blood glucose test** of 200 mg/dL or higher.

Seven Super Foods—
Delicious Ways to Fight Disease

Nearly 2,500 years ago, Hippocrates, the father of modern medicine, said, *"Let food be thy medicine and medicine be thy food."* This is still true today—the right foods help you remain healthy and are powerful disease fighters. *Here are seven of the best...*

1. Beans

Americans' consumption of beans has steadily increased over the past two decades, and that's good news because beans provide tremendous healing power. Most popular varieties include soybeans, garbanzo (chickpeas), pinto, kidney, lima, navy and black beans. Beans are a type of legume, a class of vegetable that also includes lentils and peas.

Beans are high in protein, low in fat and calories, and rich in complex carbohydrates, fiber, *phytonutrients* and several vitamins and minerals, including folic acid and other B vitamins, potassium, magnesium and iron.

In addition, beans are loaded with *soluble fiber*, the same type of gummy fiber found in the oat bran in oatmeal. This type of fiber helps bind and eliminate cholesterol and stabilize blood sugar levels.

A study conducted by the US Department of Agriculture found that beans—especially black, pinto and kidney beans—topped the list of vegetables rich in disease-fighting antioxidants.

Specifically, several studies have shown that regular consumption of beans significantly reduces the risk for cardiovascular disease. New studies are now suggesting that beans also have potent anticancer properties. Both meat eaters and vegetarians enjoy this easy-to-find food.

Recommended: Eat one-half cup of beans four times per week. Beans make an excellent addition to salads, rice dishes and soups, and they can be pureed as a dip.

Helpful: Many people avoid beans because they experience gas after eating them. If this is a problem, take an enzyme product such as Beano, available at most grocery stores and drugstores. Follow directions on the label.

2. Broccoli

I am thankful that broccoli is such a popular food in my household—all three of my children like it. This king of the *cruciferous family* (other members include brussels sprouts, cabbage, kale, cauliflower and bok choy) is an excellent source of vitamin C, vitamin A, folic acid, calcium and fiber.

Broccoli fights cancer. It contains two classes of anticancer phytonutrients—*isothiocyanates* and *glucosinolates*.

• *Sulforaphane* is an isothiocyanate that activates detoxifying enzymes in the body that prevent the formation of cancer-causing substances. Sulforaphane also has potent antioxidant properties.

• *Indole-3-carbinol* (I3C) is a glucosinolate that has been shown to benefit women with early-stage cervical cancer and helps protect estrogen-sensitive cells, such as breast cells.

Broccoli also is rich in the *carotenoid* antioxidants *lutein* and *zeaxanthin*. Both are important in preventing ultraviolet damage to the eyes and can help prevent cataracts and *age-related macular degeneration*, the leading cause of blindness in people age 65 and older.

Recommended: Eat one-half cup of raw or lightly steamed broccoli daily (buying frozen broccoli is fine). Avoid boiling—it diminishes its nutritional value.

Broccoli sprouts, which are the newly sprouted seeds of broccoli, can be added to sandwiches or salads. They contain 30 to 50 times the concentration of protective phytonutrients that are found in mature broccoli plants. Broccoli sprouts are especially rich in sulforaphane. Because broccoli sprouts can be contaminated with bacteria, people with weak immune systems should check with their doctors before consuming them.

3. Eggs

The egg is an excellent source of protein, and it contains all the *essential amino acids* that your body cannot produce on its own. In addition, it is a rich source of vitamin K, cancer-fighting selenium, vitamin B-12 and *choline*, a nutrient required by cell membranes for healthy function. Some of these nutrients are found in the yolk, so egg whites alone are not as beneficial.

In the past, the egg got a bad reputation when it came to cholesterol and heart disease. However, multiple studies have now vindicated the egg.

A study in the *Journal of the American Medical Association*, conducted at Harvard School of Public Health, found no relationship between egg consumption and cardiovascular disease in a population of more than 117,000 nurses and health professionals who were followed for eight to 14 years. There was no difference in heart disease risk between those who ate less than one egg a week and those who ate one egg a day.

In fact, the protein in eggs appears to prevent blood clots. Eggs also contain the eye-protective nutrient *lutein*—and lutein from eggs is more easily absorbed than that from spinach (one of the richest sources) or from supplements.

In addition, in one Chinese study, women who ate at least six eggs a week lowered their risk of breast cancer by 44 percent, compared with no risk reduction in women who consumed two or fewer eggs a week.

Recommended: Eat one to six organic eggs weekly. Organic eggs don't contain hormone or antibiotic residues.

Caution: All people with gallbladder disease should avoid eggs. Eggs may worsen symptoms, including pain and spasms, possibly due to the fat content.

4. Blueberries

One of nature's antiaging stars, blueberries contain a megasupply of powerful antioxidants known as *anthocyanins*, which help to protect against cell damage. Anthocyanins have been shown to enhance the effects of vitamin C, improve capillaries so they're less likely to rupture and support the body's connective tissues. Anthocyanins give blueberries their blue-purple color. Blueberries also are a good source of vitamin C and vitamin E, manganese and fiber.

Blueberries contain the anthocyanin *pterostilbene*, a powerful antioxidant compound that is known to fight cancer. Animal studies have shown that pterostilbene also reduces cholesterol, improves memory and shortens recovery time from stroke. In addition, blueberries promote good eye health—they are particularly helpful in the prevention of macular degeneration.

Like cranberries, blueberries have been found to contain substances that prevent bacteria from adhering to the lining of the urinary tract, which may help guard against urinary tract infections.

Recommended: Eat one-half cup of blueberries five times weekly. Sprinkle blueberries, fresh or frozen, on cereal or add them to muffins and smoothies.

5. Oatmeal

Oatmeal, one of the most nutritious complex carbohydrates, contains several vital minerals, including manganese, selenium, magnesium, zinc and copper.

Oatmeal also provides protein and, as I mentioned earlier, is an excellent source of soluble fiber. Because this type of fiber stabilizes blood sugar, oatmeal is an excellent choice for people with diabetes.

The best-known benefits of this super food are its cholesterol-lowering properties. A type of soluble fiber known as *beta-glucan* (which also activates immune cells) and compounds called *saponins* bind dietary cholesterol and usher it out of the body unabsorbed.

A daily bowl of oatmeal can reduce total cholesterol by as much as 23 percent. It has also been shown to decrease the "bad" LDL cholesterol without changing levels of beneficial HDL cholesterol.

In addition, oats are a rich source of *tocotrienols*. These relatives of the vitamin E family guard against the oxidation of LDL cholesterol (thereby preventing LDL cholesterol from sticking to artery walls and causing plaque buildup) and reduce the production of cholesterol by the liver.

Recommended: Eat one cup of oatmeal three to four times weekly. When possible, choose the longer-cooking variety—instant oatmeal has a weaker cholesterol-lowering effect and often has salt and sugar added. Oatmeal is even healthier when sprinkled with a tablespoon of ground flaxseed and one-half teaspoon of cinnamon, both of which help lower cholesterol.

6. Walnuts

Walnuts are the perfect snack. They are rich in *omega-3 fatty acids*, which reduce inflammation in the body. Walnuts also contain the minerals manganese and copper, both of which play key roles in the body's antioxidant network.

In addition, these tasty nuts contain *gamma-tocopherol*, a component of vitamin E that provides antioxidant protection, as well as the amino acid *l-arginine*, which improves circulation. Walnuts also contain the phytonutrient *ellagic acid*, which helps protect against cancer-causing free radical damage.

Walnuts also are a source of the sleep hormone *melatonin*. The amount is too small to promote sleep, but the melatonin in walnuts provides additional antioxidant activity.

Several studies have shown that the consumption of walnuts reduces the risk of coronary artery disease. One study found that a walnut-rich diet lowered levels of *C-reactive protein*, a marker of inflammation, which is strongly associated with *atherosclerosis* and heart disease. Walnuts not only increase levels of omega-3 fatty acids but also decrease the adhesion of cholesterol to the lining of the arteries.

One study that was done at the Lipid Clinic at the Endocrinology and Nutrition Service, Institut d'Investigacions Biomediques, Barcelona, Spain, showed that a walnut-rich diet reduced total cholesterol by 4.4 percent and LDL cholesterol by 6.4 percent.

Other studies have found that walnuts significantly increase the elasticity of the arteries, which is a marker for healthy blood vessels. The Food and Drug Administration allows walnuts to carry the health claim that "eating 1.5 ounces of walnuts per day as part of a diet low in saturated fat and cholesterol may reduce the risk for heart disease."

Recommended: Eat four to eight walnuts (approximately 1.5 ounces) per day in cereals, salads and yogurt—or eat them plain.

7. Yogurt

Yogurt is a fermented dairy product rich in "friendly" bacteria. These bacteria, such as *Lactobacillus acidophilus* and *Lactobacillus bulgaricus*, improve immune function. Yogurt also is a helpful source of calcium, phosphorus, vitamin B-2 (*riboflavin*), iodine, vitamin B-12, vitamin B-5 (*pantothenic acid*), zinc, potassium and protein. Several studies have shown that incorporating calcium-rich foods, such as low-fat yogurt and cheese, into a reduced-calorie diet is an effective weight-management technique.

Yogurt also suppresses the growth of *Helicobacter pylori*, the bacterium that causes most cases of stomach ulcer. Along with other dairy products, yogurt appears to protect against colon and rectal cancers—perhaps because of the calcium content. Studies also have found that yogurt reduces the compounds that contribute to bad breath, cavities and gum disease.

Recommended: Eat one-half to one cup of yogurt daily. Look for low-fat yogurts that list "live active cultures" or "living yogurt cultures" on the label.

Do not buy any yogurt that contains artificial color, flavoring or sweetener. Choose plain yogurt or flavored yogurt made by Horizon or other companies that do not use artificial ingredients. Opt for organic yogurt products to avoid hormone and antibiotic residues. Yogurt is delicious when used in place of milk in cereals or as part of a smoothie.

Caution: Avoid yogurt if you are allergic or sensitive to cow's milk. Goat's milk yogurt maybe an alternative, depending on your sensitivity.

New Study Shocker:
America's #1 Drug Increases Your
Risk of Diabetes by up to 80 Percent

The "greatest thing in medicine right now!"

That's what Julie's doctor called statin drugs. And it's the reason she told me she decided to take them.

It's unbelievable! American doctors—and the public—have been hypnotized by Big Pharma and its "miraculous" cholesterol-lowering statin drugs. And unfortunately for Julie, her regular doctor is no exception.

Not to mention that these days, it almost doesn't matter what your cholesterol is, you are *not* getting out of your doctor's office without a prescription. Case in point: Julie's total cholesterol was a measly 215 mg/dL ("normal" is <200 mg/dL). Let's ignore for a minute that, even by mainstream standards, it's barely elevated. Because now we know that total cholesterol alone isn't a reliable cardiovascular risk predictor.

Knowing that, I told Julie that statins have been shown to increase the risk of liver, muscle, and kidney damage; as well as inciting infection and memory problems. Then I added that some simple diet changes and supplementation with nutrients/herbal formulas would put her in the normal range.

Julie looked at me as if she was in shock, "But that's what my doctor recommended."

By the end of the visit, I had reversed her brainwashing.

Julie decided to stop her statin medication to reduce her likelihood of serious medication-related health problems. In that simple step I helped improve her health right then and there, even before we addressed the rest of her health program.

Diabetes skyrockets—even in the least likely patients

I thought about Julie again today when I saw the most recent shocker about these dangerous drugs.

A new study shows that statin use increases the risk of diabetes in some women by almost 80 percent![1] Data was analyzed from the Women's Health Initiative, a long-term survey of more than 153,000 post-menopausal women aged 50-79 years. (This is the very same study that brought HRT use to a screeching halt in 2002, when it was associated with an increase in invasive breast cancer, in addition to more women dying from lung cancer, blood clots, and heart attacks.)

The drugs being taken included all the big ones: Simvastatin (Zocor), lovastatin (Altocor, Altoprev, Mevacor), pravastatin (Pravachol), fluvastatin (Lescol), and atorvastatin (Lipitor).

Overall, the risk of diabetes associated with statin therapy was an astonishing 48 percent! The biggest jumps were seen in white (49 percent), Hispanic (57 percent), and Asian women (78 percent).

Those numbers are shocking. But here's an even bigger stunner: The study found that women with the *lowest* body mass index had a higher risk of diabetes compared with obese women. Clearly the diabetic effect can't be pinned just on overweight anymore! Imagine what is going on in your body if even thin women are susceptible to diabetes, simply from taking statin drugs.

Statins trap you in a catch-22 health nightmare

This isn't the first research showing statin drugs affect your blood sugar metabolism leading to diabetes. While people taking statins believe they are reducing their risk of heart disease, they are actually *increasing* their risk of heart disease because diabetes causes heart disease! And, of course, diabetes increases the risk of other dreadful conditions such as blindness, amputation, impotence, fatigue, and dementia.

And the list goes on. But let's stay focused on diabetes for now.

So, how *do* statins cause diabetes?

A 2010 study published in the *Journal of the American College of Cardiology* demonstrated statins **significantly** increase insulin levels.[2] This hormone, produced by your pancreas, transports blood sugar (glucose) into your cells. When your body repeatedly produces high levels of insulin, your cells become resistant to its glucose-transporting effects. This leads to further insulin spiking and, ultimately, higher blood sugar levels.

It is not understood exactly *how* statin drugs cause diabetes. Based on the research, I believe they may alter glucose metabolism of the liver or muscles. Preliminary research is also suggesting the medication may alter adinopectin metabolism. Adinopectin is secreted by fat cells and is critical for glucose and fatty acid metabolism. Whatever the mechanism—it's a major concern!

Not just a problem for the fairer sex

And if you're a man, don't think you're getting off scot-free. In fact, you are at risk, too. While this study used data only from the WHI, previous studies have shown that statin use also increases the risk of diabetes in men.

According to a 2011 study involving five statin trials, high dose statin therapy was associated with a 12 percent increased risk in new-onset diabetes.[3] And remember, the mainstream media hyped up the 2008 Jupiter trial involving statin drugs, praising the ability of the statin drug known as rouvastatin (Crestor) to reduce the risk for heart attack and stroke in people who had normal cholesterol and high levels of C-reactive protein. (Never mind that, in reality, only one person out of 120 actually would benefit from the drug.)

What did I report back then that you didn't hear from the talking heads? This statin increased the risk of diabetes by 25 percent!

The real way to a healthy heart—without all the risk

You've heard me say it before: Obesity is the biggest contributor to type 2 diabetes. And the one thing every expert agrees on is that it is out of control.

So we certainly don't need the diabetes explosion fueled even further by these overhyped statin drugs. Big Pharma has practically programmed doctors to ignore the common sense science on diet, exercise, detoxification, and stress management to treat cardiovascular disease.

Case in point: The 7.8 year EPIC study looked at 23,000 German adults and four healthy lifestyle factors among German adults (never smoking, having a body mass index lower than 30, performing 3.5 hours per week or more of physical activity, and adhering to a healthy diet including a high intake of fruits, vegetables, whole-grain bread, and low meat consumption). Surprise, surprise... they found a 93 percent lower risk of diabetes![4]

In future editions of *Health Revelations*, I will explain what *really* causes heart disease—and how you can lower your risk—without swallowing one single statin.

Because while the mainstream likes to tie it up in one easy package and declare that cholesterol is the only indicator that matters, they couldn't be more wrong. Important root causes such as LDL particle size, insulin resistance, inflammation, toxic metals, nutrient deficiencies, and the oxidation of cholesterol all contribute more to your risk of heart failure than your total cholesterol.

What else do these things have in common: Most doctors ignore them. And that's a sin, because we have the tools and technology to address these issues—naturally and without making you even sicker.

Work with a holistic doctor to avoid statin medications – and to get off of them if your doctor pulled the same stunt as Julie's.

There are some very simple yet effective dietary strategies that will help balance your lipid levels. Here is what I recommend my patients eat:

- At least two servings a week of heart healthy fish such as sardines, trout, and wild salmon

- Five to seven servings of fruits and vegetables daily

- Soluble fiber-rich foods daily such as beans, peas, apples, pears (and keep in mind that a daily bowl of oatmeal can reduce total cholesterol by up to 23 percent)

- Nuts such as almonds and walnuts. Just 1.5 ounces daily can lower LDL cholesterol by up to 10 percent

In addition to what you should add, you should also reduce simple sugars in your diet to less than 30 g daily and avoid ALL trans fat-laden foods that damage your arteries and cholesterol.

Keep in mind that 30 minutes of moderate exercise three to five times weekly balances your lipid levels. You don't have to run a marathon but working up a light sweat will do wonders for your heart.

If you need support beyond diet and exercise for lipid balance consider supplements such as red yeast rice (2,400 mg daily), plant sterols (1,000 mg with each meal), fish oil (3,000 mg of EPA and DHA combined daily), and niacin (1,000-1,500 mg daily in divided doses). You can start with red yeast rice or plant sterols and always combine with fish oil.

With this approach you will keep the drug pushers off your back and make your heart and arteries healthier, not to mention your entire body.

How an All-Natural "Bean Cure" Can Get You Off Your Diabetes Drug—For Good

When my friend called to ask what I thought about the Actos, his doctor prescribed for his diabetes, it didn't take me more than a couple seconds to answer him.

"That's easy," I warned, "You should toss that prescription in the trash!"

I explained that Actos might increase your risk of bladder cancer. Plus, it comes with a whole laundry list of other health problems.[1] He was shocked that his doctor never told him about the risks. The cancer warning was his wake up call. He followed my advice to change his diet, start exercising, and to start a supplement program. Before long his blood sugar plummeted and his days of Actos were gone.

Is diabetes becoming America's #1 export?

As the American fast-food lifestyle has invaded the rest of the world, it's easy to spot all the health problems that have spread right along with it. According to the World Health Organization, 346 million people worldwide now have diabetes![2] When you count the number of people with pre-diabetes who are *already* experiencing some organ damage, that number jumps up to about 1.7 billion people with blood sugar problems.

Here in the US, about 10 percent of Americans have diabetes and another 20 percent pre-diabetes.[3] That means that in this country alone, we're faced with over 70 million people with abnormal blood sugar levels. Looking at those numbers it's really no wonder why so many patients come to see me with blood sugar problems.

While the country debates how health insurance should work, something we can all agree on is that diabetes is destroying our health. It's a major cause of heart disease and stroke, and a leading cause of kidney failure and new cases of blindness among adults. In fact, it's now the seventh leading cause of death in the US.[4]

Warning: Your diabetes drugs may be making you sick!

Not surprisingly, the market for diabetes drugs is exploding. The pharmaceutical industry is licking its lips as it capitalizes on this new epidemic releasing one new designer drug after another. But be wary of these new wonder drugs. They're dangerous and they don't even treat the real reasons for your blood sugar problems.

A new study found that the popular class of drugs known as Thiazolidinediones, which Actos and Avandia both belong too, increases your risk of diabetic macular edema (DME) by three to six times.[5] DME is a very serious condition that causes fluid to leak from the blood vessels inside the area of the retina responsible for vision called the macula. This causes the retinas to swell and puts you at risk for blindness.

Another study earlier this year found this same class of drugs increased the risk of bone fractures by 1.5 times when compared to patients without diabetes.[6] Of course, considering their track record, we really shouldn't be surprised. The first drug in this class, Rezulin, was banned after it was reported to cause serious liver problems in some users. And thiazolidinediones are also linked with an increased risk of heart failure and heart attack![7]

Personally, I never recommend them. And the only time I can imagine using these risky drugs is for someone who simply refuses to change their diet and lifestyle habits or to use blood-sugar-balancing supplements. Because, the truth is, both pre-diabetes and diabetes can be reversed with a comprehensive natural strategy. I prove this every single day with the dramatic changes that I see in the patients at my own clinic.

Food holds the secret to finally beating your diabetes

Let's face it. We live in a hectic world filled with foods that are big on convenience and very low in nutrients. Of course, our healthy blood sugar levels suffer because of it. But risky drugs are not the answer. You can use a non-toxic approach instead. By working with your body's own healing system, you can get your blood sugar levels back to normal.

I always recommend you start with a high fiber diet that includes moderate amounts of protein and complex carbohydrates.

Getting the RIGHT kind of fiber is key to blood-sugar control

To keep your blood sugar under control it's very important to get the right *type* of fiber. I'm not talking about the kind that helps in the bathroom, called insoluble fiber. Rather it's the type most medical doctors never mention—soluble fiber. This means it dissolves in water and forms a gel like material. This "gel" blocks some of the sugars and cholesterol in your food from entering your blood stream. The result is lower insulin levels and better blood sugar control. Foods that are rich in soluble fiber include oats, peas, beans, Brussels sprouts, almonds, artichokes, apples, citrus fruits, carrots, barley, and spinach.

I should also add that soluble fiber could also help reduce your appetite. When you take it with water it expands in your stomach and digestive tract making you feel full faster. And, of course, when you eat less food you generally have better blood sugar levels.

Powerful "bean cure" helps your body *resist* your diabetes

Most doctors are clueless when it comes to the power of a group of foods that are high in what is called "resistant starches." Resistant starches balance your blood sugar levels by reducing the rate that other starches you eat at the same time are processed. This prevents spikes in blood sugar and insulin levels. Resistant starches are so powerful that they can even improve your blood sugar and insulin response for several hours after a meal and even the following day.

The best food sources for resistant starches are in the legume family, especially beans and lentils. The secret to the beans/blood sugar balancing act is a protein called phaseolamin (faze-*ahl*-uh-min). Phaseolamin restricts the digestive enzyme amylase that's needed to digest starches and sugars so that some of them pass right through your system without ever being absorbed.

A large study of 64,227 middle aged Chinese women found those who ate the most legumes were 38 percent less likely to have diabetes and those who ate the most soybeans were 47 percent less likely to have diabetes.[8] It's important to note, however, that this benefit was not seen in processed soy products including soy protein. Instead, you should get your soy from fermented foods such as miso, tempeh, tofu, and natto.

Putting your diabetes-fighting fiber plan into action

There are two soluble fiber products you should know about. The first is glucomannan, also known as Asian Konjac root. A 14-study analysis found glucomannan reduces fasting blood sugar by about six percent. It was also effective for treating elevated blood fats, cholesterol, body weight, and blood pressure.[9] You can find glucomannan in health food stores. Work up to taking four grams with an eight ounce glass of water thirty to sixty minutes before meals.

Another product that has been featured in the media recently is PGX. This very sticky soluble fiber has been the focus of several studies including one done at the University of Toronto. I'm a big fan of PGX and have used it with a number of patients. It can help you control diabetes, reduce your appetite, lose weight, and even significantly lower your total and LDL cholesterol.

The key to soluble fiber lowering your blood sugar is to use it consistently. This means eating soluble fiber rich foods with at least two meals a day and preferably all three.

Keep in mind that the better you control your glucose and insulin, the easier it is to lose weight. An interesting 15-week study followed obese or overweight women who weren't dieting but took a PGX supplement. The women all lost approximately 3.5 pounds and 1.5 inches from their waists.[10]

PGX is available in capsule and granule form. Start by taking one capsule or 1/3 of a scoop with an eight ounce glass of water 30 minutes before each meal. Increase this dose by one capsule or 1/3 scoop every three to four days until you're taking three to four soft gels or one scoop per meal.

One caution: Soluble fiber can cause gas, bloating, or constipation. You can avoid this by slowly increasing the dose and making sure to drink at least eight ounces of water every time you take it.

"Hidden-in-Plain-Sight" Toxin Rockets Your Risk for Developing Diabetes Up by 65 Percent— Read This BEFORE You Take Your Next Bite

I t's one of the world's most under-acknowledged causes of illness. Elevated levels of it are linked to heart disease, impaired cognitive function, chronic fatigue syndrome, immune system dysfunction, hormone imbalance, and even attention deficit hyperactivity disorder. Your average physician and dentist don't have a clue about the devastating damage this poison can cause in the human body. But now a bombshell study, published in the world's top diabetes journal, may finally change all that. The hidden-in-plain-sight mystery toxin I'm referring to is mercury.

Researchers from the Indiana University School of Public Health found that adults who were exposed to higher mercury levels when they were younger had a whopping 65 percent increased risk of developing type 2 diabetes later in life.[1] The study tracked 3,875 American men and women between the ages of 20 and 32 for 18 years. Even after controlling for dietary and lifestyle factors such as omega-3 fatty acids and magnesium—both of which can help with blood sugar metabolism and can help reduce the toxic effects of mercury—researchers found that the jump in risk remained.

Hidden heavy metal may wreak havoc with your pancreas

Have you ever wondered why some people who seem relatively healthy otherwise develop type 2 diabetes? Mercury toxicity could be the reason. Mercury that was unknowingly being ingested when eating fish or from decaying amalgam fillings could have caused the cells of the pancreas to malfunction allowing glucose to build up in the blood. Also, toxic metals such as mercury can disrupt normal enzyme function in all your cells.

With its link to a 65 percent increase in diabetes risk, mercury toxicity is now on the same list with the other two widely known causes of diabetes: Refined carbohydrates and high-sugar foods. My friend, make no mistake about it, this is a game changer. A poor diet, not enough exercise, and mercury exposure from the time you're in the womb is a triple whammy that can almost certainly send you down the road to diabetes.

Mercury is highly toxic to human health

I routinely screen patients for elevated body levels of toxic metals, including mercury, lead, arsenic, aluminum, and cadmium, using fully accredited medical laboratories to ensure accuracy. Elevated levels of any toxic metal can be treated with chelation and detox therapy. When these metals are removed from the body, patients typically find that good things happen: Energy improves, the mind becomes clearer, digestion improves, autoimmune response markers come down, skin conditions resolve, and pain levels are reduced.

Conventional medical doctors and dentists commonly claim that mercury had nothing to do with health problems or that lab tests are somehow inaccurate. But the countless positive heavy-metal detox experiences of my patients refute this ridiculous assertion. The fact is, there's a mountain of evidence showing that mercury is a dangerous toxin that can harm both the human body and the environment. Even the World Health Organization acknowledges this. For years they've published guidelines for acceptable mercury levels. Their publication "Exposure to Mercury: A Major Public Health Concern" says it all in its title, and clarifies the risk in the first sentence: "Mercury is highly toxic to human health."[3]

Seeking out sources of mercury exposure

Mercury occurs naturally in the environment in several different forms. Human beings can neither create it nor destroy it. It's found in the earth's crust and in rocks, including coal. According to the Environmental Protection Agency, "Coal-burning power plants are the largest human-caused source of mercury emissions to the air in the US."[4] It's also released into the atmosphere as a byproduct of gold and mercury mining, and in the manufacturing of cement, pesticides, chlorine, mirrors, medical equipment, and through dentistry (amalgam fillings), industrial leaks, and corpse and waste incineration.[5]

The most common forms of mercury are elemental mercury, methyl mercury, and inorganic mercury compounds. The elemental form is commonly (and safely) used in medical equipment such as thermometers, blood pressure cuffs, barometers, and some types of light bulbs. However, if the elemental mercury isn't enclosed in a container it will give off vapor. High levels of this vapor breathed in over a short period of time can be fatal. The two other forms are what we're most commonly affected by.

Elemental mercury is no longer safe when it's released into the environment as a byproduct of coal burning power plants. In fact, it's a major source of human exposure to the toxic metal. According to the WHO "It can stay for up to a year in the atmosphere, where it can be transported and deposited globally. It ultimately settles in the sediment of lakes, rivers or bays where it is transformed into methyl mercury, absorbed by phytoplankton, ingested by zooplankton and fish, and accumulates especially in long-lived predatory species, such as shark and swordfish."[3] And, of course, fish that eat the toxic methyl mercury pass that mercury on to humans when we eat the fish, which explains why fish are ultimately the biggest source of mercury toxicity in the human body. The more methyl mercury a fish feeds on, and the longer it lives, determines how much mercury it passes on to us.

Fish are a major source of mercury toxicity

Shockingly, a recent study found that between 43 percent and 100 percent of the fish from nine countries (including the US) contained mercury at levels so high that eating them more than once per month would be unsafe.[6] The biggest risk is to children, especially those who are still developing in the womb and being exposed to mercury when the mother consumes unsafe fish (mercury passes through the placenta into the bloodstream of the fetus). However, adults are affected, too. Richard Gelfond, the CEO of the movie company IMAX is a good example of just how dangerous mercury exposure in adults can be. Gelfond developed a balance problem that became so severe he couldn't even cross a street without his wife holding his hand. After seeing many specialists a neurologist finally thought to ask him how much fish he was eating. It turns out Gelfond, a fish fan, was eating two meals of fish a day. His diagnosis? You guessed it—mercury toxicity.[7]

Do you have a mouthful of mercury?

Dental amalgams (silver fillings), which contain approximately 50 percent mercury, are a source of exposure to the troublesome inorganic mercury. A study in *Journal of Dental Research* analyzed mercury vapor concentration in 46 people, 35 of whom had amalgam fillings.[8] Researchers found that participants with amalgam fillings produced mercury vapors that were nine times greater than baseline levels in participants with no amalgams. Chewing increased their mercury concentration by six-fold compared to non-chewing mercury levels—a stunning 54-fold increase over people without amalgam fillings.[8] (If a dentist tries to tell you silver fillings don't increase body mercury levels direct him to this study published in a reputable dental journal.) And to make matters worse some

Mercury toxicity symptoms

Exposure to elemental mercury (which usually occurs in the vapor form) can cause:[9]

- Mood swings, nervousness, irritability, and other emotional changes

- Insomnia

- Headache

- Abnormal sensations (such as numbness or tingling)

- Muscle twitching

- Tremors

- Weakness

- Muscle atrophy

- Decreased cognitive function

- Peripheral vision impairment

- Stinging or needle-like sensations in the extremities and mouth

- Loss of coordination

- Muscle weakness

- Impairments of speech and hearing

of the mercury from fillings that enters the digestive tract is transformed into methylmercury, the type of mercury commonly found in fish.

Another form of inorganic mercury compounds are known as mercury salts. They have long been used in folk medicine and in herbal formulas developed by traditional Chinese medicine or Ayurvedic medicine practitioners. It would be rare for Chinese or Ayurvedic medicine herbalists in the US to use formulas that contain this very toxic form of mercury. However, herbal supplements and teas imported from China and India have been found to contain mercury and other contaminants. Therefore I recommend using only herbal products that are harvested and manufactured in the US, or at least independently tested for toxic metals and other contaminants.

Diagnosing mercury toxicity

There are several tests that can be used to diagnose your mercury burden. These include hair, urine, stool, toenail and blood analyses. For children, hair analysis is usually the easiest test to use. For adults any of the tests… or a combination of them… can be used.

When testing finds elevated levels of mercury, especially the methyl mercury type, the first step in treatment is to eliminate the source. This means avoiding mercury-laden fish, especially tuna, swordfish, and shark. (In fact, I recommend this for everyone as a preventative measure.) And the proper removal of amalgam fillings is critical (a holistic dentist can take care of this).

Next, you should start on a chelation and detoxification program. The key to the successfully removing mercury from the body is to make sure the body's detoxification systems are working properly. The liver and kidneys are particularly important because they work to metabolize and excrete mercury out of the body. A healthy diet that contains adequate protein, fiber, and nutrients is important for these organs to work properly. Most mercury is excreted through the stool. This requires enough fiber in the diet to bind and carry the mercury out so that it's not reabsorbed through the gut right back into the blood stream. A diet high in vegetables is critical. Ground flaxseeds, chia seeds, and psyllium seeds can boost your fiber levels to aid with the elimination of mercury. Adequate filtered water is necessary for proper detoxification as well.

Glutathione helps you metabolize mercury

Glutathione is a valuable antioxidant that supports your body's ability to metabolize mercury. It works on a cellular level to help your body to detox from mercury. There are several ways to increase glutathione levels. These start with intravenous, transdermal, and inhaled or nebulized glutathione, all of which must be administered by a healthcare professional. Or you can take some additional supplements, which will naturally stimulate your own glutathione production including:

- Selenium—200 mcg daily

- N'acetylcysteine—1,000 mg daily

- Whey protein—25 g daily

- Vitamin C—1,000 mg twice daily

- Alpha lipoic acid—600 mg daily

- Milk Thistle—500 mg daily

Glutathione levels can also be increased orally. Technological advances have allowed us to make a form of the supplement, called S-acetyl glutathione, that can survive stomach acid. A typical dosage is 200 mg taken two to three times daily. There are a number of good glutathione products available from Max International.

More supplements that help with mercury detox

Several small human studies have found that chlorella, a type of algae, may support mercury detoxification. The algae appear to bind with mercury in the digestive tract helping to eliminate it. A typical adult dose is to work up to 1,000 mg twice daily. Bioray (www.bioray.com) produces a gentle detox formula that contains chlorella called NDF. For young children you can work with a healthcare practitioner.

Probiotics are the good bacteria in the digestive tract which also help to metabolize mercury. They are an important part of the detoxification activity in the gut. Take a quality probiotic daily.

Vitamin C not only supports glutathione levels, but also aids in the detoxification of mercury in several ways. It acts as an antioxidant and also increases bile production. Take 1,000 mg twice daily.

Multivitamin and mineral formulas provide a base of nutrients that aid your organs and cells in eliminating mercury. Take as directed.

For patients with high levels of mercury or conditions I feel are directly caused by their mercury toxicity I also use more aggressive protocols. This can involve the oral use of DMSA (Meso-2, 3-dimercaptosuccinic acid) which is a chelating agent shown to chelate heavy metals including mercury. It has been used for the treatment of heavy metal toxicity since the 1950's. Research has shown that it's safe and effective. I typically have patients use 250 mg to 500 mg a day for several weeks with breaks to help pull mercury out of the body. Another approach I use is the intravenous administration of DMPS (2,3-Dimercapto-1-propanesulfonic acid), which similar to DMSA works to pull mercury out of the body's tissues. I've found that one treatment every three weeks for five treatments is very effective in reducing mercury levels.

Saunas, whether they are steam, dry, or infrared, can help to eliminate mercury as well. Some practitioners also recommend colonics to support colon cleansing as part of a mercury detoxification regimen.

The length of time it takes to eliminate mercury from the body depends on many factors. This includes the health of the patient, how high the mercury levels are, type of chelation program used, genetics (people vary in their ability to detoxify mercury based on their genetics) and if the source of the mercury contamination is eliminated (such as fish consumption or amalgam fillings). For some patients it takes a few months while for others with a high body storage level it can take six months or longer.

During treatment I find that some patients have a temporary increase in their mercury levels as their body releases stored metal. This is normal and means the chelation treatment is pulling the mercury out of the tissues it's stored in. Over time the levels will drop. I very rarely see side effects with mercury chelation. If a patient's mineral levels dip too low I have him supplement with extra minerals and reduce the strength or frequency of his chelation program. Your holistic doctor can use tests to determine when you are done treatment.

It's important to avoid mercury contamination and to get your levels tested and treated if elevated. This is particularly true if you have a chronic disease including diabetes. I suspect researchers have only scratched the surface on the detrimental effects of mercury on human health. Fortunately we already have effective methods for preventing, identifying, and treating the problem.

Part VII

Alzheimer 's Disease and Memory

Recommendations for Poor Memory

Do you have a poor memory? *Dr. Stengler recommends the following seven remedies that can help make it better...*

1. Phosphatidylserine. Take 300 mg per day. This naturally occurring *phospholipid* improves brain cell communication and memory.

2. Bacopa (Bacopa monniera). This nutrient has been shown to improve memory and recall. Take 300 mg daily.

3. Ginkgo biloba (24 percent). Take 120 mg two to three times daily. It improves circulation to the brain as well as memory and has antioxidant benefits. Avoid ginkgo if you take a blood-thinning medication such as *warfarin* (Coumadin).

4. Vitamin B-12. Use 800 to 1,600 mcg daily. Consider using a sublingual form at 400 mcg. A vitamin B-12 deficiency contributes to poor memory.

5. Club moss (Huperzia serrata). Take a product standardized to contain 0.2 milligrams of huperzine A daily. This compound has been shown to increase *acetylcholine levels* in the brain and to improve memory in people with Alzheimer's disease.

6. Essential fatty acids. Take one to two tablespoons of flaxseed oil or two to five grams of fish oil daily. It supplies essential fatty acids for proper brain function.

7. Acetyl-L-carnitine. Take 500 mg three times daily. It improves brain cell communication and memory.

Internet Searches Boost Brain Power

Older adults had enhanced brain function after spending one hour a day online for a week, say researchers at University of California at Los Angeles. They found that conducting online research—which involves retaining information and picking up points from competing graphics and words—is a form of brain exercise that benefits those who are new to the Internet as well as those with experience.

Chinese Club Moss for Better Memory

Every so often, we learn that an ancient medicinal herb has new and astonishing health benefits. So it is with Chinese club moss. Perhaps you have heard of it by another name—*huperzia* or *Qian ceng ta*—but most people haven't heard of it at all. Yet as the baby boomer population ages, people will be talking a lot about Chinese club moss and its active ingredient, *huperzine A* (HupA).

New finding: HupA improves memory and slows age-related cognitive decline—even in early-stage Alzheimer's disease patients. (Neither HupA nor drugs help much in later stages of Alzheimer's.)

Chinese medicine practitioners have utilized club moss for centuries as a diuretic and an anti-inflammatory. Two decades ago, a Chinese scientist discovered that an *alkaloid* (an organic compound) in HupA could improve brain function. This sparked many studies, some ongoing, including a clinical trial at the National Institutes of Health.

HupA's cognitive benefits are due mainly to its effects on acetylcholine, a neurotransmitter critical for normal thinking, memory and attention. These mental processes falter when *acetylcholine* production drops or an enzyme known as *acetylcholinesterase* (which normally breaks down unused acetylcholine) gets overactive, degrading the much needed acetylcholine.

HupA appears to inhibit activity of acetylcholinesterase, thereby sparing acetylcholine. This also is how pharmaceuticals for Alzheimer's work—but several human clinical trials suggest that HupA may be even more effective than the drugs *donepezil* (Aricept) and *tacrine* (Cognex). Animal studies demonstrate that HupA further supports cognitive function by protecting brain cells from damage caused by free radicals (harmful negatively charged molecules), toxins and/or lack of oxygen (for instance, from poor circulation or stroke)… and by reducing formation of *beta-amyloid*, a protein that forms lesions in the brain tissue of Alzheimer's patients.

I started prescribing HupA eight years ago for patients with memory problems—and many have been delighted with their improvement. HupA seems to work better than *ginkgo biloba*, an herb that increases blood flow to the brain. For ability to improve brain function, on a scale of one to 10, I rate ginkgo at six and HupA at nine. And unlike ginkgo, HupA is safe for people who take blood thinners, such as aspirin or *warfarin* (Coumadin).

For intermittent problems with short-term memory, I recommend that adults under age 55 take 50 mcg to 100 mcg of HupA daily… and that those age 55 and older take 100 mcg twice daily. For more severe memory problems, such as in early Alzheimer's, take 200 mcg twice daily.

HupA is generally safe and can be taken indefinitely. Occasional side effects include nausea, diarrhea, dizziness and/or loss of appetite. Before starting HupA, talk to your doctor. Do not take HupA if you suffer a cardiac condition that impacts heart rate, such as *bradycardia* (slow resting heart rate) or congestive heart failure, because HupA can decrease heart rate and lead to fainting. If you take medication for Alzheimer's disease, do not use HupA, because it might worsen the drug's side effects (nausea, vomiting and sweating). If you are dissatisfied with the Alzheimer's drugs you are taking, ask your doctor about discontinuing them and trying HupA instead.

Huperzine A brands I like include Source Naturals (800-815-2333, www.sourcenaturals.com), sold at health-food stores and online (for instance, at www.iherb.com)... and Ceriva by Metagenics (800-692-9400, www.metagenics.com), available from health-care practitioners. Cost runs about $10 per month at a dose of 100 mcg daily. In my view, that is a small price to pay for improved memory and clearer thinking.

The Truth About Brain Food... And Supplements That Keep Your Memory Intact

Everyone forgets something from time to time. Some people have trouble remembering names. Others cannot keep track of their car keys. Whether we suffer everyday absentmindedness or moments of real memory loss, all of us are concerned about keeping our brain power intact.

In recent years, a great deal of research has focused on the most severe kinds of memory loss—senile dementia and Alzheimer's disease. In the US, these closely related conditions affect up to 10 percent of people over age 65 and nearly half of those over age 85.

Many studies have identified ways to lower risk of these age-related problems. Popular methods include stress-reduction strategies, such as daily exercise, positive mental imagery, biofeedback and close personal relationships, to prevent spikes in the memory-draining stress hormone *cortisol*... "brain workouts," including crossword puzzles, word games and challenging card games... and eight to nine hours of sleep each night. Good nutrition—and the right kind of supplementation—also can help protect our brains and safeguard our memories at any age. The sooner you get started with a brain-protecting regimen, the more you'll benefit.

For optimal brain function, your diet should be well-balanced with carbohydrates (40 percent), protein (30 percent) and fats (30 percent). You can accomplish this by eating meals that include whole grains, fruits and vegetables (for complex carbohydrates)… fish, poultry, lean meats, legumes, nuts and seeds (for protein)… and fish oil, olive oil, avocados, almonds, walnuts and ground flaxseed (for fats). Steer clear of dairy products and packaged and processed foods, such as cookies, white bread and pasta, which are packed with simple carbohydrates that wreak havoc on glucose levels, contributing to diabetes, stroke/vascular disease and dementia.

The value of fish

Fish provides *docosahexaenoic acid* (DHA) and *eicosapentaenoic acid* (EPA), the most plentiful fatty acids in the brain. DHA, an *omega-3 fatty acid*, is found in abundance in cold-water fish such as mackerel, sardines, salmon and herring. You also can get it from fish-oil supplements, egg yolks, DHA-enriched eggs and some algae supplements, such as Neuromins, a product that is available at most health-food stores. Foods such as walnuts… leafy, green vegetables… and supplements including flaxseed and hemp oil contain *alpha-linolenic acid*, an omega-3 fatty acid that can be converted by the body into DHA and EPA.

How essential is DHA to memory? It has been known for some years that people have a higher risk of Alzheimer's if they have low blood levels of DHA. A study in *Archives of Neurology* revealed that people who ate fish one to three times a month had a 40 percent lower risk of Alzheimer's than those who never ate fish. Those who consumed fish once a week or more had a 60 percent lower risk. Fish may be baked, broiled or grilled.

It also makes sense to take a fish-oil supplement daily. I suggest using 1,000 mg of combined DHA and EPA. Good brands are Nordic Naturals (800-662-2544, www.nordicnaturals.com) and Carlson Laboratories (888-234-5656, www.carlsonlabs.com), both available at health-food stores.

Caution: Fish oil can thin blood, so check with your doctor before using it if you take blood-thinning medications such as *warfarin* (Coumadin).

GLA is essential

Omega-6s make up another class of essential fatty acids that are necessary for good brain function. Omega-6 is found in vegetable oils, including safflower, sunflower and corn oils. Most American diets contain too much of these oils due to consumption of packaged and fried foods. However, the most important omega-6 fatty acid is *linoleic acid*, which is converted in the body to *gamma-linolenic acid* (or GLA). This essential fatty acid plays a big role in the formation of healthy brain-cell membranes, the part of the cell that stores information. Taking borage oil or evening primrose oil is a healthful way to increase GLA intake—hempseed and hempseed oil also are good sources. Another way to get GLA in the diet is by consuming flaxseed (with water to prevent constipation) or flaxseed oil.

Count on choline

Just as a car needs spark plugs, an active brain requires quick-firing neurotransmitters. As the name implies, a neurotransmitter sends a signal that jumps from one brain cell to another. Substances that act as neurotransmitters—the most important of which is a brain chemical called *acetylcholine*—are all vital components of the brain's communication system.

There is one hitch. In order for your body to manufacture enough *acetylcholine*, you need to get a closely related nutrient called *choline*. The best source of choline is *phosphatidylcholine* (PC), which occurs naturally in fish, egg yolks, legumes, nuts, meat and vegetables. It also is found in breast milk. To help prevent memory problems, you can boost your PC intake by taking a 1,500 mg to 2,000 mg PC supplement daily. (Doses of more than 3,000 mg can cause digestive upset, including diarrhea, nausea and stomachache.)

PC is only part of the neurotransmitter equation. To turn PC into brain-friendly *choline*, you also need to get healthy doses of vitamin C and certain B vitamins. You can get plenty of these vitamins in your diet by eating red, yellow and green peppers, citrus fruits and cantaloupe for vitamin C and sweet potatoes, tuna and avocados for B vitamins. Also, I recommend taking a balanced daily multivitamin/mineral supplement.

Deficiencies of folic acid and other key B vitamins have been associated with an increased risk of Alzheimer's disease. These nutrients help to lower levels of *homocysteine*, a harmful by-product of protein metabolism that is increased in people who are genetically susceptible. That's why it is important to have your blood levels of homocysteine, folic acid and B-12 tested by your doctor to see if you need additional supplementation of folic acid and/or B-12.

The European cure

For years, European doctors have recommended the supplement called *L-alpha-glycerylphosphorylcholine* (GPC) to promote mental acuity (the ability to respond quickly and appropriately to mental challenges). GPC actually is used by the brain more effectively than PC to form *acetylcholine*—but it costs twice as much and is less widely available in the US. A good GPC supplement by Source Naturals is sold in some health-food stores under the brand name Alpha GPC (to locate a retailer, go to www.sourcenaturals.com). Take two 300-mg capsules twice daily for the first four weeks, then two 300-mg capsules once daily as a maintenance dosage. Side effects are rare, but take GPC with a meal if it seems to interfere with your digestion.

PS: Be sure to get more

Phosphatidylserine (PS) is a fat that the brain needs to preserve the key brain chemicals *serotonin* and *dopamine*. It also has been shown to reduce levels of the stress hormone cortisol. PS is found in fish, soy and leafy, green vegetables. As we age, PS levels in the body start to decline, so most people need to take a supplement once they're past age 50.

A normal daily diet has about 70 mg of PS. You will need about four times that much if you have memory problems. Nearly anyone can benefit from a 300 mg daily supplement of PS. You're likely to notice improvements in mental alertness after four to eight weeks. A small percentage of people have digestive upset, such as bloating and diarrhea, but you can reduce the dosage if this is a problem. PS is available at health-food stores and pharmacies. Make sure you buy a product that lists "phosphatidylserine" on the label. (Some supplements contain "phosphorylated serine," a nutrient complex that doesn't provide the same benefits as PS.) A high-quality PS supplement is made by Jarrow Formulas (to find a retailer, call 310-204-6936 or go to www.jarrow.com).

Help from ALC

When it is taken as a supplement, a nutrient known as *acetyl-L-carnitine* (ALC) has been shown to improve cognitive function and memory in older adults. Researchers also have found that ALC slows the progression of early-stage Alzheimer's disease. By improving communication between the two main hemispheres of the brain, ALC helps enhance the interplay of creative and cognitive brain activity.

For people with mild memory problems, I recommend taking 500 mg of ALC daily on an empty stomach. For those with more severe problems such as dementia, I suggest the same dose three times daily. Cut back if you have digestive upset. Most health-food stores carry a reliable ALC formula produced by Now Foods (888-669-3663, www.nowfoods.com).

Add antioxidants

With all likelihood, Alzheimer's disease and other types of dementia are related to excessive damage by free radicals (normal by-products of metabolism that can destroy cells, organs and tissues). Free radicals irreversibly injure our cells and contribute to accelerated aging, but studies have shown that this damage can be warded off by getting enough antioxidant nutrients to help guard our brain-cell membranes.

There's ample evidence that a daily dose of 2,000 IU of the powerful antioxidant vitamin E can slow the decline of cognitive function in people who have moderate to severe Alzheimer's disease. There have been controversial vitamin E studies that seemed to show a link to worsening chronic disease. However, I don't have much confidence in those studies because they were performed on unhealthy people. When it comes to Alzheimer's, results of vitamin E studies have been quite good.

All fresh fruits, vegetables and other plant foods provide multiple naturally occurring antioxidants. Juices are an especially concentrated source of antioxidants. In fact, a study of nearly 2,000 Japanese Americans found that those who reported drinking fruit and vegetable juices at least three times a week had a 75 percent lower risk of developing dementia than those who drank juices less than once a week. The most nutritious fruit juices include cranberry, pomegranate, apple and blueberry. I also like mixed vegetable juices containing any combination of spinach, celery, lettuce, parsley, watercress, carrot and tomato.

If there is a strong family history of dementia or you have beginning signs of it, take up to 2,000 IU of vitamin E daily. Green tea also is an excellent source of antioxidants. I recommend drinking two to four cups of green tea daily and eight ounces of fresh juice.

Ginkgo—the brain pleaser

Ginkgo biloba is an herbal remedy that has been shown to improve memory and cognitive processing by promoting blood flow to the brain. I recommend a 24 percent *flavoglycoside* extract. Start with a dose of 120 mg to 240 mg daily, and increase to 360 mg daily over a four-week period. Some people begin to see results in four to eight weeks. If you're already taking a blood-thinning medication such as aspirin or *warfarin*, consult your doctor before taking ginkgo.

Breakthrough Jellyfish Treatment

Scientists have found that a naturally occurring protein in one of the planet's oldest sea creatures—the jellyfish—might hold the key to improved memory and comprehension. The substance, *apoaequorin* (a-poh-ee-kwawr-in), found in the *Aequorea victoria* jellyfish species, has a unique way of working in the brain that is different from other natural memory enhancers. Many of my patients already are benefiting from it. Apoaequorin not only seems to reverse some of the effects of aging on the brain but also might help alleviate the effects of serious neurodegenerative diseases such as Alzheimer's disease, Parkinson's disease and ALS (Lou Gehrig's disease).

The jellyfish connection

Scientists first discovered apoaequorin and its companion molecule, *green fluorescent protein* (GFP), in the Aequorea jellyfish, found off the west coast of North America, in the 1960s. The natural glow of GFP enables researchers to observe microscopic processes within cells that were previously invisible, such as how proteins are transported or how viruses enter cell membranes.

Apoaequorin, which binds to calcium and becomes luminescent once it does, has been used since the 1990s in a similar way to track the activity of calcium in the body's cells. In 2008, three researchers who played key roles in developing these chemical markers were awarded the Nobel Prize in Chemistry.

Apoaequorin's value as a memory-boosting supplement also depends on its properties as a calcium binder but in a different way. In the brain, calcium plays an important role in the chemical process that allows nerve cells to recharge before firing. It has to be present in just the right amounts. If too much calcium builds up inside a nerve cell, it interferes with the nerve-firing process and causes the cell to die. One of the key roles of calcium-binding proteins is to prevent the toxic buildup of calcium by removing excess calcium from the nerve cells. In the normal course of aging, starting at around age 40, the number of calcium-binding proteins in our brain cells starts to decline, resulting in the gradual buildup of toxic calcium inside these cells. This leads to impaired cellular function and eventually brain damage as the toxic calcium kills off brain cells.

The symptoms of this age-related deterioration start slowly but then accelerate as we get older. Because apoaequorin is similar to the naturally occurring calcium-binding proteins in the brain, the theory is that by taking daily supplements, you can replace the calcium-binding proteins that are lost through the aging process—allowing your brain cells to function optimally again while also preserving them from the long-term toxic effects of excess calcium.

A "Eureka" moment

The jellyfish protein went from "scientific" discovery to "supplement for the brain" because of the efforts of Mark Underwood, cofounder of the biotech firm Quincy Bioscience, the company that makes Prevagen (888-565-5385, www.prevagen.com), the only commercially available form of apoaequorin. Underwood's "eureka" moment came when he was reading about an Australian swimmer who developed multiple sclerosis–like symptoms after being stung by a jellyfish. Underwood wondered what protected the jellyfish from its own venom… and whether apoaequorin's calcium-binding abilities could have neuroprotective properties.

His company conducted a number of studies in conjunction with the University of Wisconsin–Milwaukee that found that apoaequorin did seem to have a powerful protective effect on brain cells. In one study, 56 people ranging in age from 20 to 78 showed significant improvements in memory after taking 10 mg of Prevagen daily for 30 days. More than half the group reported gains in general memory and information retention… two-thirds did better at word recall… and 84 percent showed improvement in their ability to remember driving directions.

Most of my patients and others report that taking Prevagen helps them feel mentally sharper, improves their memory and gives them more mental energy. Some even say that their mood is enhanced and that they sleep more soundly.

How to use it

Prevagen is best taken in the morning (because cognitive function is more important during the day than at night), with or without food. I recommend it for anyone over age 40 who wants to improve memory and focus. While 10 mg daily is the recommended starting dose, apoaequorin also is safe at higher doses. I recommend that my own patients who have suffered a noticeable decline in cognitive function start out with 10 mg daily for four weeks. If they don't notice an improvement in memory and focus, they can increase to 20 mg daily.

Most of my patients benefit from taking 10 mg or 20 mg daily. Research has shown that Prevagen is safe to take with other memory-enhancing supplements, such as omega-3 fish oils, or medications, such as *donepezil* (Aricept). People with allergies to fish or shellfish can use it because jellyfish is neither.

All About Underactive Thyroid, Not Dementia

It is my experience that many cases of hypothyroidism are undiagnosed. A common scenario is the patient who has several hypothyroid symptoms but no abnormal blood test results. Their doctor refuses to treat the patient for hypothyroidism without abnormalities in their tests. Many of these patients are what is termed sub-clinical hypothyroidism. That is to say they exhibit symptoms of low thyroid but their blood tests have not revealed a deficiency. Many of these patients' symptoms improve tremendously from thyroid support with natural therapy (including nutritional supplements) or carefully monitored bio-identical thyroid hormone replacement.

Prescription medications for hypothyroidism are very common in the US. According to the American Association of Clinical Endocrinologists studies have shown that as many as 10 percent of women and three percent of men have hypothyroidism (low thyroid activity). The thyroid gland is located at the base of your neck below your Adam's apple. It secretes thyroid hormones that have pronounced effects on the cells of your body.

The two main thyroid hormones include T3 (liothyronine) and T4 (L-thyroxine). Another thyroid hormone known as thyroid stimulating hormone (TSH) regulates the secretion of T3 and T4. This hormone is secreted by the pituitary gland when it senses blood levels of thyroid hormones are getting low. It also receives messages from the brain (hypothalamus) that influences TSH secretion. When the hypothalamus senses blood levels of thyroid hormones it signals the pituitary gland to release more TSH. It is secreted by the pituitary and then signals the thyroid gland to release more of T4 and T3 hormone.

Thyroid hormones control the metabolic activity in every cell. This is important for temperature control, weight regulation, heart rate, and energy production. Thyroid activity even influences one's mood and neurotransmitter balance and affects the balance of other hormones in the body. Hypothyroidism occurs when the thyroid gland is under active. This leads to a shortage of thyroid hormones. The most common cause is a disease known as Hashimoto's thyroiditis. This is an autoimmune condition where the body's immune system produces antibodies to the thyroid gland. This attack on the thyroid gland leads to the suppression of thyroid hormone production and secretion. Other reasons for hypothyroidism may include iodine and other nutritional deficiencies, stress, pregnancy, medications such as lithium or estrogen therapy, and an under functioning pituitary gland.

Hypothyroidism is most common in middle-aged and older women. It can occur at any age though, including infants and teenager. Untreated hypothyroidism can be life threatening.

Symptoms of Hypothyroidism

Common symptoms of hypothyroidism include fatigue, weight gain, dry skin, hair loss, constipation, intolerance to cold, and poor memory. Since thyroid hormones affect all cells of the body there are many other signs and symptoms including:

- Anxiety

- Arthritis

- Brittle nails

- Cold hands and feet

- Eyebrow loss (especially outer 1/3)

- High cholesterol

- Heart palpitations

- Infertility

- Headaches

- Depression

- Low libido

- Low body temperature

- PMS

- Fluid retention

- Raynaud's phenomenon

- Carpal Tunnel Syndrome

- Anemia

- Slow healing

- A puffy face

- Hoarse voice

- Muscle aches, tenderness and stiffness

- Muscle weakness

- Heavier than normal menstrual periods

A blood test is often used to diagnose hypothyroidism. However, this test often does not catch mild to moderate cases of the disorder. If your basal body temperature is consistently low and if you experience the symptoms described above, but a blood test does not reveal hypothyroidism, I would suggest meeting with a holistic doctor for preventative care. It may be more effective to run a saliva or urine thyroid test, in addition to measuring basal body temperature.

Here are some natural remedies for Hypothyroidism:

1. *Bladderwrack* (Fucus vesiculosus). Take 100 mg or one milliliter twice daily.

2. *Thyroid glandular.* Take one tablet/capsule three times daily on an empty stomach or as directed.

3. *Pituitary glandular.* Take one tablet/capsule three times daily on an empty stomach or as directed.

4. *L-tyrosine.* Take 500 mg twice daily on an empty stomach. It is used in the synthesis of the thyroid hormone.

5. *Natural progesterone.* This can be effective for women experiencing low thyroid hormones and progesterone levels.

6. *Guggul* (Commiphora mukul). Take 25 mg of guggulsterones three times daily.

7. *Homeopathic thyroidinum 3X or 6X.* Take three pellets three times daily.

Protect Your Brain with the Two MUST-HAVE Nutrients for Fighting Alzheimer's

Most times when you are treating Alzheimer's, it's the family that sees the improvement—or decline—not the patient. And for one in eight of those families, the drugs promoted by Big Pharma are especially disappointing. The truth is there's little the medical community has to offer to prevent or treat this disease.

But, as I always say, "when in doubt try a natural solution *first*." You don't need to take an ineffective drug with side effects when two natural ingredients that you can find at your local health food store are so great at fighting Alzheimer's. And unlike those drugs they actually *target* the core of this terrible disease.

Oh, and I should also mention that they do it at a fraction of the cost of those over-hyped Alzheimer's meds. I'll tell you more about these natural brain-savers in just a moment, but first let me explain what's happening inside someone's head when they develop Alzheimer's disease.

Alzheimer's is a progressive brain disorder. It begins with memory loss and eventually leads to dementia and death. Once you reach age 85, you have almost a 50 percent chance of having this dreadful disease. It targets the part of the brain known as the hippocampus, the area responsible for memory and intellect. In a person with Alzheimer's, the brain nerve cells essentially die. Protein pieces called beta-amyloid clump together and form plaque. This plaque blocks nerve signals and is thought to cause inflammation. This is where those natural brain-savers that I mentioned earlier come into play. These compounds help to clear away the brain-attacking plaque.

Defend against Alzheimer's with this superstar vitamin

The connection between vitamin D and Alzheimer's risk isn't new. In fact, according to a study published in *Archives of Internal Medicine* in 2010 people with low vitamin D levels are also likely to have cognitive problems.[1] Now exciting new research, published in the *Journal of Alzheimer's Disease*, shows the path that vitamin D and turmeric use to clear beta-amyloid from the brain!

Work done in the researchers' lab showed that vitamin D3 and turmeric extract can help open a specific channel within immune cells. Once the channel is open the beta-amyloid can be swallowed up and removed. Vitamin D is able to open these channels in two types of immune cells and curcuminoids in one type.[2] This is nothing short of amazing and these exciting findings will fuel the next generation of Alzheimer's research.

My experience through testing thousands of patients is that most people require 5,000 IU of extra vitamin D daily. Your doctor can monitor your levels. It's certainly one nutrient you don't want to run low on, especially in light of this new research on Alzheimer's disease.

Protect your brain with this treasure from India

Turmeric is a natural subject for Alzheimer's research. It has compounds in it called curcuminoids that fight inflammation. And, in fact, research on how the spice might be able to protect the brain began over a decade ago.

Alzheimer's is much less common in India. The country has one of the lowest rates of the disease in the world. US researchers felt that something in the diet might be the reason for the lower rates.

The researchers looked at people in a town in India who were over 65 and that had signs of the disease, and compared them to a group in a Pennsylvania town, where most people eat little—or no—turmeric. The results were startling: In India, just 4.7 per 1,000 person-years (a common measure of incidence rate) showed signs of Alzheimer's, compared with a rate of 17.5 per 1,000 person-years in Pennsylvania.[3]

Another study, from the National University of Singapore, involved 1,010 people over age 60. Those who ate curry "often or very often" or even "occasionally" scored higher on mental performance tests than those who rarely or never ate it.[4]

Turmeric is good for your brain and entire body. I encourage my patients, especially those over age 50, to eat one or two teaspoons a day. There are many ways to use this spice in your regular diet. Sprinkle it into egg salad or over vegetables while sautéing... add it to soups or broths... put it on fish or meat... use it to flavor rice or a creamy vegetable dip... or add it to your favorite protein shake. Be sure to look for an organic source such as, one of my favorites, Great Organic Spices (www.greatorganicspices.com).

If you're not a fan of the flavor of turmeric I've got good news. You can get even more bang for your turmeric buck by taking it as a supplement. In my clinic I usually recommend a time-release formula. Take one tablet two times daily for prevention. And if you or a loved one is already taking a prescription drug for Alzheimer's, you'll be happy to know there's no known risk in mixing turmeric with these medications. Of course, if you're on any meds you should always consult with your doctor before adding something new.

Revitalize brain cells with... rosemary?

A study published this year in the journal *Therapeutic Advances in*

Psychopharmacology didn't focus on Alzheimer's, but is still worth mentioning. Researchers found that healthy volunteers performed better on mental math tasks when exposed to one of the main components of rosemary essential oil.[5]

Volunteers were asked to complete math questions while sitting in a cubicle that smelled of rosemary. It turns out that those volunteers who absorbed more of the rosemary into their bloodstreams were able to complete the questions faster and with more accuracy than those who absorbed less.

I will keep my eyes open for any new research on using rosemary to promote brain health. I have a hunch that it will soon join vitamin D and turmeric on my "must have" nutrients for fighting Alzheimer's. You can find rosemary essential oil in health food stores.

Keep your mind super sharp with exercise

My final brain-sharpening tip *is* all natural, but it's not a food or supplement. According to studies keeping your brain active with reading, crossword puzzles, and other mentally stimulating activities also can help keep it firing on all cylinders.

Cognitive stimulation therapy (CST) is one interesting brain exercise that mainstream medicine often overlooks. Despite the scary name, CST is simply good old-fashioned group talk therapy. The sessions usually revolve around a theme like food, current affairs, or childhood. The conversations are designed to challenge the participants and exercise their brains, but be enjoyable too.

One group of people with dementia (not necessarily Alzheimer's) took part in seven weeks of initial CST plus up to six more months of weekly CST sessions saw benefits. The therapy helped improve their cognitive function. And both the patients and their caregivers reported a big jump in their quality of life.[6]

I believe natural medicine will be the key to Alzheimer's prevention and treatment. Start using vitamin D and turmeric in your daily routine. Try scenting your home or workplace with rosemary oil. And be sure to exercise your noggin daily with brain-stimulating activities.

How You Can Boost Your Brainpower and Revitalize Memory with a Powerful Nutrient You've Never Heard Of

Your brain weighs only three pounds but this vital organ is far more complex in design than any supercomputer. Mental activities require a lot of energy—scientists estimate that your brain consumes 20 percent of your body's energy when at rest. Just like you would not expect a computer to run without electricity, your brain needs a constant supply of energy so you can maintain focus and memory. A unique nutrient, you've probably never even heard of, called citicoline has a remarkable ability to provide that energy.

Citicoline is a natural nutrient found in all the cells of the body, but is especially important for brain function. It improves energy production within your brain cells. Just like in other cells of your body, the production of ATP—the energy molecule—is critical to brain function. Natural substances such as citicoline support this vital energy production for maximum brainpower without the unwanted side effects of stimulants such as anxiety, increased blood pressure, and chest pain.

Powerful brain booster

Citicoline has benefits beyond support of energy production in brain cells. First, it protects brain cells, known as neurons, against the destructive effects of free radicals and inflammation. Next, it's broken down by the body into the nutrients choline (a B vitamin) and cytidine (a natural molecule involved in cell division) that make up phospholipids. That's important because your cell membranes are composed of phospholipids that help transport information between neurons. So better phospholipid production means healthier brain cells, and healthier brain cells, of course, means better focus and memory!

You may have heard of the dietary supplement lecithin before. Lecithin is rich in the phospholipid phosphatidylcholine, which has been shown to help memory. Similarly, the phospholipid phosphatidylserine is a popular supplement for improving memory, and studies back up its use. Citicoline helps the body produce phosphatidylserine, supporting repair of the pathways between brain cells.

Citicoline is also important for the production of acetylcholine. This is a key brain chemical (neurotransmitter) involved in memory. Many dementia and Alzheimer's disease drugs are targeted at increasing acetylcholine levels in the brain. Unfortunately they can come with a lot of nasty side effects and their benefits don't last very long, which is not the case with citicoline. Plus citicoline increases blood flow to the brain.[1]

Seeking a source of "brain food"

It's difficult to get enough citicoline through diet alone because food only contains small amounts. Two of the best dietary sources are liver and brains, but I don't recommend eating either of these. Rather, the best way to get more citicoline… and to improve mental function while you're at it… is to take it as a supplement. Studies have shown that citicoline supplements are safe.[2]

Although citicoline has been available as a supplement for several decades its new reputation as a cognitive-function booster has made it

much more popular recently. Several human studies have shown it helps improve learning and memory.

Fight Alzheimer's and improve memory

For example:

- When citicoline was given to groups of elderly people they saw improvements in memory, attention, behavior, reaction time, relational life, independence, and cooperation.[3]

- In a study of older adults with memory deficits but without dementia, citicoline supplements significantly improved immediate and short-term memory. This suggests beneficial effects on the underlying cognitive processes of memory retrieval and storage.[4]

- A review of double-blind, randomized human trials on citicoline and cognitive function found that citicoline modestly improves memory and behavioral outcomes.[1]

- Three months of citicoline supplementation was found to improve verbal memory in a group of healthy older adults who were free of any medical, neurological, or psychiatric illness but who had relatively inefficient memories.[5]

Citicoline has been shown in small human studies to have benefits for those suffering with Alzheimer's disease. In one study of 19 people with Alzheimer's, 1,000 mg of citicoline was taken daily for 30 days. The supplement significantly improved the cognitive function for those with early-onset Alzheimer's and overall there was a trend of improvement in all the participants.[6]

Another study of people between 57 and 87 years old who had been diagnosed with Alzheimer's disease found 1,000 mg daily of citicoline resulted in improved mental function, particularly for those who were suffering with early onset of the disease. This study *also* found improved blood flow in one of the main brain arteries.[7]

Citicoline can be helpful for learning, memory, and early stage Alzheimer's disease. You can find citicoline supplements under the trade name Cognizin from various supplement manufacturers. A typical dose is 500 mg to 1,000 mg daily.

much more popular recently. Several human studies have shown it helps improve learning and memory.

Fight Alzheimer's and improve memory

For example:

- When citicoline was given to groups of elderly people they saw improvements in memory, attention, behavior, reaction time, relational life, independence, and cooperation.[3]

- In a study of older adults with memory deficits but without dementia, citicoline supplements significantly improved immediate and short-term memory. This suggests beneficial effects on the underlying cognitive processes of memory retrieval and storage.[4]

- A review of double-blind, randomized human trials on citicoline and cognitive function found that citicoline modestly improves memory and behavioral outcomes.[1]

- Three months of citicoline supplementation was found to improve verbal memory in a group of healthy older adults who were free of any medical, neurological, or psychiatric illness but who had relatively inefficient memories.[5]

Citicoline has been shown in small human studies to have benefits for those suffering with Alzheimer's disease. In one study of 19 people with Alzheimer's, 1,000 mg of citicoline was taken daily for 30 days. The supplement significantly improved the cognitive function for those with early-onset Alzheimer's and overall there was a trend of improvement in all the participants.[6]

Another study of people between 57 and 87 years old who had been diagnosed with Alzheimer's disease found 1,000 mg daily of citicoline resulted in improved mental function, particularly for those who were suffering with early onset of the disease. This study *also* found improved blood flow in one of the main brain arteries.[7]

Citicoline can be helpful for learning, memory, and early stage Alzheimer's disease. You can find citicoline supplements under the trade name Cognizin from various supplement manufacturers. A typical dose is 500 mg to 1,000 mg daily.

Stop Alzheimer's BEFORE it Starts— With the Breakthrough Brain-Saving "Penny Cure"

I f you've seen it once, you've seen it a hundred times; the mainstream media… once again suckered by Big Pharma's brilliant publicists… transforms into a puppet. It typically, goes something like this, "Exciting new research has found new drug prevents or reverses X disease!"

These breathless announcements are always met with much excitement and fanfare. And trust me, if they *were* true I would be among those cheering the loudest. But when details of the studies finally come out we inevitably find out that this miraculous benefit has only been found in animal studies.

Billions spent on Alzheimer's drug development

Far too many times I've heard similar headlines only to be disappointed—like so many others—when the human studies never pan out. Case-in-point, the drug companies have literally spent billions trying to develop effective treatments for Alzheimer's, but have been met with utter failure.

According to a joint US and European Union task force report released in 2011, "Despite enormous financial and scientific efforts, still no approved disease-modifying therapies exist for Alzheimer's disease (AD). During the last decade all Phase III clinical trials on disease modifiers in AD have failed."[1]

So you will no doubt appreciate the irony when I tell you that naturopathy, the David of medicine, has uncovered an effective natural solution for preventing Alzheimer's disease that Big Pharma Goliath, was unable to find… despite that colossal budget. And unlike its counterpart, the natural solution is non-toxic and costs just pennies a day.

B vitamins reduce brain shrinkage

The study, detailing this unprecedented discovery, was published in the prestigious journal *Proceedings of the National Academy of Sciences.* The two year trial at Oxford University followed 156 people, 70 years and older, who showed signs of cognitive impairment (a precursor to Alzheimer's) and elevated levels of the protein metabolite known as homocysteine.

Patients were given vitamins B6, B12, and folic acid. They had MRI scans of their brains done to check for shrinkage and blood levels of homocysteine both at the beginning of and at the end of the trial.[2]

The study revealed that B vitamins reduce brain shrinkage in the areas of the brain associated with Alzheimer's by up to 90 percent and slashing homocysteine levels. Dr. David Smith, professor emeritus of pharmacology at Oxford, who led the study, was reported to have said: "It's a big effect, much bigger than we would have dreamt of. I find the specificity of this staggering. We never dreamt it would be so specific."[3]

Homocysteine causes blood vessel inflammation

As I've explained before, vitamin B12 deficiency can lead to significant brain shrinkage. The key to this current study however, lies with those elevated homocysteine levels.

Homocysteine is produced when an amino acid called methionine

is broken down in the body. It's normal to have some homocysteine in our blood. However, elevated levels (also called hyperhomocysteinemia) can cause inflammation of the blood vessels and is a risk factor for the buildup of plaque in the arteries resulting in a heart attack or stroke. It's also associated with an increased risk of Alzheimer's. But, it turns out that B12 can naturally lower homocysteine levels.

Simple blood test reveals high homocysteine

Research shows that up to 20 percent of the population has elevated homocysteine levels. Elevated levels are easily detected with a simple blood test. I test my patients' homocysteine levels once a year to make sure they are not elevated. Less common reasons for high levels, like kidney disease or low thyroid function, can be discovered through regular testing as well. A good value is less than 10 micromoles per liter. All the major blood laboratories can test this marker so make sure you get your level tested. Unfortunately, most doctors *don't* routinely screen for it.

If it turns out that you *do* have elevated homocysteine levels the culprit is often a genetic abnormality. The *MTHFR* gene (you will hear a lot about it in the next few years, it's big stuff) produces an enzyme that helps regulate homocysteine levels in the body. Metabolism of the B vitamin folic acid is affected by the gene. If there's a mutation (genetic abnormality) in the MTHFR gene, homocysteine levels can increase.

Up to 50 percent of people have this gene mutation

Everyone has two of these genes… one inherited from each parent. You could have a genetic mutation in one MTHFR gene (heterozygous for the mutation) or both genes (homozygous for the mutation). In the general population, up to 50 percent of people could have one gene mutation, while up to 20 percent have two mutated genes. Obviously, those with two mutations have more of a problem with folic acid metabolism and end up with higher homocysteine levels.

There are two components of MTHFR testing. One is the MTHFR C677T and the other is MTHFR A1298C. The C677T is the gene associated with cardiovascular and dementia problems such as homocysteine metabolism. The A1298C is important in other ways such as predisposition to neurotransmitter imbalance and conditions like depression. Laboratories such as Quest Labs, LabCorp, or Spectracell can perform this genetic testing.

Beef up folic acid levels with leafy greens

If you have the mutation, especially homozygous C677T, then you should concentrate on getting folic acid from uncooked leafy green vegetables or activated folic acid known as methylfolate (L-5 Methyl Tetrahydrofolate). One word of warning, however, the folic acid that is often added to foods, and found in many supplements, is a synthetic version of folate, which is not optimal for human cell function. That's why I prefer the natural, activated form. You also need vitamin B2, B6, and B12 for optimal folic acid metabolism. I typically start with 400 to 800 mcg of activated folic acid (or L-5 Methyl Tetrahydrofolate) and 1,000 to 2,500 mcg of methylcobalamin.

If you're serious about reducing your Alzheimer's risk be sure to speak with your doctor about getting your homocysteine levels checked and MTHFR genetic testing. Knowledge is power!

PART VIII

Allergies, Digestion and Nutrition

Breakthrough Treatment for Sinus and Lung Problems

I have developed a special treatment for patients with sinus and/or lung problems, including acute sinusitis… asthma flare-ups… and chronic obstructive pulmonary disease (COPD), a condition in which patients have trouble breathing. This incredibly effective treatment involves three natural substances in liquid form administered through a nebulizer, a small machine that transforms liquid medications into mists that can be inhaled through a mouthpiece or mask. *The treatment includes the following…*

• **Glutathione**. This potent antioxidant appears to reduce inflammation of the lungs.

• **N-acetylcysteine (NAC)**. This antioxidant thins mucus and stimulates the immune system. It has long been used to treat chronic bronchitis and emphysema. Many doctors know it best as *acetylcysteine* (Mucomyst).

• **Glycyrrhizin**. This is the sweet-tasting compound extract from licorice root. It has anti-inflammatory effects on the respiratory tract.

I first provide patients with this 15-minute treatment in the office to make sure that they can tolerate it, although I've never known anyone to have an allergic or negative reaction to it. If a patient requires further treatments, we send him/her home with vials of the solution and a nebulizer. With reduced dosage, this nebulization therapy also is gentle enough to use with children.

If you are interested in this treatment, your doctor can order these nutrients from a compounding pharmacy. (Because it's prepared in a sterile liquefied solution and tested for microbes, you cannot assemble this treatment on your own.) The solution consists of glutathione (100 mg), N-acetylcysteine (100 mg) and glycyrrhizin (four milligrams). One nebulized treatment consists of two milliliters of the nutrient solution combined with two milliliters of distilled water. This nutrient solution can be ordered by your doctor from ApothéCure, Inc. Nebulizers can be purchased online or at drugstores for about $40 to $60.

Shocking News About Allergies and Asthma

Millions of people are walking around suffering from respiratory allergies… asthma… recurring colds… and bronchitis—and they don't have to be.

Let me give you an example: Pam, a woman in her 40s, had three colds in a row that turned into bronchitis. Another doctor had given her an asthma diagnosis. When she came to see me, she told me that she had been struggling with allergies and persistent fatigue for most of her adult life. I see so many patients with this combination of symptoms that I immediately suspected that she had an altogether different problem. It is called adrenal fatigue (AF), a collection of symptoms that occur when the adrenal glands, which produce stress and inflammation-fighting hormones, no longer function properly.

You might wonder what AF has to do with these other conditions.

My answer: Everything. What's really going on is that AF is masquerading as allergies or asthma. Once AF is properly diagnosed and treated, these other conditions quickly clear up. I prescribed a treatment plan for Pam designed to get her adrenal glands functioning normally again. After just two months on the program, her respiratory problems disappeared and her energy level was higher than it had been in years.

What you need to know: AF is most often associated with a wide range of symptoms, including lack of energy, insomnia, blood sugar swings, cognitive impairment and depressed mood. But AF also can have a significant impact on your immune system. In addition, it often is not recognized by conventional physicians because it doesn't show up on regular lab tests. As surprising as it may sound, if you suffer from a respiratory allergy to dust, pollen, ragweed, pet dander or other environmental allergen—or if you have asthma that recurs despite treatment— there's a chance that your real problem is improperly functioning adrenal glands. (I have even found that AF is associated with asthma in some children, although it is more common in adults with asthma.)

AF can be the root of other problems

The adrenal glands are responsible for producing the hormone cortisol (released into the bloodstream in response to stress) and *dehydroepiandrosterone* or DHEA (a precursor to hormones such as estrogen and testosterone). AF usually occurs when patients undergo extended periods of stress, which cause levels of DHEA and cortisol to become elevated for long periods of time, usually four months or longer (although this varies by patient). The surplus production of DHEA and cortisol overtaxes the adrenals, resulting in a sharp drop in DHEA and cortisol levels.

What AF does to the immune system: Both cortisol and DHEA modulate the immune system's inflammatory response. When the glands no longer produce sufficient amounts of these hormones, the immune system becomes overactive, producing inflammatory responses even when there's no real threat or infection looming.

Result: Allergic responses… respiratory infections… and asthma. Most conventional medical doctors treat these conditions by prescribing antihistamines for allergy symptoms and corticosteroids to ward off asthma. In other words, they treat the symptoms, not the disease.

Diagnosis and testing

If you suspect that you have AF, it's best to see a naturopathic physician and have your adrenal function tested. My preference is a saliva test, which is more accurate than a blood or urine test. Your physician will retest you three or four months after treatment begins to see if your levels have improved.

How to heal the adrenals

My treatment protocol for AF involves supplements to boost adrenal function and/or increase resistance to stress. Patients follow the protocol for four to six months, which is the time it usually takes to get the adrenals working properly again. Most patients begin to feel better within the first month or two. When patients are doing well, I help wean them off their allergy or asthma medications during this time. People with very severe cases usually stay on my regimen for eight to 10 months. After treatment, patients either take lower doses or stop taking these supplements altogether, depending on their overall health. The supplements that I recommend below include herbs (which are most important in helping this condition) and B vitamins. There are no side effects except as noted.

• **Ashwagandha**. This herb, used in Ayurvedic medicine to treat inflammation, is a potent adaptogen, an herb that helps to bring physiological processes into balance and enhances the body's ability to handle stress. It has a strong effect on the adrenal glands and normalizes production of cortisol.

Dose: 250 mg daily of ashwagandha standardized to contain eight percent of the active ingredient *anolide*.

• **Rhodiola**. Another adaptogen, rhodiola is an herb that has been used for centuries in Eastern Europe and Asia as an energy and mood enhancer. It boosts adrenal function, and studies show that it also improves the body's resistance to stress.

Dose: 300 mg daily of rhodiola standardized to contain three percent of the active ingredient rosavin.

• **Siberian ginseng** (*Eleutherococcus*). Another adaptogen, this herbal extract has been used for centuries in Russia and Asia to boost energy and fight stress.

Dose: 150 mg to 200 mg daily of Siberian ginseng extract standardized to contain 0.8 percent *eleutheroside.*

Side effects: Can cause insomnia if taken before bedtime and can affect some diabetes drugs. Should not be used during pregnancy.

• **Vitamin B-5 (pantothenic acid).** Vitamin B-5 helps adrenal function and is used by the body to manufacture cortisol.

Dose: 250 mg to 500 mg of vitamin B-5 daily.

• **Vitamin B-12.** This vitamin helps boost resistance to the effects of stress.

Dose: 50 mcg to 100 mcg of vitamin B-12 daily.

Finally, I advise my patients to take steps to reduce stress in their daily lives.

Recommendations: Get enough sleep (seven to eight hours a night)... take a 30-minute midday nap, if possible... eliminate all refined sugars from your diet... take regular vacations... and minimize daily stress by exercising or participating in relaxing activities, such as listening to calming music.

My "Identify and Conquer" Plan for Beating Asthma and Breathing Better

I hadn't seen Joyce, a 55-year-old patient of mine for nine months. When I last saw her, she was managing her asthma symptoms very well. But this visit, as we talked in the office, she was interrupted by coughing fits, one of the signs of asthma. She admitted that she had been eating wheat, one of her asthma triggers that we had confirmed with testing. Also, she had stopped taking several of the nutritional supplements that had worked well to help her control her asthma.

When I listened to her lungs and heard pronounced wheezing. I suggested we see how she would respond to a nutritional IV. For the next hour Joyce received an intravenous infusion of vitamin C, B vitamins, glutathione, and magnesium. When I checked on her near the end of her treatment she was smiling. Her breathing was back to normal and the coughing had stopped. When I listened to her lungs again the wheezing was barely noticeable any more. Such is the power of nutrition-based therapies.

Here are some sobering asthma statistics. The number of people with asthma continues to grow every year. Approximately one in 12 people in the US have the condition and an estimated 300 million people worldwide suffer from the airway narrowing disorder with 250,000 annual deaths attributed to this respiratory disease. On average, US costs associated with asthma run about $3,300 per year in medical costs, missed school and work days, and early deaths.[1]

Common types of asthma drugs[2,3]

Short-Acting Beta-Agonists (SABAs): Relax airway muscles to give prompt relief of symptoms. Examples include: Albuterol (Pro-Air HFA, Ventolin HFA, others), levalbuterol (Xopenex HFA), and pirbuterol (Maxair Autohaler)

Inhaled Corticosteroids: Used for long-term control. Examples include: Fluticasone (Flovent Diskus, Flovent HFA), budesonide (Pulmicort Flexhaler), mometasone (Asmanex), ciclesonide (Alvesco), flunisolide (Aerobid), beclomethasone (Qvar)

Long-Acting Beta-Agonists (LABAs): They are used in combination with inhaled corticosteroids for long-term control. Examples include: Fluticasone and salmeterol (Advair Diskus, Advair HFA), budesonide and formoterol (Symbicort), and mometasone and formoterol (Dulera).

Cromolyn and Theophylline: Alternative medications used to prevent and control asthma.

Leukotriene Modifiers: Alternative control medications. Examples include: Montelukast (Singulair), zafirlukast (Accolate) and zileuton (Zyflo, Zyflo CR)

Oral Corticosteroids: Steroid medications taken internally for a short term. Examples include: Prednisone and methylprednisolone.

Immunomodulators: Medication that modifies the allergic immune response. Omalizumab (Xolair) is an example.

Reduce the need for drugs

There are a number of medications used to treat asthma. Most are inhaled drugs that relax the airway, which becomes inflamed and constricted with a flare-up of asthma. (See the sidebar on page 424 for details on the most commonly prescribed asthma medications.) There are two basic approaches. One approach is controller medications that are inhaled daily to keep the bronchial tubes relaxed and open. The second approach is quick relief or rescue. These drugs are used to quickly relax and open the airways and relieve symptoms *during* an asthma attack. They may also be taken before exercise. Potential side effects of some asthma drugs include osteoporosis, anxiety, and sore throat as a result of fungal overgrowth.

The truth is these medications work extremely well for relieving acute respiratory distress. If a patient is having an acute asthma flare-up I tell him it's fine to use a prescribed inhaler medication (since most are not at my clinic when the flare up occurs). However, NONE of these medications work at the root cause of the asthma. Holistic medicine is superior in its ability to treat the underlying triggers of asthma. The goal is to remove the triggers and balance the body so that the inflammatory reaction is prevented in the first place and medication is rarely required.

To gain control start with the cause

It is important to know what the cause or trigger(s) of your asthma are. For many children and adults it involves allergies. Common environmental allergies include pet dander, dust mites, pollen, and mold. Other environmental triggers include smoke, pollution, and exposure to cold air or changes in weather.[4]

Obviously you need to avoid triggers you have control over such as pet dander, smoke, and indoor mold. A high-energy particulate filter (HEPA) in the home, especially the bedroom, is very helpful to reduce pollen exposure. Remember to keep windows shut at night. At my clinic we use a computerized test for identifying patients' environmental (and food) sensitivities. We then use desensitization drops over several months to reduce the body's immune reaction to the offending substance. This helps keep their allergies and asthma better controlled.

Research has shown that asthma affects many more city dwellers than residents in non-urban areas. Urban air has higher levels of pollution from vehicle exhaust, industry, and sewage treatment plants. For example, studies out of the Columbia University Center for Children's Environmental Health show that black carbon from street traffic comes indoors. In fact, machines that measure pollution placed in homes showed nearly the same amount of black carbon *inside* homes as is found outside.

Indoor pollutants are a problem for many asthma sufferers. If you live in an apartment building you're likely more exposed to secondhand smoke and heating fuels. Researchers have found indoor pollutants known as PAHs (polycyclic aromatic hydrocarbons) increase the risk of asthma as well as cancer. PAHs get into the air when fuel is burned. Examples include heating fuels, cooking blackened foods, and burning candles and incense. Besides using a HEPA filter in the home, make sure to not burn, char, or blacken food. Also, use a kitchen fan while cooking and limit the use of candles and incense.

The asthma triggers you won't hear about in your doctor's office

There are many asthma triggers that go beyond the typical allergies and weather changes But these root causes aren't ones that you are likely to hear about from your conventional doctor. And, of course, without addressing the root causes of your asthma you're simply putting out fires, but not keeping them from flaring up in the first place.

Start with the stomach: Digestive problems can be an often-overlooked underlying cause of asthma. A hiatal hernia where the stomach comes up through the diaphragm opening is a trigger for some. The inability to break food down and absorb it properly can be an issue, as can acid reflux.

Focus on the food: Unlike allergies, food sensitivities are an often overlooked asthma trigger. Although food sensitivities don't cause an immune response in the body like allergies do, they can wreak havoc with your health and can be the culprit behind asthma symptoms. The most common food sensitivities for asthma are wheat and dairy products. Avoid these foods for six to eight weeks and you will likely notice improvement.

Blame the belly: Surprisingly, the obesity epidemic has had an impact on asthma as well. Insulin resistance—the elevation of the hormone insulin in response to high blood sugar levels—creates inflammation. And that inflammation includes the respiratory tract. For some patients, especially the obese, losing weight can make a dramatic difference in asthma control.

The hormone heavy: Hormonal issues such as low thyroid have been shown to be an asthma trigger as can the drop of hormone levels that are seen with menopause. I also find adrenal fatigue—low levels of stress hormones—predispose a person to asthma because these hormones help reduce inflammation.

A fungus among us: Another one you won't hear much about is fungal overgrowth in the body. The use of antibiotics and a high-sugar diet leads to the overgrowth of this microbe that can also thrive in the respiratory tract. I have seen many asthma patients respond well to anti-fungal treatments.

Spotlight on the spine: There can be a structural aspect to asthma. The structure of the spine—especially from the neck to the midback is—critical to proper nerve signaling to the respiratory tract. A good chiropractor or osteopath can help assess and treat imbalances that can result in asthma improvement.

The emotional element: Emotional distress is a common trigger. For example, divorce can lead to an increase in asthma attacks for both adults and children. Homeopathic remedies and counseling can help resolve these triggers.

Super supplements for asthma

If you're currently using asthma medications you should know that there are nutritional therapies that may be able to help you reduce your dependence on those drugs. These supplements can be used to reduce your symptoms and susceptibility to asthma. If you decide to give any of them a try be sure to let your doctor know.

Pine bark extract, also known as pycnogenol, has helped many of my asthmatic patients over the years. It has powerful anti-inflammatory effects and I have yet to see any side effects from it.

It has been proven in studies to be effective. For example, a randomized, placebo controlled, double blind study (in other words a high quality study) involving 60 people ages 6 to 18 years over three months. Researchers found that those who took the supplement had significantly improved lung function and asthma symptoms as well as decreased need for rescue medications compared to those who took a placebo.[5] The standard dose for children and adults is one milligram per pound of body weight daily.

Magnesium relaxes the bronchial muscles of the respiratory tract. Studies show that children with higher blood levels of magnesium have a lower risk of asthma.[6]

Some holistic doctors, like myself, (and the occasional emergency room physician) will use it for acute asthma. Studies confirm intravenous magnesium to be effective, including a recent one that found "intravenous infusion of magnesium sulfate during the first hour of hospitalization in patients with acute severe asthma significantly reduced the percentage of children who required mechanical ventilation support."[7,8,9] Unfortunately, few medical institutions use this valuable mineral to help people with acute asthma. Most people with acute asthma will not have access to intravenous magnesium. However, you can find a nutrition-oriented physician who uses intravenous nutrients as part of a preventative program.

I find an intravenous formulation combining magnesium, vitamin C, glutathione, and all the B vitamins to be effective in helping people with chronic asthma improve their lung function. One to two treatments a week for five weeks can work wonders along with a maintenance treatment as needed.

I recommend that both children and adults supplement magnesium. For children a typical dose is 250 to 500 mg daily and for adults 500 to 1,000 mg daily. Reduce the dosage if you get loose stool. Magnesium glycinate is one form that is less likely to cause loose stool. If you have chronic kidney disease consult with your physician before using magnesium.

Vitamin D plays a powerful role in two ways to prevent asthma. First it optimizes your immune function, which reduces your likelihood of a respiratory tract infection. And since both colds and the flu are common triggers for asthma vitamin D can be the difference between having an asthma attack and breathing easy. Second, vitamin D reduces inflammation and allergy response. This is critical for preventing asthma.

Several studies have linked low vitamin D levels and asthma symptoms in children.[10,11,12] There have also been studies done with adults that show an association between decreased blood vitamin D levels and decreased lung function and response to asthma medications.[13,14,15]

Vitamin D deficiency or low levels of vitamin D are very common here in the US. People have been scared into avoiding the sun for fear of skin damage. They smear on UV blocking sunscreens and stay indoors. But in order for your body to make vitamin D your skin must get some UV exposure. And if you're a darker complexion the pigment in your skin makes you naturally more prone to deficiency, which can make the problem even worse. Obesity, another common and growing problem, has also been linked with low vitamin D levels.

Have your vitamin D blood levels tested. I like to see a value between 50 to 80 ng/mL. My average patient requires 5,000 IU of vitamin D3 daily. (There is no reason to fear vitamin D3, concerns about this nutrient stem from a flawed study conducted over 40 years ago.)

Astragalus is a popular Chinese herb readily available in North American health food stores. It has historically been used for the prevention and treatment of allergies, respiratory tract infections, and asthma. I often recommend it to my asthma patients during the winter months to reduce their risk of respiratory tract infections such as the common cold, flu, and bronchitis—all common triggers of asthma.

Astragalus works by stimulating the production of an antiviral chemical in the body known as interferon, which prevents viruses from replicating. Studies confirm that it reduces the risk of respiratory tract infections.[16] A typical dose for children is 10 drops of the liquid form for adults 20 to 30 drops or 500 mg of the capsule two to three times daily.

Lycopene is a supplement that anyone who has exercise-induced asthma needs to know about. This antioxidant nutrient is found in foods like tomatoes and watermelon. To reduce your asthma symptoms caused by exercise you will need the supplement form. A double blind trial found that more than half of people with exercise-induced asthma had significantly fewer asthma symptoms after taking 30 mg of lycopene per day (Lyc-O-Mato brand).[17]

Say Good-Bye to Hay Fever

O h, the sneezing! Close to 35 million Americans suffer from upper respiratory tract symptoms due to airborne allergies. One of the most common is hay fever, which results from a reaction to pollen.

Pollen enters the nasal cavity and triggers a cascade of reactions that lead to the release of *histamine* and other inflammatory chemicals. This can cause sneezing, coughing and postnasal drip, a runny or congested nose and itchy, watery, red eyes with dark circles underneath. Hay fever can keep you awake at night, making you feel fatigued and generally terrible all day long.

The most widespread pollen allergen is *ragweed*. One plant can generate a million grains of pollen a day. Other offenders include sagebrush, *redroot pigweed, lamb's quarter, Russian thistle* (tumbleweed) and *English plantain*.

Even if none of the plants that cause hay fever are found in your area, you are still susceptible to exposure because the small, light, dry pollen grains are easily transported by wind. Scientists have found ragweed pollen two miles high in the air and up to 400 miles away from its original source.

Prevention strategies

Pollen season occurs during the spring, summer and fall, when pollen is released by trees, grasses and weeds. Pollen amounts tend to be highest in the morning, especially on warm, dry, breezy days, and lowest during cool, rainy periods. The pollen concentration is available for most urban areas—check your newspaper. Another resource for pollen counts is the American Academy of Allergy, Asthma & Immunology's National Allergy Bureau at www.aaaai.org/nab. You can monitor pollen levels and plan accordingly. For example, allergy sufferers should try to stay indoors with the windows closed when pollen levels are high.

You can wear a dust and pollen mask designed to stop pollen from entering the nasal passageways (available at most pharmacies). You can use a *high-efficiency particulate air (HEPA) purifier* in your house, especially in your bedroom since pollen counts increase during the night.

Drug therapies

Several pharmaceutical medications can be used to treat hay fever, all of which can have side effects.

We all know about antihistamines, which are used to control excess mucus and reduce itching and sneezing. Examples include the prescription drugs *fexofenadine* (Allegra) and *desloratadine* (Clarinex) and the over-the-counter (OTC) medications *cetirizine* (Zyrtec), *loratadine* (Claritin) and *diphenhydramine* (Benadryl). *Cromolyn sodium* (Nasalcrom) is an OTC nasal spray antihistamine.

Potential side effects of oral medications can include drowsiness and impaired coordination. The nasal spray can cause cough, nasal congestion or irritation, nausea, sneezing, throat irritation and wheezing.

Decongestants are used for nasal congestion. A common OTC oral form is *pseudoephedrine* (Sudafed). *Phenylephrine* (Neo-Synephrine, Sinex) is a widely used nasal spray. Decongestants may raise blood pressure, cause insomnia and irritability and inhibit urinary flow. They should be avoided by people with high blood pressure and/or glaucoma (they can increase the eye's intraocular pressure). Decongestants should be taken for only a few days—long-term use causes increased blood vessel constriction, which worsens blood pressure.

Corticosteroid treatments contain small doses of steroids to reduce nasal inflammation and swelling. They prevent and treat most allergy symptoms. Common examples of prescription nasal corticosteroids include *fluticasone* (Flonase), *mometasone* (Nasonex) and *triamcinolone* (Nasacort). These nasal corticosteroid sprays can cause fungal infection of the sinuses and mouth.

Sometimes oral steroids are used for severe allergies. These are very powerful prescription medicines that should be used for only a short time (up to a few weeks). Short-term side effects may include weight gain, water retention, high blood pressure, mood swings and depression. Long-term side effects include increased risk for diabetes, cataracts, osteoporosis and muscle weakness.

I know firsthand the miseries of hay fever. *Fortunately, the natural approaches I describe below have worked extremely well for me and for my patients...*

Nasal rinse

An effective technique for people prone to hay fever and/or sinusitis is nasal irrigation. This involves rinsing the nasal passages with a warm saline solution to reduce the concentration of pollen, dust and other allergens. It also helps to clear excess mucus from the nasal passageways. This is typically done with a *neti pot*, a small ceramic container with a narrow spout that allows you to pour water into your nostrils and sinus cavities. Neti pots are available at health-food stores for about $20.

To use a neti pot, mix one-quarter teaspoon of salt in a cup of warm water. Pour the solution into the neti pot. Tilt your head to the side, and insert the spout into the upper nostril. The solution will flow into the upper nostril and out the lower nostril. After a few seconds, remove the pot. With your head still tilted, blow through both nostrils. Do not cover one side of your nose—this will force the mucus and bacteria up into your sinuses. Repeat the rinse on the other side. It's messy, but it works. Use once daily for low-grade allergies and twice daily for acute allergies.

An easier alternative is Sinus Rinse. You open a packet of premeasured saline and baking soda, pour it into the bottle that comes with the kit and add warm water. Push the tip of the bottle into one nostril, and squeeze the bottle so the solution comes out the other nostril. Repeat with the other nostril. Do this once or twice daily. Sinus Rinse kits are available at www.natlallergy.com or by calling 800-522-1448.

Important: To avoid introducing bacteria into your nasal passageways, clean the tip of the neti pot (or Sinus Rinse bottle) with alcohol between uses.

Homeopathic help

Homeopathy treats hay fever by desensitizing the immune system to the offending pollen(s)—or the symptoms they trigger. This is based on the principle that "like cures like"—that is, substances that cause allergy symptoms can be used in a highly diluted form to alleviate those same symptoms.

For example, ragweed, oak and grasses can be taken as individual remedies or as part of a combination remedy. If you know that you are allergic to ragweed pollen, you can take homeopathic ragweed to minimize your response. An allergist can do skin testing to determine which allergens affect you.

Homeopathic remedies are somewhat similar to conventional allergy shots, in which minute doses of the substances you're allergic to are injected under the skin. The advantage of the homeopathic approach is that it is convenient (it requires dissolving some pellets or a liquid solution under your tongue) and relatively inexpensive ($10 to $20 a month).

Researchers working at the Southwest College of Naturopathic Medicine and Health Sciences in Tempe, Arizona, conducted a four-week, double- blind clinical trial comparing homeopathic preparations with a placebo during the regional allergy season from February to May. Participants included 40 men and women, ages 26 to 63, diagnosed with moderate to severe seasonal allergy symptoms. Those taking the homeopathic preparations had a 38 percent reduction in symptoms, such as watery eyes and sneezing, compared with a 26 percent decline for those using the placebo.

There are two homeopathic remedies that I recommend for the treatment of hay fever. Which one you take depends on your symptoms. They are available at most health-food stores. The dosage is two pellets of a 30C potency twice daily.

• **Allium cepa** (from onion) is for those with watery and burning eyes… runny nose… headache … sneezing.

• **Euphrasia** (from the eyebright plant) is for hay fever that mainly affects only the eyes, causing burning, tearing and redness.

If you don't know which homeopathic remedy to use, try Sabadil Allergy by Boiron, available at health-food stores for about eight dollars. This formula contains six remedies commonly used for hay fever. The typical dose is two tablets dissolved in the mouth every 15 minutes for one hour, then two pellets three times daily.

Choosing supplements

The right supplements also help control hay fever. *My recommendations…*

• **Quercetin**, a type of plant pigment known as a *flavonoid*, is a natural antihistamine, with anti-inflammatory and antioxidant characteristics. It is found in onions, apples and green tea. It works best at a starting dosage of 1,000 mg three times daily for five days, followed by a maintenance dosage of 500 mg two or three times daily. Quercetin is very safe, and side effects are uncommon. Quercetin also works well when combined with vitamin C, which may help reduce allergy symptoms in some individuals. A typical dose for hay fever is 3,000 mg to 5,000 mg of vitamin C daily. Reduce the dosage if you develop loose stools. If you have a history of kidney stones, consult your doctor before taking vitamin C supplements.

• **Stinging nettle leaf** is a popular herbal treatment for the relief of hay fever. I have seen it help some patients when used at the first sign of hay fever symptoms. A randomized, double-blind study conducted at the National College of Naturopathic Medicine in Portland, Oregon, involved 69 people with hay fever who took 300 mg of a stinging nettle leaf supplement or a placebo daily. Researchers found that after one week, 58 percent of those who took stinging nettle leaf had a reduction in symptoms, such as sneezing and itchy eyes, compared with 37 percent of those who received a placebo.

Interestingly, nettle leaves are a natural source of vitamin C and quercetin. Stinging nettle leaf supplements should be avoided by those with kidney disease because they have a diuretic (water- excreting) effect. The type of stinging nettle leaf used in the study mentioned above is available from Eclectic Institute and can be found at health-food stores.

• **N-acetylcysteine (NAC)** is a great supplement to use if you are suffering from postnasal drip or coughing as the result of mucous formation. I find that 500 mg twice daily is helpful for patients. Side effects, such as nausea, constipation and diarrhea, are rare.

Getting started

When using homeopathic remedies and supplements, it's best to start two weeks before allergy season and then continue until the end of the season if the treatment is helping. Try quercetin first. If you do not get relief within one week, try stinging nettle leaf, NAC and/or a homeopathic treatment.

A book that I especially like is *Sinus Survival: A Self-Help Guide*, by Robert Ivker, DO (Tarcher).

Answer from the Natural Physician— Bitter Herbs for Your Stomach

My chiropractor told me I have low stomach acid and therefore cannot digest protein well. Is there anything I can take besides hydrochloric acid supplements to increase my stomach acid?

Yes, bitter herbs such as gentian (pronounced *gen-shun*) root work well to increase stomach acid. In Europe, gentian root is often used to help digest large or fatty meals, and to "increase the digestive powers" of the elderly or those with chronic disease. Gentian root contains a class of bitter compounds, one of which is called amarogentin. Bitter-tasting herbs such as gentian have a very interesting mechanism of action. Historically, bitters have always been taken in the form of liquid, so that one would taste the bitterness. This makes sense because the tongue contains bitter receptors (as with all the different tastes). Gentian happens to be one of the most bitter substances known. According to Rudolf Weiss, MD, "the bitter taste (of gentian) persists even in a dilution of 1:20,000. It is the most important of all European bitters…" It is believed that when bitter receptors are stimulated, a reflex occurs where the vagus nerve becomes stimulated. *This nerve is known to stimulate the digestive organs including…*

- **Stomach** (hydrochloric acid and pepsin)

- **Pancreas** (digestive enzymes for protein, carbohydrates, and fats)

• **Liver and gallbladder** (digest fats)

Studies have also found that gentian stimulates stomach function without being tasted. This is an important issue for those who take gentian root by capsule. I have used gentian root in capsule form with good results as it is a good tonic for the digestive system. One study involving 205 people found that gentian-root capsules gave quick and dramatic relief of constipation, flatulence, appetite loss, vomiting, heartburn, abdominal pain, and nausea.

The dosage for gentian is 10 to 20 drops in a small amount of water (two ounces) or 300 to 600 mg of the capsule form five to 15 minutes before meals (allows the digestive juices to kick in before you eat). I have found that gentian is still helpful to stimulate the digestive system when taken with or shortly after meals. Gentian should be avoided for those who have active ulcers and for pregnant or breastfeeding women.

The Stomach-Turning Trouble That Could Be Lurking in Your Next Meal

Millions of Americans will be eating out at restaurants or at loved one's homes this holiday season. But be careful, you may be gobbling down more than just turkey dinner!

More on that dinner-time disaster later, but first let's talk tummy troubles.

Sam, a pleasant forty-five year old attorney sought my help for a decade old struggle with irritable bowel syndrome (IBS). His problem was bloating, gas, and an uneasy sensation in his abdomen. These symptoms were a source of stress for him in an already stressful environment—the courtroom.

I explained to Sam that IBS is a very common condition. It affects approximately 30 percent of the US adult population.[1] Common symptoms include abdominal cramping, gas, bloating, loose stool or constipation (or an alternation of both), and sometimes mucus in the stool. Now according to conventional wisdom IBS can't be cured, but symptoms can be reduced.[2] My experience is that symptoms can be relieved *and* the condition can be cured when the root causes are treated.

Pinpointing a cause

There are many different causes of IBS. For example, food intolerances can cause havoc in the digestive tract. One of the most common is the milk sugar, known as lactose. By age twenty about 30 million American adults have some degree of lactose intolerance. Another common... and growing... intolerance I see with patients is gluten, especially wheat. I believe the genetic modification of wheat has changed its molecular structure so much that for many it's now recognized as a foreign invader in the digestive tract. Milk and wheat ate just two of countless foods that can cause IBS symptoms. Your local holistic doctor can give you tests to pinpoint your own trigger foods.

Not getting enough fiber in your diet can also cause uncomfortable IBS symptoms to kick in. But with fiber it always takes a little bit of trial and error to get the balance right. Some patients with IBS respond well to increased fiber in their diet while others need to increase the amount

---

The shocking connection between parasites and suicide

A recent study published in the journal *Archives of General Psychiatry* reported that women infected with the parasite Toxoplasma gondii (T.gondii) were more likely to attempt suicide than women who were not infected. More specifically, they found infected women were 81 percent more likely to have a violent suicide attempt than non-infected women.[3]

T. gondii infection is most commonly caused by eating undercooked meat. It's also transmitted from handling infected cat feces, consuming unwashed produce, and handling contaminated soil.

A previous study suggested that T. gondii increases the risk for schizophrenia.[4] It's thought that this parasite increases inflammation of the brain which disrupts brain chemistry. And it is estimated that 10 to 20 percent of the American population unknowingly are carrying this parasite.

slowly or else their symptoms worsen.

Vegetables, fruits, nuts, and seeds are all good sources of fiber. But be careful when it comes to nuts, especially peanuts since they're highly allergenic. Good supplemental sources of fiber include chia seeds, Psyllium, and ground flaxseeds. Make sure to ingest a good amount of water… around eight to 10 oz per serving of fiber… so you don't plug up your bowels!

Avoid getting sick from the stress

As is the case with most conditions, stress can be a big factor when it comes to how well your gut is doing its job. Stress can have a negative effect on your digestion. So it's important to tune into the factors in your life that are causing you stress and to look for ways to reduce those sources of strain.

But, let's face facts. No one's life is 100 percent stress free. So it's *also* important to have outlets that can help you reduce your stress level like exercise or other activities. The activities you choose to get involved in for stress relief aren't nearly as important as how they make you feel. Just make sure yours don't involve overeating or other unhealthy activities.

Shine a light on overlooked infections

An undiagnosed intestinal infection can lead to IBS. In fact, it's quite common. Take candida albicans for example. This yeast lives in the digestive tract of virtually every human being walking this earth. Normally candida doesn't cause problems, but if you introduce an antibiotic the tables can suddenly turn. The problem, of course, is that the antibiotic doesn't just destroy the bad bugs it destroys the good ones too. And once your gut flora is out of balance the candida can overgrow and become infectious. A high sugar diet or chlorine laden water supply also contributes to candida overgrowth.

The same type of overgrowth can happen with other bacteria in your small intestine as well. But no matter the bug, bacteria, or yeast that triggers it the results are the same... the classic IBS symptoms of gas, abdominal pain, and distention.

Your doctor can easily diagnose this problem with a procedure known as the Hydrogen Breath Test. You will be given a sugar... either lactulose or glucose... to eat. Then a number of breath samples are stored in a special bag and sent off to the lab for analysis. If it turns out that you have a hidden candida or bacterial infection then herbal antibacterial

---

Common IBS symptoms to look out for[5]

- Constipation

- Diarrhea

- Mucus in stools

- Flatulence and abdominal rumblings

- Nausea

- Headache

- Abdominal pain and cramping, usually either relieved by going to the bathroom or brought on by it

- Intolerance to certain foods

- Gurgling and rumbling of the abdomen

- Burping

- Heartburn

- Alternating constipation and diarrhea

- Occasional vomiting

- Painful sexual intercourse (dyspareunia)

- Fatigue

- Feeling full easily

- Depression

- Anxiety

- Frequent urination

- Painful periods

- Irritation of the rectum

- Insomnia

- Mental "fog"

- Unpleasant taste in mouth

agents and probiotics can be used to reduce the level of the bacteria in your small intestine.

Look what came with dinner

Now let's get back to that unwelcome dinnertime surprise I hinted at earlier. I admit it's not a popular topic… but it's an important one. I'm talking about parasites that can infect you in a number of ways, including hitching a ride inside on your fork.

Not surprisingly parasites are the number one thing that's guaranteed to gross my patients out when I review their stool test results. Until that point most people think of parasites as a third world problem, and it certainly is with hundreds of millions of people harboring parasitic infections, especially poorer nations because of poor sanitation. However, the uncomfortable truth is that in America they're a lot more common than you would expect. In fact, they affect millions here every year.

Most people who have parasites are unaware of their infection. They, and their doctors, assume that since they don't have extreme digestive symptoms such as gushing diarrhea, blood in their stool, fever, or weight loss that it's not a possibility. They're wrong. And, unfortunately, relying on traditional lab tests alone can be tricky because unless it's a severe infection the traditional test can miss detecting the parasites. You see the bugs often attach to the wall of the digestive tract and this means that they may not always be present in the stool.

I have had good results using a newer technology which utilizes DNA analysis to identify a variety of parasites. It's a much more sensitive test than what laboratories currently use in their analysis. In the case of Sam that I told you about at the beginning of this article we found he had two different parasites, one of which was a type of worm. Using a combination of medications, anti-parasitic herbs, and a probiotic we were able to eliminate Sam's ten-year-old problem in just four weeks!

Peppermint Oil Eases Irritable Bowel Syndrome (IBS)

IBS is a chronic digestive disorder that can cause abdominal pain and bloating… diarrhea or constipation… and urgent, painful, gassy and/or incomplete defecation. In a recent Italian study, 57 IBS patients were given 450 mg of peppermint oil capsules twice daily or a placebo.

Results: Compared with the patients taking a placebo, those who took peppermint oil had significantly fewer and milder symptoms at the end of the four-week study and four weeks after therapy was discontinued.

My view: Previous studies showed that peppermint oil relieves IBS symptoms, and now we know that improvement can be achieved in four weeks. Use *enteric-coated* capsules, which pass through the stomach, then dissolve in the small intestine to allow for direct antispasmodic and gas-relieving effects. They are sold in health-food stores and generally are safe. Take 450 mg one hour before breakfast and dinner.

Castor Oil—
Quick Fix for Constipation?

One of my readers recently told me that he had begun taking *castor oil* for his chronic constipation. He asked me if it was harmful.

Castor oil comes from the seeds of the castor bean and has long been used to treat constipation. It aids elimination by preventing absorption of liquids from the intestinal tract, but prolonged use can lead to a depletion of minerals, especially potassium. It should be used as a laxative only for a few days. Repeated use contributes to a "lazy" digestive tract, which can worsen constipation in the long run.

If constipation is a frequent problem for you, consult your doctor to make sure that there is no medical cause, such as thyroid disease or a tumor in the digestive tract. Also, I have found that taking two tablespoons of ground *flaxseed* with 10 oz of water each morning helps many patients. Flaxseed has other benefits, too—it is rich in healthful *omega-3 fatty acids* and offers you cancer-preventing properties. In addition, be sure to drink water throughout the day—ideally one-half ounce per pound of body weight up to 64 oz a day. Regular exercise also encourages bowel regularity.

When Gas Won't Quit

Despite cautious dietary practices (you do not have carbonated drinks, coffee and beans, plus you regularly supplement with Beano and Gas-X), you might continue to find that gassiness can't be avoided.

The problem may lie with your medication. Ask your doctor if any of the drugs you take commonly cause flatulence or digestive upset. Gas may result when digestive bacteria fail to break down foods sufficiently. To fix this, stimulate stomach acid secretion with the herb *gentian root*. Take 10 to 20 drops of liquid extract (in one ounce of water) or 300 mg in capsule form about 10 minutes before meals. (Do not use gentian root if you have an active ulcer.) Also take an equal dose of gingerroot, which acts as a *carminative* (gas reducer) and improves stomach function. For much improved digestion, restore the friendly bacteria to your digestive tract by eating sauerkraut, kefir and/or yogurt, or by taking a *probiotic* supplement that contains at least five billion colony-forming units (CFU) of *lactobacillus acidophilus* and/or *bifidobacterium*. If gassiness persists after three weeks, consult a holistic doctor for food-intolerance testing—you may have a sensitivity to dairy, grains or other foods.

Can Bread Make You Sick?
The Answer is Yes!

Millions of people endure chronic symptoms including abdominal distress and episodes of fatigue—but they may not have to.

For you (or someone you love), the solution to these and many other troubles might be shockingly simple—*if* you and your doctor are willing to do a little unusual sleuthing.

When Bonita, age 60, came to see me, she complained of daily abdominal pain and flatulence. She told me that she had suffered frequent waves of fatigue since she was a child. Numerous visits to doctors and specialists over the years turned up a variety of problems. Bonita had been diagnosed with *chronic anemia* (a low red blood cell count) and *hypoglycemia* (low blood sugar). Those conditions could help account for her fatigue.

There were other issues as well. Osteoporosis had set in—a bone density scan indicated loss of bone mass. Bonita also had lost too much weight. Examinations revealed that she also had fatty liver (fat buildup in the liver cells) and inflammation of the pancreas. Typically, when I see such signs in the liver and pancreas, I suspect excessive alcohol consumption—but Bonita didn't touch a drop!

These signs pointed to *celiac disease* (CD), also sometimes called by its older name, sprue. If you don't know much about this condition, you're not alone. It took medical researchers many years to unravel its root cause—and even today, lots of people have it and don't know it.

When I ran some additional blood tests on Bonita, my suspicions proved correct. I immediately put her on a diet free of *gluten* (a protein complex found in wheat, barley and rye), meaning she could have absolutely no bread, crackers, cake, cereal or other foods containing these common grains. Within weeks, there was a noticeable improvement in Bonita's energy. Her abdominal pain diminished. Blood tests showed that her anemia was improving, as were liver and pancreatic function. She felt much better, gained some weight and looked vibrant!

The curse of the grain

Celiac disease, the cause of Bonita's lifelong discomfort, is an auto-immune condition, which means that the immune system—designed to prevent infection and fight off disease—turns traitor and harms the body.

With CD, the body recognizes gluten as a harmful foreign substance. When someone with CD consumes gluten, a big problem develops in the small intestine—specifically with the multitude of soft, tiny, finger-like projections called villi that line the intestinal walls. *Villi* are responsible for absorbing nutrients.

In people who have CD, the villi are damaged and can't do their job properly. They're caught in a cross fire between the immune system and the gluten that's traveling through the small intestine. For some reason, in certain people—this is the part we don't fully understand—the immune system attacks the gluten, and the fragile villi get mauled in the autoimmune battle.

When a CD sufferer stops eating foods that contain gluten, the turn-around can be remarkable —and often within a matter of weeks. For people who have suffered with this condition for years without knowing the cause, eliminating gluten can seem like the beginning of a new life.

Many doctors do not pay much attention to CD's all-too-common signs. That's a big mistake because recent studies have shown that it is much more prevalent than previously suspected. At a conference held by the National Institutes of Health in 2004, researchers reported that CD affects as many as three million Americans, or about one out of every 100 people.

Malabsorption mayhem

CD leaves plenty of clues. When inflamed villi can no longer absorb nutrients as they should, you end up with a condition called *malabsorption*, which results in nutritional deficiencies.

Other possible damage can occur as well, including a condition called *increased intestinal permeability*. This type of intestinal-wall damage can be compared to holes punched in a screen door—larger-than-normal molecules can escape through holes in the small intestine and enter the bloodstream. Among those larger molecules are portions of protein compounds (*gluten fractions*) that are not supposed to penetrate the intestinal wall.

Result: The body, sensing the presence of these fractions, begins to intensify the autoimmune reaction.

If an infant or a child has CD, malabsorption takes a cruel toll. Some infants display signs of "failure to thrive" (slowed growth in a number of the body's systems). Older children may have physical and behavioral development problems.

The longer CD goes undetected and a person continues to eat gluten, the more likely he/she is to develop other autoimmune diseases—*insulin-dependent type 1 diabetes, thyroiditis* (inflammation of the thyroid) and *hepatitis* (inflammation of the liver). People with untreated CD also have an elevated risk of certain types of cancer, especially *intestinal lymphoma*. While CD exists in sufferers from birth through adulthood, the symptoms may start to show up at any time.

The tests—what's involved?

CD can affect anyone, but it is more prevalent in people of European (especially Northern European) descent. Studies also show that it affects Hispanic, black and Asian populations.

Because neglecting CD can be life-threatening, I recommend that screening begin in early childhood. If you have any of the symptoms or suffer from lupus, type 1 diabetes, rheumatoid arthritis or thyroid disease, then it is even more critical to be screened for CD. Genetics is a factor, so if a parent, sibling or child of yours tests positive for CD, I recommend that you also get screened.

CD is detected by a group of blood tests referred to as a *celiac panel*. These tests, which generally are covered by health insurance, measure your immune system's response to gluten in the foods you eat. If blood tests point to a diagnosis of CD, your doctor may recommend that you see a gastroenterologist for a biopsy of the small intestine.

The biopsy involves the use of an *endoscope* (a long, thin tube with a tiny periscope and cutting tool at the end), which is inserted through the mouth and manipulated through the small intestine. If the extracted villi are severely damaged, it confirms CD.

Caution: Don't stop consuming gluten before a celiac blood test or biopsy. This could throw off your test results. (Fortunately, the blood tests now used to diagnose CD are so accurate that a biopsy usually isn't necessary.)

Gluten sensitivity

If you have a number of symptoms that suggest CD but your test results are negative, there's a chance that you have a less severe form of the condition, called *gluten sensitivity*. In my own practice, I have found that gluten sensitivity is much more common than CD.

Some patients complain of bloating, headache, rashes or other symptoms that might be related to CD or to allergies, but traditional skin-scratch or blood antibody tests don't point to a single diagnosis. To find out whether gluten is a factor, I recommend reducing (or better, eliminating) intake of wheat and other gluten-containing grains. If symptoms improve, it's a strong indication of gluten sensitivity.

Some people with gluten sensitivity can eat grains as long as they "rotate" among different kinds—that is, consuming different grains instead of the same ones all the time—to reduce symptoms and provide a wider variety of nutrients. This plan is not appropriate for people who have CD—they must completely eliminate gluten from their diets, permanently, period.

What the future holds

Continuing research shows that we still have much to learn about CD, but there is good reason to be hopeful that prevention might one day be possible. In identical twins who live in the same household, for example, sometimes only one has CD—raising the question of what role environment plays.

A study published in *American Journal of Clinical Nutrition* showed that the more gluten- containing foods introduced to an infant, the greater the risk of developing CD in childhood. However, breast-feeding during this time cuts the risk of developing CD in childhood. We do not yet know whether these findings hold true throughout life.

And, based on Dutch research, there may be a connection between the overgrowth of *Candida albicans*, a yeast normally found in the digestive tract, and the onset of CD, perhaps because of chemical similarities between Candida and gluten. The idea that infections of the gut and autoimmune conditions are linked continues to gain acceptance—and I will keep you up to date.

Additional reading

Wheat-Free, Worry-Free: The Art of Happy, Healthy, Gluten-Free Living, by Danna Korn (Hay House).

Going Against the Grain: How Reducing and Avoiding Grains Can Revitalize Your Health, by Melissa Diane Smith (McGraw-Hill).

Signs of CD

CD is associated with a wide range of symptoms, including...

•**Diarrhea.**

•**Feeling or looking bloated.**

•**Unexplained fatigue.**

•**Unexplained abdominal pain.**

•**Gassiness.**

•**Skin redness, rash, itchy skin.**

•**Loss of tooth enamel.**

•**Unexpected hair loss.**

•**Low body weight.**

•**Infertility or irregular menses.**

•**Premature osteoporosis.**

If you have any of these symptoms, ask your doctor about CD—the sooner, the better.

How to Go Gluten-Free

As restricted diets go, gluten-free is not bad. You can eat meat, seafood, fruits and vegetables. There are zero restrictions against nuts, peas, beans, soybeans and items made out of them, such as tofu made from soybeans. You also are allowed to have rice, corn and a variety of other grains, including amaranth, buckwheat (kasha), millet, quinoa and sorghum, and anything made from them, including rice pasta. Over recent years, researchers have stated that oats also can be consumed. Dairy products, wine and sweets are safe, too. All of the above assumes that these foods haven't been processed or cooked with any gluten-containing ingredients.

Here is the slightly tricky part. In avoiding wheat and the other grains listed below, it's easy to forgo obvious gluten-containing foods, such as bread (and most things that are breaded), cookies, pancakes, etc. But you must watch out for the many food products that aren't grains per se but that contain gluten because they are produced with grain derivatives, such as wheat starch or malt (from barley). Less obvious gluten-containing ingredients are commonly used in condiments... sauces (including soy sauce)... salad dressings... meat products such as sausage and cold cuts... processed seafood products... processed cheese products... etc. Even some dietary supplements and medications contain gluten. The basic rule with CD is, when in doubt, don't eat it. Call the manufacturer to find out for next time.

Now more good news. The food industry is waking up to CD, and you will find a growing number of gluten-free ingredients for cooking. Many chain supermarkets now have a gluten-free section. Even restaurants are starting to offer gluten-free choices, and several national chains—including Legal Sea Foods, Outback Steakhouse and PF Chang's China Bistro—have developed gluten-free menus.

For more on gluten-free eating, go to the Celiac Disease Foundation's site at www.celiac.org, and the Celiac Sprue Association's site at www.csaceliacs.info.

Foods to avoid

• **Wheat**, including wheat flour, wheat germ, wheat bran, cracked wheat, einkorn wheat, emmer wheat.

• **Couscous**.

• **Kamut**.

• **Spelt**.

• **Semolina**.

• **Rye**.

• **Triticale** (wheat-rye hybrid).

• **Barley**.

Cooked Broccoli and Thyroid Function

I have advised readers and patients to avoid cooking broccoli, but this may not be the best way to go if you have thyroid problems.

Broccoli contains *goitrogens*, substances that can interfere with the functioning of the thyroid gland. Other foods that contain goitrogens include brussels sprouts, cabbage, cauliflower, kale, kohlrabi, mustard greens, rutabagas and turnips, as well as soy, millet, peaches, peanuts, radishes and spinach.

There is little data on the effect of these foods on human thyroid function. I advised readers to eat broccoli raw or lightly steamed and avoid boiling it so it does not lose its vitamin C and phytonutrient content. But I recommend that all people with an existing thyroid problem, especially low thyroid function (*hypothyroidism*), or those with a family history of hypothyroidism, consume these foods raw only in moderation (a maximum of two to three servings a week will give you the full benefit of the food's vitamin C and *phytonutrients*). Cooking these foods appears to inactivate the goitrogens, allowing you to eat them more than two or three times a week if you choose to do so.

Save Your Eyesight...
With the Right Foods
and Supplements

Vision is an amazing gift. The nutrients we absorb from our food enhance and maintain circulation to keep the tissues and structures in our eyes healthy. Without proper nutrition and eye protection, we run the risk of developing eye disease.

Cataracts and *age-related macular degeneration* affect about 29 million Americans age 40 and older. Both can lead to partial vision loss or blindness.

Cataracts develop slowly, causing a clouding of the eye lens that impairs vision. About half of all Americans over age 65 have some degree of cataract formation. Cataract surgery has a high success rate, but it's better to prevent cataracts from forming in the first place.

Macular degeneration is more serious. It occurs when the *macula* (the part of the eye that allows us to see detail in the center of our vision field) becomes damaged and deteriorates. This leads to the loss of central vision and makes it difficult to read and see small objects, such as buttons on a cuff.

The two main types of macular degeneration are dry and wet. The dry type accounts for about 85 percent of cases and can be prevented and treated with proper nutrition. The wet type is caused by abnormal blood vessel growth under the retina (the light-sensitive layer lining the interior of the eye). Laser treatments can improve this type but won't cure it.

To help prevent eye disease, you must avoid the formation of free radicals. These harmful molecules can come from a variety of sources, including exposure to smoke (from tobacco, fireplaces, etc.) and toxic metals, such as lead, which are found in some water supplies, as well as from fried foods.

In addition, it is crucial to wear sunglasses that block 100 percent of *ultraviolet A* (UVA) and *ultraviolet B* (UVB) rays. UVA rays are associated with the development of macular degeneration, while UVB rays are linked to the formation of cataracts. Not all sunglasses block both types of rays, so read the label carefully to find a pair that does. Wear them anytime you're out in the sun. If you already have cataracts or macular degeneration, wear sunglasses whenever you're outside during daytime, even when it is overcast.

Best choice: Wraparound sunglasses, which prevent damaging rays of sun from entering from the sides.

Eye-protecting nutrients

A number of nutrients can help you prevent—and even treat—cataracts and macular degeneration. Although fresh foods are the best source of most eye-protecting nutrients, supplements help ensure that you're getting adequate amounts. If you already have been diagnosed with one of these eye conditions, you should be taking supplements, even if you are undergoing conventional treatment. Adults who are concerned about developing eye disease also should consider taking eye-protecting supplements.

Each nutrient listed below can be purchased individually or as part of a vision formula. Individual supplements typically provide higher dosages, but people who don't like to bother with a lot of bottles may prefer a vision formula that combines many key nutrients. Good eye formulas include Vision Optimizer by Jarrow Formulas (to find a retailer in your area, call 310-204-2520 or go to www.jarrow.com) and Visual Eyes Multinutrient Complex by Source Naturals (to find a retailer in your area, call 800-815-2333 or go to www.sourcenaturals.com).

The most important eye-protecting nutrients...

• **Lutein** is part of the carotenoid family (fat-soluble pigments found in plants). This antioxidant helps filter all types of light, including UV rays, that damage cells of the eye, particularly the macula. Population studies have found an association between a high dietary intake of lutein and a decreased risk of developing macular degeneration and cataracts.

Lutein-filled foods: Egg yolks, spinach, broccoli, kale and corn. Most Americans have only one to two milligrams of lutein in their daily diets, but eye-disease prevention requires higher levels of this nutrient. People with macular degeneration or cataracts should take a supplement that contains 15 mg of lutein daily. To prevent these diseases, take two to five milligrams of lutein daily as part of a high-potency multivitamin or eye formula. Because lutein is fat soluble, it should be taken with a meal for best absorption. Lutein has no known side effects.

• **Zeaxanthin** also is in the *carotenoid* family. Like lutein, zeaxanthin protects the eye from the damaging effects of UV rays. Zeaxanthin is found in the same foods as lutein, as well as oranges and tangerines. Supplemental eye formulas and mixed carotenoid complexes contain zeaxanthin. People with macular degeneration should take a supplement that contains three milligrams of zeaxanthin daily with a meal. For prevention, take 500 mcg to one milligram daily. There are no known side effects.

• **Vitamin C** protects against cataracts and macular degeneration. As people age, vitamin C levels in the eye decrease. That's why it is so important to eat foods that are rich in vitamin C and take a supplement that contains this nutrient. Population studies have found that people taking multivitamins or any supplements containing vitamins C and E for more than 10 years had a 60 percent lower risk of developing cataracts. To prevent cataracts and macular degeneration, take 500 mg of vitamin C daily. People who already have eye disease, especially cataracts, should take 2,000 mg to 3,000 mg daily in divided doses.

Note: If you experience loose stools from this dose, reduce your intake by 500 mg daily until symptoms subside. People with a history of kidney stones should check with a doctor before taking high-dose vitamin C.

• **Bilberry** contains antioxidant compounds known as *anthocyanidins*. These *phytonutrients* protect the lens and other eye tissue against the free radical damage associated with both cataracts and macular degeneration. Those who have cataracts or macular degeneration should take 160 mg two to three times daily of a 25 percent anthocyanoside extract. Take the same dose for prevention. Bilberry has no significant side effects.

• **Vitamin E complex**, taken at a dose of 400 IU with 80 mg of zinc, 500 mg of vitamin C and 15 mg of beta-carotene daily, has been shown to reduce the risk of visual acuity loss by 27 percent and curb by 25 percent the risk for progression of macular degeneration in people with an advanced form of this disease. Researchers have estimated that 300,000 of the eight million Americans with macular degeneration (in one or both eyes) could prevent their eye disease from advancing and avoid any associated vision loss during the next five years by taking this supplement combination. For eye-disease prevention, take 200 IU of a mixed vitamin E complex that contains the vitamin E subgroups *tocopherols* and *tocotrienols*. People diagnosed with macular degeneration or cataracts can try 400 IU of a mixed vitamin E complex daily, along with the other nutrients listed in this section, all under the close supervision of a doctor.

• **Zinc** promotes the activity of enzymes in the retina. When used alone or in combination with other antioxidants, such as beta-carotene, vitamin C or vitamin E, zinc has been shown to reduce the risk of vision loss associated with macular degeneration. If you have cataracts or macular degeneration, take 45 mg to 80 mg of zinc daily, along with one to two milligrams of copper (zinc supplements can lower copper levels in the body). For prevention, take 15 mg to 30 mg of zinc daily and one to two milligrams of copper. Side effects, such as occasional digestive upset, are rare.

• **Betaine hydrochloride (betaine HCl)** supports healthy digestion and absorption. Not only do many older adults not consume enough fruits and vegetables to get ample nutrition for their eyes, but their digestion is too terrible to make efficient use of what they do eat. Stomach acid levels are believed to decrease as people age, which can hinder mineral absorption from foods and supplements. Betaine HCl mimics the *hydrochloric acid* normally produced by the stomach. I highly recommend that anyone with cataracts or macular degeneration take one or two 500-mg or 600-mg capsules of betaine HCl with each meal. Use the same dose to help prevent eye disease. People taking antacid medications and those with reflux or active ulcers should not use betaine HCl. It can aggravate those conditions.

• **B vitamins**, such as vitamin B-1 (*thiamine*), vitamin B-2 (*riboflavin*) and vitamin B-3 (*niacin*), are associated with a decreased risk of cataracts when consumed at high levels. These B vitamins, especially riboflavin and niacin, are believed to help regenerate *glutathione*, a powerful antioxidant found in the body's cells, including the eye lens. Most high-potency multivitamins contain these B vitamins in adequate amounts (2 mg of B-1, three milligrams of B-2 and 40 mg of B-3) to help prevent eye disease. For people diagnosed with cataracts, take an additional 50 mg B complex daily.

• **N-acetylcarnosine** has recently received a great deal of attention from nutrition-oriented doctors as a treatment for cataracts. Its parent compound, *L-carnosine*, is a molecule that is made up of the two amino acids *histidine* and *alanine*. N-acetylcarnosine acts like an antioxidant and has been shown to protect cell membranes from oxidative damage. A 2001 Russian study involving two randomized, double-blind, placebo-controlled trials reported that N-acetylcarnosine eyedrops improved visual acuity and glare sensitivity in 26 of 41 cataract patients (average age 65). The dose used in this study was two drops twice daily of a one percent aqueous solution. The same type of eyedrops used in the study are available for $39.95 in a product that's called Can-C, manufactured by Smart Nutrition (858-270-7907, www.smart-nutrition.net). Cataract patients who use these drops should be monitored by a doctor.

Intravenous therapy

The most aggressive natural therapy for people with macular degeneration is *intravenous (IV) therapy*, which involves the infusion of nutrients in a solution directly into the bloodstream via a needle inserted into a vein in the arm. This method provides a much greater therapeutic dose of nutrients to the cells of the macula, since it bypasses the digestive tract.

Jonathan Kalman, ND, who practices at my clinic, specializes in IV therapy for serious diseases. He routinely administers IV nutrients such as glutathione, zinc, vitamin C, B vitamins and mineral complexes. In many cases, this type of treatment can halt the progression of the dry form of macular degeneration and often improves vision. Dr. Kalman recommends an initial series of 15 twice-weekly treatments. To find a doctor who offers IV therapy, consult the American College for Advancement in Medicine (949-309-3520, www.acamnet.org). IV therapy costs $100 to $125 per treatment. It's not covered by insurance, but it can be well worth the investment.

Eye nutrients

Here is a summary of my recommendations for people diagnosed with eye disease. Preventive doses appear in parentheses.

Cataracts

• **Lutein**. 15 mg daily (two to five milligrams daily in a high-potency multivitamin or eye formula).

• **Vitamin C**. 2,000 mg to 3,000 mg daily (500 mg daily).

• **Bilberry**. 160 mg two to three times daily of a 25 percent anthocy-anoside extract (same dose).

• **Vitamin E complex**. 400 IU daily (200 IU daily) with a doctor's approval.

• **Zinc**. 45 mg to 80 mg daily with one to two milligrams of copper (15 mg to 30 mg daily with one to two milligrams of copper).

• **Betaine hydrochloride**. One to two 500- to 600-mg capsules with each meal (same dose).

• **Vitamin B complex**. 50 mg daily plus a high-potency multivitamin (high-potency multivitamin).

• **N-acetylcarnosine eyedrops**. Two drops twice daily of a one percent aqueous solution, used under a doctor's supervision.

Macular Degeneration

Take the first six supplements listed above, plus...

• **Zeaxanthin**. Three milligrams daily (500 mcg to one milligram daily).

• **Beta-carotene**. 15 mg daily (same dose).

Grocery Cart Smarts— What to Buy... and Why

Friends sometimes tease my wife, Angela, and me for being health-food fanatics, feigning amazement at our "exotic" meals. But then they ask, in all seriousness, for hands-on instruction in healthful food shopping. Going to the market with our family of five—including Angela (who is also a naturopathic doctor) and our three children, ages nine, six and four—they marvel at how much our kids know about nutrition.

That's why I thought it would be fun to take readers shopping, too. So come along for a tour of the market.

Very healthful veggies

The fresher the food, the more nutritious it generally is, so we like to shop several times per week. We go to a nearby health-food store for locally grown produce (which hasn't spent days in transit) and organic products (which aren't contaminated with pesticides) and head straight for the vegetables.

• **Eggplant,** which Angela adores, is often the first item in our cart. The skin is a rich source of *nasunin*, a potent antioxidant (a substance that neutralizes disease-causing molecules called free radicals). Eggplant provides minerals that promote good circulation and/or strong bones, including potassium, manganese, copper and magnesium... plus B vitamins for heart health, including B-1 (*thiamine*), B-3 (*niacin*), B-6 (*pyridoxine*) and B-9 (*folate*). This versatile vegetable can be diced and stir-fried... thin-sliced and grilled... or cut in half, oven-baked until tender (about 20 minutes at 350 degrees), then topped with cottage cheese.

Note: Avoid eggplant if its *alkaloids* (organic compounds) aggravate your arthritis.

• **Beets** help to detoxify the body by raising levels of the antioxidant *glutathione* in the liver... improve gallbladder function by thinning bile (a digestive fluid)... and provide folate and manganese for joint health. Red beets provide the most *betacyanin*, a plant pigment that protects against colon cancer. Beets can be combined with carrots and juiced... grated and added to salads... or cut into chunks and roasted.

• **Broccoli** contains the antioxidants *sulforaphane* and *chlorophyl*... vitamins A, C and E, which strengthen the immune system... calcium and vitamin K for bone health... folate for normal cell division... and *lutein* (a plant pigment) for eye health. Cauliflower provides many of the same *phytonutrients* (beneficial plant chemicals) as broccoli.

• **Carrots** pack easily into lunch boxes. We love baby carrots dipped in salad dressing, so we buy dressings with no unhealthful hydrogenated fat, high-fructose corn syrup or *monosodium glutamate* (MSG), a salty additive. For carrot juice, we peel large carrots and put them in our Vitamix (from $449, 800-848-2649, www.vitamix.com), a high-power blender that preserves the fiber-rich pulp of fruits and vegetables.

• **Cabbage** is a super source of vitamin K (for bone health)... vitamin C (for tissue growth and repair)... and organic compounds called *indoles* (for cancer prevention). Red cabbage has more healthful plant pigments than white. Since its juice has a very mild flavor, Angela adds red cabbage to almost everything we make in the Vita-Mix. Our kids get a kick from the looks on their friends' faces when we add cabbage to a fruit sorbet or fruit smoothie—and it's even more fun when their friends love the taste!

• **Cherry tomatoes,** rich in vitamins A and C, taste great with slices of low-fat mozzarella cheese.

• **Salad greens** we consume daily include romaine, red- or green-leaf lettuce and fresh spinach. They provide vitamin K, as well as fiber for bowel regularity.

Favorite fruits

We love fresh fruit for snacks and desserts.

• **Mango,** one of my favorites, is rich in fiber, beta-carotene, magnesium, potassium and vitamins B-1, B-2 (*riboflavin*), B-3 and B-6. Sweet, tangy and juicy, mangoes make a delicious (if messy) snack when peeled and sliced. Mango slices also can be added to green salad and fruit smoothies or baked in pies.

• **Kiwifruit**—fuzzy brown outside and brilliant green inside—is packed with vitamin C. The kiwifruit is a natural blood thinner that reduces blood levels of *triglycerides* (fats). Peel and slice to eat alone, add to a fruit salad or blend into a smoothie.

• **Apricots** are rich in vitamin A and healthful plant pigments called *carotenoids* (such as *beta-carotene* and *lycopene*), which aid vision. Lycopene also may combat heart disease and prostate problems.

• **Apples** provide fiber plus heart-healthy *quercetin*. Slice and spread with almond butter (for protein), or sprinkle with cinnamon (to balance blood sugar).

• **Bananas** are rich in potassium, to maintain normal blood pressure and heart function... and provide B vitamins, which help to balance brain chemicals called *neurotransmitters*. Our after-dinner snack often consists of bananas with cinnamon or peanut butter.

• **Blueberries** contain purplish pigments called *anthocyanins* (also found in red grapes and cranberries), which fight urinary tract infections and may protect the brain from oxidative stress, reducing the effects of dementia. Blueberries have vitamin E and other nutrients that strengthen blood vessels.

• **Oranges** have more than 170 phytonutrients and more than 60 *flavonoids* (healthful plant pigments) that fight inflammation, blood clots and various cancers. Other citrus fruits provide similar benefits.

• **Avocados** are rich in *oleic acid*, a monounsaturated fat that lowers LDL "bad" cholesterol. Peel and slice them into salads, add them to burritos, or mash as a sandwich spread.

Body-building proteins

Protein is required for muscle and tissue repair, blood sugar balance and proper immune function.

• **Eggs** we buy are organic (laid by chickens that eat grains free of chemicals and that are not treated with hormones or antibiotics) and enriched with *omega-3 fatty acids* for cardiovascular health. We each have three to five eggs weekly—boiled, poached or scrambled with cheese.

• **Poultry** (skin removed) is typically lower in saturated fat than red meat and therefore is healthier for the cardiovascular system. We select poultry labeled *free range* (meaning the animals were not constantly caged and were not fed antibiotics). From the deli counter, we buy cooked, sliced turkey and chicken breast for sandwiches, opting for low-sodium, preservative-free brands. Favorite dinner entrées include turkey loaf (ground turkey can be substituted for beef and pork in meat loaf recipes) and pan-fried or broiled turkey burgers. We also love Angela's baked chicken breasts, seasoned with rosemary, lemon and poultry seasoning. We seldom barbecue meat or poultry because doing so triggers cancer-causing compounds called *heterocyclic amines* (HCAs).

• **Wild ocean salmon** (which some consider to be more healthful than farm-raised) in season is delicious baked or broiled with olive oil and lemon. In addition to being low both in calories and saturated fat, salmon is high in protein... omega-3s... vitamins B-3, B-6 and B-12 (*cobalamin*)… phosphorous… and magnesium. We avoid tuna—including canned—due to concerns about mercury contamination. However, canned ocean salmon packed in water is healthful, as are canned sardines—though I confess that we do not enjoy the taste (or smell) of sardines.

• **Cheeses** we enjoy in moderation include Colby and string cheese for snacks and shredded cheddar on burritos. Along with protein and calcium, cheese provides the amino acid *tryptophan*, which promotes thyroid function and positive moods.

Cans, cartons and jars

Packaged goods can be healthful, provided they don't have added preservatives, oils, sugars or salt.

• **Beans** are a must for Mexican-style tostados. Their soluble fiber promotes proper cholesterol and blood sugar levels. Black beans are rich in antioxidant anthocyanins. Pinto beans have magnesium, potassium, manganese, copper and *molybdenum*, which help the liver with detoxification.

• **Almond milk** is rich in potassium. Blue Diamond's unsweetened almond milk tastes great in cereal and scrambled eggs. A sweetened brand called Almond Breeze has seven grams of sugar per eight-ounce serving. We pour it over hot oatmeal and drink it as a snack. We also buy oat milk and rice milk. (We avoid drinking cow's milk because it can cause allergic and immune reactions and digestive distress.)

• **Peanut butter** is a passion for our kids (and our dog, Blast). We buy pure peanut butter (in a glass container to avoid chemicals that may leach from plastics) that has no added sugar or *partially hydrogenated fat*. Peanut butter has heart-healthy *monounsaturated fats*, vitamin E, niacin, folate, manganese and *resveratrol* (the same antioxidant found in red wine). We also like almond butter, which is similar in nutrient content.

Great grains and other goodies

Selecting grains can be complicated for people who—like my youngest son and me—experience nasal congestion, bloating and diarrhea after consuming foods with *gluten* (a protein complex). Wheat, rye and barley all contain gluten.

• **Gluten-free grains** include corn, amaranth, rice, buckwheat and quinoa. Of the gluten-free breads we have tried, those from Kinnikinnick Foods Inc. (www.kinnikinnick.com) taste best. Pastas, cereals, pretzels, corn chips, tortillas and tostado shells also come in gluten-free varieties.

• **Cereals** we select have no more than three grams of sugar and provide at least two to three grams of fiber per serving. Our big favorites include Rice Crunch-Ems from Health Valley… Amazon Frosted Flakes from Nature's Path… and Kix and Cheerios from General Mills. We also have oatmeal—a source of energy-sustaining complex carbohydrates, as well as *manganese, selenium* and *silicon*, which promote bone and cartilage health. The slow-cooking kind has the most fiber.

• **Seeds and nuts** are on our list, too. I grind up two tablespoons of *flaxseeds* each morning, place them on my tongue, and wash them down with water. Flaxseeds provide fiber and essential fatty acids, and may combat cancer. Hemp seeds are high in protein and omega-3s. Almonds and walnuts are rich in antioxidants and omega-3s, respectively. Angela and I eat one-quarter cup daily, and we try to get our kids to eat a few.

• **Chips** are big hits, especially bruschetta chips. A brand called Jensen's Orchard can be ordered from Amazon.com. Made with potatoes, tomatoes, basil and olive oil, they provide protein and fiber but no sugar or trans fat.

• **Oils** are important to good cooks (like Angela). Extra-virgin olive oil is what we use when cooking fish and chicken or roasting vegetables. Its monounsaturated fats promote cardiovascular health. To scramble eggs, we use organic canola oil, which contains vitamin E and omega-3s. Macadamia nut oil is best for stir-frying because it has a higher *smoke point* (the temperature at which a cooking oil breaks down and smokes, giving food an unpleasant taste).

• **Fun foods** we enjoy without guilt include Rice Dream Bars (ice cream bars made from rice milk)… Newman's Own brand fig cookies… Ghirardelli semisweet chocolate chips… and SunSpire carob chips.

Eating healthfully comes at a premium. The price of organic foods is about 25 percent higher than the cost of foods that may have been grown using pesticides or made with unhealthful processing methods. We are happy to pay the price because our family's health is worth it. I suspect you feel the same way.

What we won't buy

We check labels and stay away from…

• **Artificial sweeteners** (*sucralose, aspartame* and *saccharin*), which may trigger headaches, rashes and mood changes.

• **High-fructose corn syrup,** which contains many calories but no nutritional benefit.

• **Monosodium glutamate (MSG),** a salty "flavor enhancer" that can cause headaches and/or digestive upset.

• **Partially hydrogenated fats,** also called trans fats, which harm the cardiovascular and immune systems.

• **Sodium nitrate and potassium nitrate,** preservatives that are linked to cancer.

What I Do to Stay Healthy and Live Longer

Terry Grossman, MD, founder and medical director of Frontier Medical Institute, an internationally renowned antiaging and longevity clinic in Denver, www.fmiclinic.com. His books include The Baby Boomers' Guide to Living Forever (Hubristic).

We are on the verge of radically extending human life. Within a few decades, a single drop of blood will detect cancer at its earliest stages or reveal preventable diseases that we might otherwise develop later in life. Medicine will be customized, with drugs and therapies that match our genetic makeup. It will be common to maintain a high quality of life into our 90s and 100s.

Our challenge today is to stay healthy so that we can benefit from this revolution. We all know how important it is to watch our weight, cholesterol and blood pressure, but that's not enough. I counsel patients on optimal management of the aging process—and I practice what I preach. *Here's what I'm doing to increase my chances of living longer…*

Take advantage of genetic testing

For about $500 (not covered by insurance), you can get tests that show your predisposition to such conditions as high blood pressure, heart attack, Alzheimer's disease and osteoporosis.

What I do: I'm in my 60s, and genomic testing revealed that I have a gene that gives me a 250 percent greater risk of Alzheimer's than the general population. The results depressed me for several days, but they motivated me to fine-tune my health. For example, I take supplements* to nourish my brain. I recommend these supplements to most of my patients, but especially those who are at higher risk for Alzheimer's. Always check with your doctor before taking any supplement.

Brain nutrients I take daily: 20 mg of *vinpocetine* (it's pronounced *vinn-POH-seh-teen*), a nutrient derived from the periwinkle plant that increases blood flow to the brain and has memory-enhancing effects… 100 mg of *phosphatidylserine*, a substance that slows memory loss and is found in the cell membranes of body tissue… 500 mg twice a day of *acetyl-l-carnitine* (it's pronounced *ah-SEE-til-el-CAR-nih-teen*), an amino acid that boosts brain metabolism… 100 mg of ginkgo biloba, a tree leaf popular in Chinese medicine that increases cerebral circulation (ginkgo should be avoided by people on blood thinners, such as aspirin or Coumadin).

To find a doctor or facility that performs genetic testing and offers counseling, contact the American College for Advancement in Medicine, 949-309-3520, www.acamnet.org.

Get body fat under 15 percent

Some fat tissue is necessary. Fat is the body's primary form of energy and is necessary to cushion vital organs. Too much fat, however, secretes inflammatory chemicals that age your body. Reducing body fat is more important than losing weight.

To determine your percentage of body fat, you can purchase a…

• Body-fat test caliper, such as the Accu-Measure Fitness 3000 Personal Body Fat Caliper, available for $20 at www.accumeasurefitness.com or 800-866-2727. This is fairly accurate.

• **Some scales also measure body fat.** They are more accurate than a caliper but also more expensive. See the Body Composition Monitor with scale HBF-510W at www.omronhealthcare.com or 877-216-1333.

What I do: At six feet tall and 178 lbs, I score very well on all the height/weight charts, but my body fat percentage is 17.9 percent. I would like to lose eight more pounds to reach my target of 15 percent body fat.

I keep my carbohydrate intake under 30 percent of total calories and emphasize fish, lean meats, vegetables, tofu and miso soup. This is similar to the diet of people in the Okinawa region of Japan, which has more 100-year-olds than any place in the world and very little serious disease.

Helpful book: *The Okinawa Program: How the World's Longest-Lived People Achieve Everlasting Health—and How You Can Too*, written by Bradley J. Willcox, D. Craig Willcox and Makoto Suzuki (Three Rivers).

Increase alkalinity

Our bodies continually produce toxic waste in the form of acid (*lactic acid, uric acid* and *fatty acids*), which needs to be removed from the blood or neutralized.

Example: While many people believe that kidney stones are caused by excess calcium, the real culprit is a high level of phosphoric acid, a primary ingredient in carbonated soft drinks.

What I do: Drink four cups of green tea daily for its alkalinizing effect and antioxidants… and avoid soda.

Eliminate sugar

All sweets, fructose, corn syrup and *high-glycemic-load carbohydrates* (pasta, doughnuts, etc.) are the biggest villains in the aging process. Sugar creates a vicious cycle that wears down the body's cells—it spikes the level of insulin in your blood, which causes an intense craving for even more sugar. I don't recommend artificial sweeteners because of the negative long-term effects.

What I do: Use *stevia*, a noncaloric herb that lowers blood sugar and kills the bacteria that cause tooth decay. It has been used in Paraguay for centuries with no health dangers and can be found in health-food stores as a dietary supplement. The FDA now recognizes stevia as safe, and it can be found in a growing number of soft drinks.

Optimize toxin removal

Methylation is a simple biochemical process that the body uses to rid itself of dangerous toxins. Between 10 percent and 44 percent of the population has a problem with proper methylation, which can lead to cancer, stroke and other conditions. In a healthy person, methylation neutralizes *homocysteine*—a toxic by-product that forms after you eat protein. Homocysteine can damage arteries, and high levels are associated with heart attack, Alzheimer's, stroke and cancer.

What I do: I get tested for homocysteine (the test costs $50 to $100). My level is excellent—below 7.5—but if it should rise, I would lower it with daily supplements, including 50 mcg to 100 mcg of vitamin B-6... 100 mcg or more of vitamin B-12... and 800 mcg or more of folic acid. These dosages are much higher than the FDA recommendation, so check with your doctor.

Reduce inflammation

Whenever its equilibrium is disrupted by injury or infection, the body responds with acute inflammation, such as in muscles and tendons. While this acute inflammation usually subsides quickly, "silent" inflammation can smolder in your body for decades without causing any obvious problems.

Example: Silent inflammation in the coronary arteries is the reason why so many seemingly healthy people suddenly drop dead of heart attacks. People with high inflammation readings suffer more than twice the rate of heart attacks as those with low readings.

What I do: Take a blood test (less than $50) for *high-sensitivity C-reactive protein* (or CRP). CRP is made in the liver and released into the blood in response to inflammation in the body. A normal CRP level is under three, but for optimal health, it should be under one. To achieve that, I eat at least four servings of fish per week. Fish and shellfish, such as sole, halibut, catfish, cod, flounder, crab, salmon and shrimp, are rich in omega-3 fatty acids and help reduce inflammation. Other foods that decrease inflammation include walnuts, spinach, broccoli, kale and such spices and herbs as turmeric and rosemary. I also take fish oil capsules (2,100 mg of *EPA* and 1,500 mg of *DHA* a day).

Invoke the relaxation response

That's what Harvard Medical School researchers call the meditative state that reduces blood levels of stress hormones, such as cortisol and adrenaline. Long-term exposure to these hormones can lead to osteoporosis, high blood pressure, cataracts and other health problems.

What I do: I attend an hour-long yoga class three times a week. The relaxing stretches help lower my blood pressure and improve my sleep and gastrointestinal functioning.

Part IX

Immune System

Glutathione… Your Body's Master Antioxidant

There's an antioxidant in your body, *glutathione* (pronounced glue-tuh-THIGH-own), that does more for you than any other. And as you already know, antioxidants do a lot. One of the primary roles of all antioxidants is to neutralize free radicals that damage cell DNA. Glutathione performs this main function and more—repairing DNA… preventing cell damage (which causes cancer and other diseases)… enhancing immune function… and breaking down toxins.

Your body makes glutathione in every cell, but many people still don't have enough glutathione in their bodies. One study published a decade ago in *The Lancet* found that healthy young people had the highest levels of glutathione… healthy elderly people had lower levels… and sick elderly people, even lower levels.

In addition to aging and illness, other factors that deplete our body's reserves of this important antioxidant include environmental toxins, medications and alcohol use.

What you may not know: Glutathione supplementation can help people who have chronic diseases feel better and help people who are healthy prevent disease.

Here's more on how glutathione helps you…

What glutathione does

• **Kills free radicals**. Free radicals (unbalanced oxygen molecules) attack cells, damage DNA and contribute to aging. They also are involved in every disease. While vitamins such as C and E help to neutralize free radicals, glutathione deactivates the most destructive free radicals.

• **Revitalizes other antioxidants**. When vitamins such as C and E neutralize free radicals, their "free-radical poison" gets used up. Glutathione works to restore the activity of these antioxidants so they can tackle more free radicals. Glutathione also helps to recycle *coenzyme Q10*, an enzyme found in the energy-producing mitochondria of all cells, back to full strength after it neutralizes free radicals. This is important work, since every cell in your body suffers about 10,000 free-radical hits daily.

• **Helps detoxification**. The vast majority of glutathione is found in the liver, where it plays a crucial role in the breakdown and removal of environmental toxins (such as food additives and pesticides) from the body. These toxins are known to cause cancer if they are left to roam freely through the body. Glutathione also helps dispose of hazardous by-products of normal metabolism, such as cellular waste products and excess hormones.

• **Protects the liver**. An example of glutathione's ability to protect the liver comes from two recent studies of children with acute lymphoblastic leukemia who were treated with chemotherapy. Like many drugs, whether prescription or over-the-counter, chemotherapy drugs increase the risk for liver damage and hepatitis. But studies published in *Advances in Hematology* and *Cancer* found that either of two glutathione boosters—*N-acetylcysteine* (NAC) combined with vitamin E… or *silymarin*, the active ingredient in the herb milk thistle—protected against liver damage in these patients. Glutathione enables the liver to break down these drugs and to bounce back from its own toxic exposure.

Benefiting from glutathione

Glutathione is available in several types of healthy foods, although not in therapeutic amounts. Because of this, I generally have patients improve their glutathione levels through supplementation rather than diet. Still, it's helpful to know that certain foods contribute to increased glutathione levels. These include proteins that contain the amino acids *glutamate*, *cysteine* and *glycine* (fish, turkey, eggs and whey protein, but not other dairy products that have been pasteurized because pasteurization breaks down the protein).

While I believe that everyone can benefit from supplementing with glutathione, the best way to determine how deficient you are is with a blood test. This can be helpful if you are ill and not getting better. Low glutathione levels may be preventing your recovery.

Depending on your health, there are different ways to boost your glutathione levels.

• **For patients with chronic diseases**. Most patients with chronic diseases (such as chronic fatigue, Parkinson's disease, mercury and lead toxicity, and immune system problems, including those due to cancer and chemotherapy) can be helped by glutathione supplementation. I often prescribe a pure form of glutathione delivered via an intravenous (IV) solution. Glutathione delivered directly into the bloodstream enables the body to get higher levels of this nutrient, compared with ingesting it. Patients who have had chronic fatigue for several years often improve their strength and vitality after just one or two treatments. These patients have about 10 treatments, either once a week or once every other week. Treatments have a cumulative effect—and the results can last from weeks to months, depending on the patient's condition.

• **For patients who are temporarily ill, have liver disease or take lots of medications**. Take any combination of the supplements below to boost your glutathione levels. This can include, for example, people who have colds, flu or asthma flare-ups.

• **For healthy patients**. Patients at any age who are healthy can benefit from taking any one of the supplements below daily. I usually have healthy patients start out by taking NAC, since it is a great all-around antioxidant.

Supplements that can help

A variety of supplements work to boost glutathione levels. All of these supplements are safe to take—on their own and in combination. There are no side effects, except as noted.

• **Liquid glutathione**. After IV glutathione, the most effective form of this antioxidant comes in liquid form. (I don't recommend glutathione in capsules because it is not well-absorbed.)

Brand to try: Vitamin Research Products Lipoceutical Glutathione (800-877-2447, www.vrp.com).

Dose: One teaspoon daily.

For patients who want a less expensive way to boost glutathione, there are several supplements that help the body make glutathione on its own. These supplements are not as effective as the IV and liquid forms of glutathione, but they do provide a huge health benefit by boosting glutathione levels…

• **N-acetylcysteine (NAC)**. This antioxidant, which helps prevent flu and reduces the severity of respiratory infections, contains cysteine and sulfur, which increase levels of glutathione. Take 500 mg to 1,000 mg daily.

• **Alpha-lipoic acid (ALA)** is another sulfur-rich antioxidant that boosts the liver's glutathione levels. Take 100 mg to 300 mg daily. ALA can reduce blood glucose levels, so patients with diabetes should be monitored by a physician.

• **Silymarin**, the active ingredient in milk thistle, helps liver function and increases glutathione levels. Take 100 mg to 200 mg daily.

Echinacea—The Best-Selling Immune Booster

I t is not unusual to get calls at my office from patients wondering what to do about the cold or flu that just hit them. My first thought is, *What natural supplements can they get quickly, right off the shelf?*

Well, just about anyone can find *echinacea* (pronounced *eck-in-ay-sha*) at a nearby store. It is one of the five top-selling herbs in North America. In fact, it's a worldwide best-seller, as herbalists and physicians in Europe have been prescribing echinacea for decades. Carrying the popular name of purple coneflower (so-called because of its beautiful, purple, daisylike petals), echinacea is renowned as an herb that enhances the immune system. It's commonly used to treat a number of conditions from flu and the common cold to a range of other infectious diseases.

The snakebite connection

Native Americans of the Plains are believed to be the first to use echinacea. It was a remedy for colds, coughs and sore throats, but also toothaches, battle wounds and even rattlesnake bites.

During the latter part of the 1800s, Plains settlers adopted the purple coneflower as a common remedy; and by the 1920s, echinacea was being sold as a commercial product and prescribed by the many physicians who were comfortable with herbal medicines.

Dr. H.C.F. Meyer of Pawnee, Nebraska, was a keen commercial promoter. Adding his own recommendations to what he had learned from Native Americans, Dr. Meyer sold echinacea as a cure-all for various ailments. His reputation was considerably enhanced by the claim that he had successfully treated 613 cases of rattlesnake poisoning. *One doctor gave the following candid account of Dr. Meyer's own, personal echinacea experiment...*

"With the courage of his convictions upon him, he injected the venom of the crotalus (rattlesnake) into the first finger of his left hand; the swelling was rapid and in six hours up to the elbow. At this time he took a dose of the remedy, bathed the part thoroughly, and laid down to pleasant dreams. On awakening in four hours, the pain and swelling were gone."

Infection fighter to the rescue

I can't say I have had any patients come to me for the natural treatment of rattlesnake bites. (If I did, I would quickly hurry them off to a hospital emergency room for a dose of up-to-date antivenom.) But it's interesting to note that echinacea does have the special property of preventing the spread of infectious substances to tissues.

Echinacea as a healing remedy was introduced to Europe during the 1930s. Since then the preponderance of scientific research on echinacea has been done in Western Europe, especially Germany, where the government plays an active role in funding natural-medicine research. But Canadian and American researchers have recently made similar strides in echinacea research, with clinical studies and biochemical analysis of the healing herb.

Over 400 studies to date have looked at the pharmacology and clinical uses of echinacea. Not all studies have shown efficacy of the herb, but most of the research indicates that echinacea helps reinforce the immune system.

Echinacea is consistently one of the best-selling herbs in North America and Europe. Over 10 million units are sold annually in Germany alone.

Though there are nine species of echinacea, *Echinacea purpurea* and *Echinacea angustifolia* are the two most often used commercially. Most clinical studies are done with these species, especially purpurea.

Tongue-tingling chemicals

Scientists have not reached a consensus about the active ingredients in echinacea. Though researchers acknowledge that this herb has many immune-boosting properties as well as anti-inflammatory and antimicrobial effects, they are not certain what chemicals or combination of chemicals are responsible.

It's known, however, that echinacea contains caffeic acid derivatives such as *cichoric acid* and *polysaccharides*. The plant also has compounds known as *alkylamides* that are believed to be important. (Alkylamides are the substances that make your tongue tingle and go numb if you take a hefty dose of straight echinacea.)

Some of these compounds are water-soluble and some are alcohol-soluble. When tinctures, pills or tablets are being created from echinacea, the manufacturer must go through an elaborate process to extract the compounds. Recent research done at the University of British Columbia in conjunction with the University of Alberta has shown that the ratio of the actives in echinacea is important for optimal immune response. So in other words, not only is it important to have active constituents in echinacea products, but also to have them in a specific ratio or blend.

Arousing immune cells

Echinacea doesn't work like the pharmaceutical antibiotics that "kill" off microbes like bacteria. Instead, echinacea arouses the immune cells that patrol and defend the body against these invaders. It increases the number and activity of disease-fighting white blood cells, and it activates antiviral chemicals such as interferon. Echinacea can even activate the immune cells that fight tumors. In addition, research has shown that the chemicals in echinacea have the power to inhibit an enzyme released by bacteria, called *hyaluronidase*. Bacteria normally produce this enzyme to penetrate into human tissue. Echinacea prevents this from happening.

Researchers in a German study found clear evidence that echinacea helps to promote good immune cells, called *phagocytes*. One group of people were given 30 drops of echinacea three times daily for five days, while people in the control group were given a placebo. The level of phagocytes was measured at the beginning and throughout the study. At day three, the phagocyte activity of those taking echinacea increased by 40 percent. By the fifth day, phagocyte activity had increased 120 percent. Whenever people stopped taking echinacea, immune-cell activity dropped off sharply. After three days, there was no difference in immune-cell activity between the group taking echinacea and the control group.

Leading researchers now feel that echinacea may actually be more of an immune-modulating herb, meaning it has a balancing effect on the immune system. As research continues, this may mean that echinacea may be more valuable than just boosting immune function.

Virus slayers

While there are a host of modern antibiotics for killing bacteria, modern medicine has a limited arsenal of weapons to defeat viral infections. This presents a problem for the many doctors who rely on conventional pharmaceuticals in their medical practice. Over 65 million people in the US each year "catch" the common cold, while another 108 million get the flu—and these are just two of the infectious diseases caused by viruses. Others include genital herpes, which affects an estimated 45 million people, as well as hepatitis C, which afflicts 170 million people in the world. Even a simple viral infection like a viral sore throat poses a challenge for any doctor who relies exclusively on antibiotics and other conventional prescription medications.

Echinacea, like some other immune-enhancing herbs, has a direct antiviral effect. Even better, it seems to summon all the resources of the immune system to help destroy viral invaders.

It also works well in combination with other antiviral plants and herbs. I like to prescribe echinacea in a formula called the "virus cocktail," which is comprised of echinacea, *lomatium, astragalus, reishi* and *licorice root*. The synergistic blend of these herbs tends to be more effective than any one herb by itself.

Bacteria and fungus

Since echinacea enhances the action of your immune cells, it is also effective against bacterial, fungal and yeast infections. This is especially helpful if you're fighting a bacterial infection, because many bacteria are now resistant to antibiotics (because they're overprescribed by doctors for things like viral infections). If needed, there is no problem using echinacea in combination with antibiotics. As a matter of fact, I find when people are on antibiotics for a bacterial infection and use echinacea simultaneously, they recover more quickly.

At least one study—which included 4,190 patients—confirmed this observation. Researchers divided the patients into two groups and gave almost half the subjects an antibacterial mixture that included echinacea (along with two other herbs—*thuja* and *baptisia*). Along with that formula, the patients received antibiotics that were chosen by the doctors. For comparison, the rest of the patients received only antibiotics, with no herbal formula.

The results showed the effectiveness of taking herbal antibacterial agents along with antibiotics. In the group that got an echinacea-based formula plus an antibiotic, people were cured significantly faster and there was a lower incidence of recurring infection than in the group of people who just got an antibiotic. Also, the symptoms of "sore throat" and "difficulty in swallowing" were improved much more efficiently in the first group than in the second group.

Dosage: Echinacea is generally available as a tincture, capsule, tablet or cream in the US. It's also possible to take it in the form of an injection, though this method is mainly used in Germany.

Glycerine (alcohol-free) tinctures are available. These are good for kids, who especially like the berry-flavored varieties.

• **Tincture.** I recommend 20 to 60 drops of the tincture every two to three hours for acute infections or twice daily for long-term use.

• **Capsule.** I recommend 500 to 1,000 mg every two to three hours for acute infections or twice daily for long-term use.

Note: High-potency, quality echinacea products are standardized to contain additional active ingredients such as alkylamides, cichoric acid and polysaccharides.

Some controversy surrounds the length of time one can use echinacea. Many authors state that echinacea should not be used on a long-term basis. However, there are no studies showing that long-term use is harmful or that echinacea loses its effectiveness.

I generally recommend patients use echinacea for acute infections until they are completely over the illness. For those who are very susceptible to infections, especially during the winter, and do not want to change their lifestyle, echinacea can be used on a long-term basis (although it is not so effective as improving diet, reducing stress and exercising). Long-term use of echinacea throughout the winter season is common in European countries.

What are the side effects? There has been no reported toxicity with echinacea, but two patients of mine have had allergic reactions, with some throat swelling after they started taking echinacea. Such a reaction has the potential of being life-threatening. In both cases, I recommended that my patients avoid using echinacea and switch to other immune-enhancing herbs instead.

Recommendations for…

•**Autoimmune conditions**. There is some controversy about prescribing echinacea to patients who have autoimmune diseases—that is, conditions that become worse when the immune system is overactive. The German Commission E, the government-backed medical board from Germany that helps regulate herbal medicine, recommends that echinacea should not be used in those who have tuberculosis, leukosis, collagenosis, multiple sclerosis, AIDS and HIV, lupus, rheumatoid arthritis and other autoimmune conditions. The assumption is that echinacea will worsen the hypersensitivity of the immune system, causing a flare-up of problems.

While I often agree with many of the Commission E recommendations, many physicians point out that there have not been any studies showing that echinacea is harmful for autoimmune conditions. I have not seen or read any reports where a patient with one of these conditions was made worse from using echinacea, despite the fact that millions of people take it every year.

That said, echinacea would not be my first choice for a condition such as multiple sclerosis, rheumatoid arthritis or other autoimmune diseases. But when my patients with these conditions have an acute infection, such as a cold or urinary-tract infection, I often recommend echinacea and other immune-enhancing herbs to fight off the infection. Usually these herbs are helpful; in any case, they don't seem to aggravate the autoimmune disease.

Interestingly, German physicians commonly use echinacea as a topical cream to relieve rheumatoid arthritis symptoms. These same doctors also frequently recommend echinacea be taken internally for its natural anti-inflammatory effects. Furthermore, newer research is showing that many autoimmune conditions are due to the immune system reacting to infectious agents, and cross-reacting with the body's own tissue at the same time. In theory, this would make echinacea helpful for these conditions. More studies are needed to tell us exactly what effect—both good or bad—echinacea has for people with inflammatory or autoimmune conditions.

• **Common cold**. I have found that echinacea can help prevent the common cold as well as reduce the symptoms and shorten the duration—but results differ. Some people respond almost miraculously, while others get no benefits at all. Overall, though, echinacea is more effective than over-the-counter medicines, which only help to reduce some of the symptoms of a cold and do nothing to assist the immune system or battle the infection.

One clinical study looked at the effectiveness of Echinacea purpurea for 120 patients who had the initial symptoms of the common cold, with "acute, uncomplicated upper airways infection." When these patients took 20 drops of echinacea every two hours for the first day—and thereafter three times daily—they fared much better than another group that took a placebo. At the end of the 10-day study, patients were questioned about the intensity of their illness and the time it took them to improve. In the echinacea group, people averaged four days to recover, while those in the placebo group took an average of eight days to recover.

• **Flu**. Yes, there are a few antiviral drugs that can help treat the flu. However, the clinical data on these drugs does not impress me very much. The most commonly prescribed drug, amantadine, isn't at all effective in the first two or three days. This is a real drawback because most people experience their worst symptoms during the first 72 hours of a flu attack.

Fortunately, my clinical experience has shown that herbs like echinacea can often help with symptoms the first 24 hours. This is supported by research—but research studies also suggest that the size of the dose is an important factor. In a study of 180 men and women between the ages of 18 and 60, researchers compared three different groups. The first group took a placebo. The second got 90 drops of Echinacea purpurea every day, which is the equivalent of a 450-mg dose, while the third group received double that, or 900 mg daily. Symptoms of all participants were evaluated after three to four days and again after eight to ten days. The results showed that 90 drops of tincture had little effect, but the people who took 180 drops were significantly better off, with less-severe symptoms that lasted for a shorter time.

• **Skin conditions**. In North America, echinacea has not quite caught on as a topical treatment for skin conditions. But many European makers of skin products are including the herbal ingredient.

A review of 4,958 clinical cases focused in on the effectiveness of echinacea ointment. The main researcher for the study concluded that the ointment was highly effective for many skin conditions. These included 1,453 patients with wounds, 900 with varicose ulcers, 629 with eczema, 26 with burns, 222 with herpes simplex and 212 with inflammatory skin problems. More than 90 percent positive results occurred when the ointment was used to treat burns, wounds and herpes.

• **Vaginitis**. Reoccurring vaginal yeast infections can be quite troublesome for women. One German study looked at 203 women with this condition. Of the 60 women taking echinacea (while the rest took a placebo or other medicines), only 10 had recurrences of yeast infections.

A boon in pregnancy

Pregnant women have to be careful about anything they eat, which includes supplements, so I am often asked whether echinacea is safe to use throughout pregnancy. My answer is yes. Echinacea has a long history of use by herbalists and naturopathic doctors for the treatment of acute infections during pregnancy. If a pregnant woman has a cold, flu or urinary-tract infection, I would not hesitate to recommend echinacea. Side effects or problems with the pregnancy or health of the baby have not been reported. In fact, my wife used echinacea during her entire first pregnancy with no adverse effects.

One study by the Hospital for Sick Children, Toronto, done in association with the Canadian Naturopathic College, has confirmed the safety of echinacea use during pregnancy. A group of 206 women who used echinacea during pregnancy for upper-respiratory-tract infections were analyzed along with a control group of 198 pregnant women who had upper-respiratory-tract infections but never used echinacea. The researchers found no association with the use of echinacea and birth defects. There were also no differences in the rate of live births or spontaneous abortions between the two groups.

Benefits for athletes

Sports medicine specialists studied the effect of echinacea on men who participated in triathlons—those grueling events that involve long-distance swimming, running and cycling. It is well known that triathletes are at an increased risk for infection because they train so exhaustively for each event. Among the participants of the study, some took a placebo, others were given a mineral supplement (43 mg of magnesium), while a third group took eight milliliters of Echinacea purpurea daily. All three groups of athletes took the supplements for 28 days before a triathlon.

During training, one-quarter to one-third of the athletes taking a placebo or mineral supplement winded up getting colds. (Athletes taking magnesium missed 13 days of training, while those in the placebo group missed a total of 24 days.) None of those who were taking echinacea showed any cold symptoms, and none missed any training days.

Nature's Virus Killers for Colds and Flu

D o you have to get a cold or the flu this coming season? No! This year can be different. With the right preparation, quick intervention and a lineup of powerful, natural virus fighters, there is a good chance that you can enjoy fall and winter without getting sick. *Here's how...*

Know your enemy

Colds and flu are both caused by viruses. They are spread through the air by coughs and sneezes and through contact with contaminated objects, such as a doorknob or a hand that has been used to cover a cough. A virus is little more than a clump of genetic material (DNA or RNA) inside a packet made of protein. Stray viruses constantly land on your body. The trouble starts when they attach to cell receptors and get inside your cells. Viruses use the cells' own reproductive equipment to duplicate themselves—damaging more and more cells as they churn out millions of look-alikes.

It actually is a good sign when you begin to get a stuffy head or a runny nose. Your body is fighting back. Your immune system picks up signals from the by-products of viral activity—pain, redness, swelling, heat, fever and rash are results of your immune system launching a counterattack. Mucus is produced to help expel viral intruders.

Flu viruses are a lot more powerful than typical cold viruses. Cold symptoms are mainly confined to the head, neck and chest. Flu causes more generalized symptoms, such as fever, body aches, nausea, cramping, vomiting and severe fatigue. Flu also can develop into bronchitis. In the worst cases, it can lead to pneumonia and other severe respiratory diseases that are sometimes fatal, especially in the elderly or others with weakened immune systems.

Recent threat: The H1N1 virus, which affected large numbers of young people.

I don't recommend the H1N1 vaccine for anyone, because far too little is known about it and its long-term side effects. I would recommend the same natural approach that can be used for the regular flu.

Start with prevention

I'll tell you about great ways to feel better if you get a cold or flu, but prevention should be your first line of defense…

• **Avoid spending time around people who already are sick**, particularly if they're coughing or sneezing. If you live with someone who is sick, sleep in separate rooms. Wash your hands frequently during cold-and-flu season, and don't share towels—assign one to each family member or use paper towels. Keep your hands away from your face, especially your nose, mouth and eyes.

• **Take vitamins**. A good multivitamin/mineral supplement provides a base of nutrients to support a healthy immune system. A formula that I recommend as a preventive against viral infections is Source Naturals Wellness Formula (to find a retailer near you, call 800-815-2333 or go to www.sourcenaturals.com). It contains vitamins A and C, which are involved in the formation of antibodies… the minerals zinc and *selenium*… and immune-supportive herbs, such as *garlic, echinacea* and *astragalus,* which increase the activity of virus-fighting white blood cells. The dosage used to prevent infection is two capsules daily during cold-and-flu season, taken in conjunction with your year-round multisupplement.

• **Reduce exposure to toxins**. You are more vulnerable to viral infection when your body is "distracted" by having to deal with toxins that can damage or suppress the immune system. Toxins aren't necessarily exotic—they could include sugars and alcohol consumed to excess, fast food and other unhealthy food laced with artificial preservatives and/or pesticides. Smoking and secondhand smoke injures the respiratory tract and makes you and your children more susceptible to colds and flus. Toxins also include small but significant amounts of metals —mercury, arsenic and lead—that you can get from food, water and air pollution.

It is even more vital to eat healthfully during cold-and-flu season because you're indoors more and are exposed to higher concentrations of germs. Go easy on holiday sweets and other treats, and you will be less likely to get sick.

Many people cut back their exercise regimens in winter months—a big mistake, since exercise strengthens your immune system. Also consider sitting in a dry sauna once or twice a week for 20 to 30 minutes… or a wet sauna for 10 to 15 minutes. Saunas increase sweating, which excretes toxins. Be sure to check with your doctor first if you have diabetes or heart disease.

For those who get colds or the flu every year, I recommend taking a super-greens formula in the fall to remove toxins from the colon, liver and lymphatic system. It also can be taken year-round for gentle continuous detoxification. One good product is Greens+ (800-643-1210, www.greensplus.com), which contains chlorella, wheat grass, super-green foods and detoxifying herbs such as milk thistle. The dosage is one scoop a day dissolved in water or juice.

Do not forget the impact that toxic emotions can have on the immune system. Anger, anxiety, resentment, loneliness and other chronic emotional difficulties trigger the release of hormones that suppress immune function. Seek support to overcome these problems if they linger.

Do conventional therapies help?

At the first sign of a runny nose or scratchy throat, some people head straight to the drugstore for cold and flu remedies. However, there are no conventional drugs—available either by prescription or over the counter—that help cure the common cold. Nasal decongestants and pain medications may make you feel better, but they don't address the actual viral infection. Natural remedies also can help you to feel better—with fewer potential side effects—and they simultaneously improve immune function.

For flu, on the other hand, a number of effective prescription antiviral drugs are available that may reduce the flu's severity and duration (by one or two days) if taken within 48 hours of the first signs of illness. Such medicines include *amantadine* (Symmetrel), *rimantadine* (Flumadine), *zanamivir* (Relenza) and *oseltamivir* (Tamiflu). Possible short-term side effects range from central nervous system problems, including anxiety and light-headedness, to decreased respiratory function and digestive upset. These antiviral drugs are not approved for children under age one.

All of these antiviral drugs except zanamivir also are approved for *preventing* the flu during outbreaks. These may benefit individuals who are *immunocompromised*—for example, those who have AIDS or have had organ or bone transplants. I prefer to have my otherwise healthy patients focus on effective natural therapies since they work so well and rarely cause side effects.

Rely on nature's virus killers

If you start to come down with a cold or the flu, my first recommendation is to change your diet. Eat lightly so that your body can focus on healing. For the first 24 hours, consume filtered water, broths and soups with lots of garlic, onions and spices, such as turmeric and cayenne, which relieve congestion, promote circulation and have a natural anti-inflammatory effect. Herbal teas (especially ginger, cinnamon and peppermint) and steamed vegetables also are good choices. When you're feeling better, move toward a more normal diet.

I have found several supplements to be effective for treating colds and flu. Consider taking these when people around you are sick or when you first feel cold and flu symptoms that can include fever (flu), headache (flu), fatigue, stuffy nose, sneezing, sore throat, chest discomfort, coughing and general aches and pains. You can use one or any combination until you feel better.

• **Lomatium dissectum** is a plant once used by Native Americans to fight Spanish flu. Preliminary research indicates that lomatium has the ability to prevent viruses from replicating and to stimulate white blood cell activity. With colds and flu, I often see improvement within 24 hours. In my experience, the only side effect has been an allergic reaction in the form of a measleslike rash in a small percentage of users. This rash will disappear a few days after lomatium is discontinued.

Eclectic Institute makes a potent product called Lomatium-Osha (800-332-4372, www.eclecticherb.com), which soothes the respiratory tract. This product is 50 percent alcohol, so take only the dosage that's recommended on the label. Women who are pregnant or nursing should not use lomatium.

• **Elderberry**, as shown by research in Israel, can stimulate the immune system, enhance white blood cell activity and inhibit viral replication. Flu patients have reported significant improvement within 48 hours of taking elderberry. It also helps with colds. A reliable brand is Sambucus Bio-Certified Black Elderberry Immune Syrup from Nature's Way (to find a retailer, call 800-962-8873 or go to www.naturesway.com). Adults should take two teaspoons four times daily… children, one teaspoon four times daily.

• **Echinacea**, contrary to recent media reports, can be effective for treating colds and flu. Echinacea makes the body's own immune cells more efficient in attacking viruses. The key is using a product that has been processed to contain a high level of active constituents. Ground-up echinacea root or leaves will not do much. The use of alcohol and water by the manufacturer to extract active components is critical to the product's potency. Also, be sure to use enough (many people don't).

Two potent, well-researched products include Fresh Alcohol-Free Echinacea Extract, the Natural Berry Flavor, and Echinamide Anti-V Formula Softgels, both by Natural Factors (to find a retailer, call 800-322-8704 or go to www.naturalfactors.com). This echinacea has been shown to reduce the length and severity of the common cold.

If you feel a cold or the flu coming on, take 20 drops of liquid extract or two capsules every two waking hours for 24 hours, then cut back to every three waking hours until the illness has passed.

The same company produces a liquid preparation known as Anti-V Formula, which contains *Echinamide*, *lomatium* and other virus fighters. It is the most aggressive product for cold and flu from the Natural Factors line and can be used instead of the other supplements. Take 1.5 milliliters every two waking hours for the first 48 hours and then every three waking hours until the illness is gone.

• **Homeopathic influenzinum** is an intriguing remedy that I have used with success. Made from active flu strains, it stimulates the body's own defense system to resist infection. It works along the same lines as an oral vaccine, but since it is homeopathic, none of the flu particles are left in the preparation. It can be used for prevention or treatment of flu and has no side effects.

Take two 30C-potency pellets twice daily for two weeks at the beginning of flu season (in early November). Take two pellets four times daily when exposed to flu sufferers or if you start to have symptoms. It is available from health-food stores and The Vitamin Shoppe (866-293-3367, www.vitaminshoppe.com).

• **Oscillococcinum** is another great homeopathic remedy for flu, which is also available from The Vitamin Shoppe, health-food markets and pharmacies or by phoning 800-264-7661 or visiting www.oscillo.com. It can be taken at the first sign of flu and is the number-one–selling homeopathic flu remedy in the US.

• **N-acetylcysteine** (NAC) helps thin the mucus that may accompany a cold or the flu. In addition to making you feel better, NAC helps to prevent sinus and more serious chest infections. A study at University of Genoa, Italy, showed that NAC, when taken as a supplement, could help prevent as well as treat flu. The nutrient increases amounts of the powerful antioxidant *glutathione* in the body, which, in turn, improves immune function. NAC is available at any health-food store and many pharmacies. If you tend to get the flu every year, take 600 mg twice daily when you are around people who have the flu or if you start feeling sick yourself.

• **Vitamin C** enhances the activity of white blood cells. I have found that taking 3,000 mg to 5,000 mg daily helps fight viral infections. However, some people get diarrhea from this amount. For immediate treatment of symptoms, start with 5,000 mg in divided doses. If loose stools occur, cut back to 3,000 mg (or even less).

Revealing the REAL Truth Behind the Flu Vaccine: How to Dodge the Flu Bullet This Year, and Every Year—Naturally

It's the time of year when my patients, and *Health Revelations* readers like you, ask me how they can avoid becoming the flu's next target. Each year I fine-tune my recommendations based on the most recent science. December is the perfect time to follow an aggressive natural approach for preventing the flu. Historically, flu activity peaks in the US in January or February.[1] So now is the time to get serious about shoring up your immune system to prevent this bug from moving in for a while.

By now you will have been bombarded for months by corporate-driven media, the medical establishment, and schools (if you have children) about the dire consequences of not getting the flu vaccine. In fact, the flu vaccination propaganda has gotten so darn strong these days that if you refuse the flu shot you get labeled "negligent, uneducated and a reckless member of society." I firmly believe, that in reality, the opposite is true. Those who have done their research and understand the limitations and potential adverse effects of the flu vaccine—and have sought credible NATURAL methods for preventing the flu—are ahead of the curve.

Let me explain why, starting with what the flu vaccine is *really* about.

Flu vaccine roulette

The truth is the yearly flu vaccine is nothing more than the product of a guessing game. Take the 2012-2013 flu vaccine for example. This year's vaccine is designed to protect against three of the common influenza (flu) viruses. This includes specific strains of influenza B virus, influenza A (H1N1) virus, and influenza A (H3N2) virus. But for vaccines to be manufactured and delivered in time for peak season in the US, they must be mass produced early. So months before the start of flu season they're playing a game of pick the virus strain out of a hat.

Now, to be fair there are *some* criteria they're using to make their choices, including the activity of flu strains in other parts of the world. However, the problem with this game of vaccine roulette lies in the very nature of viruses. You see, viruses mutate; that is, they change their structure, so a premade vaccine may not be identical to the strains that ultimately affect our country.

On its website, the Centers for Disease Control and Prevention (CDC) states, "It's not possible to predict with certainty which flu viruses will predominate during a given season," and "Because of these factors, there is always the possibility of a less than optimal match between circulating viruses and the viruses in the vaccine."[2] I wholeheartedly agree.

Does the flu shot work?

Getting the truth about the effectiveness of the flu vaccine from mainstream medicine is tricky. When you talk with so-called "flu experts," much like with politicians you *do* get an answer, but it often comes with very little detail.

I believe the flu vaccine is of limited value at best. The first major stumbling block for the flu shot is the one I've already mentioned, which is that the flu strains are selected many months ahead of time. Viruses can mutate quickly, meaning that it's simply not possible for the strains

The two types of conventional flu vaccines[3]

1) The regular "flu shot" is an inactivated vaccine (containing killed virus) that's given intravenously using a needle, usually in the arm. It's approved for people older than 6 months, including healthy people and people with chronic medical conditions.

In addition to the regular flu shot, two other flu shots are available:

- A high-dose flu shot approved for people 65 and older, and

- An intradermal flu shot approved for people 18 to 64 years of age.

2) The nasal-spray flu vaccine is made with live, weakened flu viruses and is given as a nasal spray. It's approved for use in healthy people 2 through 49 years of age who are not pregnant.

chosen for the current year's vaccine to always be correct. So, in the end, you're really just taking a literal shot in the dark.

According to CDC data from January and March 2012 the 2011-2012 flu shot was 52 percent effective in preventing illness.[4] Now, even if you give the CDC the benefit of the doubt on how they came to this effectiveness rate (do keep in mind this is the same agency that took the stance that mercury-containing vaccines are not a health hazard!) there's an important factor missing here. You must also take into account that all the experts agreed that 2011-2012 flu season was a relatively *mild* one. And when you factor this into the equation, suddenly the 52 percent effectiveness rate isn't overly exciting. And here's why.

Suppose we have a very nasty flu strain that was making a lot of people extremely sick... so many that it becomes an epidemic infecting 60 million Americans or more. (This is entirely possible considering that CDC statistics state that within an average season five percent to 20 percent of the population gets the flu.[5]) If the flu shot ends up being about

50 percent effective, then you would have no hope of controlling the epidemic. There would still be 30 million or more people very sick with the flu. Remember, during 1918-1919 the influenza pandemic (meaning worldwide epidemic), known as the Spanish flu, killed up to 40 million people worldwide. It was the most devastating epidemic in recorded world history. An estimated 675,000 Americans perished.[6]

Is the flu shot even safe?

Now let's talk about the issue of side effects. One of the hushed-up embarrassments for the flu manufacturers comes to us from Canada. Influenza experts at the British Columbia Centre for Disease Control noticed something strange. People who got the 2008-2009 flu shot seemed *more* likely to get infected by the virus than people who hadn't received a flu shot at all.[7]

Reports from other provinces showed the same odd result. So the Canadian influenza experts decided to recreate the situation using ferrets to see if they could figure out the mystery. Surprisingly, the ferrets that received the flu shot and were then exposed to the flu virus got *sicker* than the animals that were exposed to the virus without first being inoculated.[8]

As you may have already discovered for yourself, one of the common side effects of the flu vaccine is flu-like symptoms including achiness and a low grade fever. Frankly, I've heard this complaint so often over the years from people who have experienced this unfortunate side effect first hand, that I've lost count. And when you consider how widespread the reports of this side effect are, there's no doubt that what we're seeing is an immune reaction to the vaccine.

Feeling like you *have* the flu after taking a shot to *prevent* it is bad enough, but it gets worse... much worse. The flu vaccine often contains thimerosal, a preservative that's laced with toxic mercury. Mercury can damage the brain, central nervous system, immune system, thyroid, and other vital organs.

Now you've probably heard that the flu shot *doesn't* contain mercury anymore. This is misleading! Although thimerosal *has* been eliminated from most vaccines for childhood diseases, it's *still* being used in many flu shots.

The truth is that while single-dose vials are mercury-free, multi-dose vials (a vial that can be used for many doses) still contain thimerosal… a fact that can easily be confirmed on the CDC website.[9] And, of course, since it's much less expensive for pharmacies and doctor's offices to carry the multi-dose vial many do. So should you choose to get the flu vaccine make sure it's thimerosal-free from a single-dose vial. Confirm it with your own eyes before allowing the injection!

But I'm not done with unwelcome additions to the vaccine yet. There are more potentially dangerous ingredients which are being used as pre-servatives and stabilizers to extend the shelf life of the flu shot. This ap-palling list includes antibiotics, the steroid hydrocortisone, monosodium glutamate (MSG), and formaldehyde.[10]

The CDC's *own* website lists formaldehyde as a "toxic substance" and states that it's "known to be a human carcinogen."[11] And the other ingredients have their own checkered pasts. Yet we're willingly injecting ourselves, and our loved ones, with these toxin-laced shots year after year. And the biggest victims of all are our children who, by the tender age of two, have been subjected to over thirty vaccines and, of course, right along with them a laundry-list of dangerous contaminants, preservatives, and stabilizers![12]

Flu vaccine failure

Ultimately, the case for pressuring Americans to get the flu vaccine is weak. Some holistic doctors believe it just doesn't have any effectiveness at all—period. The truth is that some years it probably does offer some limited protection. The problem is that it doesn't have a *consistent* record of high protection rates. And that poor record has to be weighed against potential exposure to mercury as well as other toxins and contaminants. In addition, there are no long-term safety studies on the flu vaccine so we simply don't know how it affects our health over the long haul. Or what effect over-stimulating the immune system may have.

The fact is there are safe and effective natural methods for preventing the flu that outperform the vaccine. And these natural methods are surely safer.

And keep in mind that you're being exposed to hundreds of other viruses that cause upper respiratory tract infections as you go about your daily life. The flu vaccine doesn't offer you a lick of protection against those other viruses. Yet many natural therapies used for flu prevention are designed to improve your *overall* immune system, which gives you added protection against all those other infections too.

Prevent the flu naturally

One of the most effective and cheapest methods to prevent the flu is to use a homeopathic remedy known as Influenzinum. It works on the same principles as a vaccine, but without the toxic preservatives or potential immune damage you see with conventional vaccines. Influenzinum is an extremely diluted homeopathic preparation that is thousands of times more dilute than a conventional vaccine. According to modern homeopathic research it works by introducing a "vibratory frequency" of the flu strains to the body's immune system. This kicks your body's immune system into action and essentially creates a memory for the flu strains. Yet because it's so dilute it poses little possibility of adverse reactions.

In my files I have a very interesting survey from the French Society of Homeopaths. Keep in mind that thousands of French medical doctors are practitioners of homeopathy. In the survey of 23 homeopathic doctors it was found that 90 percent of 453 people who took Influenzinum didn't get the flu. I've used the treatment for over 15 years in my own practice and my own informal studies have shown a similar success record.

I have patients take one milliliter of the liquid form or two pellets of either a 30C or 200C potency once monthly during the flu season (November to April). You can purchase this homeopathic remedy at health food stores, online, or directly from holistic doctors at their offices.

Defend with D

There's good evidence that vitamin D reduces the risk of developing and dying from the flu. When flu season peaks people are indoors more, which not only exposes them to other people with the flu, but also comes at a time when they're exposed to fewer of the ultraviolet rays from the sun that are needed to boost vitamin D production. We know that vitamin D improves immunity by increasing white blood cell activity. It also boosts the levels of two microbe-killing compounds known as cathelicidin and defensins. One randomized controlled trial using daily doses of 1,200 IU of vitamin D for school children in Japan found that only 10.8 percent of children taking vitamin D caught type A influenza compared with almost twice that number of children taking a placebo.[13]

I find most adults do well taking 5,000 IU of vitamin D daily with a meal. For children and infants a typical dose is 1,000 to 2,000 IU daily. Have your doctor check your blood level of this nutrient. In my view an optimal level is 60 to 80 ng/mL.

Help prevent flu with probiotics

A healthy gut is required for a healthy immune system that protects you against infections. Part of that protection comes from hidden patches of "lymphoid" tissue in your gut. These patches, called "gut associated lymphoid tissue," produce disease-fighting factors, including antibodies. (By the way this includes the appendix, once thought by some to be a nonfunctioning remnant of evolutionary processes. Of course, every organ of the body was designed for a specific purpose. But that's a story for another time.)

Probiotics—the trillions of flora varieties that live throughout your body, but mainly in your digestive tract—are especially important for keeping those gut lymphoid tissues healthy. One study on seniors over the age of 70 found significant increases in antibodies to the flu virus in those who got the vaccine plus a probiotic versus those who got the vaccine and a placebo.[14]

Amino acid ally

Next up in your flu-fighting arsenal should be N'acetylcysteine (NAC). NAC is an amino acid-like substance that's been used in conventional medicine for the treatment of bronchitis and emphysema. It thins mucus, making it easier to excrete.

NAC has been shown to help prevent the flu and also reduce the severity of your symptoms if you get the virus. A landmark study found that only 25 percent of older people who were injected with flu virus after taking NAC for six months experienced flu symptoms versus 79 percent who took a placebo.[15] A preventative dose is 600 mg twice daily on an empty stomach.

Astragalus goes antiviral

Thousands of years of Chinese medicine experience and success is worth paying attention to. The Chinese herb *Astragalus membranaceus* is used by many practitioners of Traditional Chinese medicine, Naturopathic doctors, and herbalists to prevent respiratory tract infections like the flu.

The herb boosts production of white blood cells as well as the body's powerful antiviral chemicals known as interferons. Plus research suggests it boosts the levels of antibodies in the blood that bind to foreign invaders and signal the immune system to destroy viruses and bacteria. A typical preventative dose is 500 mg twice daily.

What to do if you get the flu

When patients come to my clinic suffering with the flu I start them on a variety of treatments. One of the first things I do is administer an intravenous treatment of vitamin C. When given in high doses intravenously vitamin C not only optimizes immune function, but directly kills the flu virus. I use doses ranging from 20,000 to 60,000 mg per treatment.

The results are nothing short of amazing and patients tolerate the treatment extremely well. I remember a few years back when there was a bad swine flu season and patients would come to the clinic with severe fatigue and muscle aches. Two days in a row of intravenous vitamin C made dramatic improvements in their recovery. Since you can't absorb high doses of vitamin C into the blood stream using oral vitamin C, supplements just can't compare to the intravenous form.

To help with aching and fatigue I also give them intravenous nutrients such as B vitamins, calcium, magnesium, trace minerals, and other antiviral nutrients including zinc and selenium. Another, similar option I use is intravenous pharmaceutical-grade hydrogen peroxide, which has a direct antiviral effect in the blood stream.

These treatments keep my patients comfortable while helping to prevent more serious problems such as bronchitis and pneumonia from developing. Intravenous treatments also have a side benefit of hydrating you, which is very important when you are suffering from the flu. Obviously only a doctor trained in nutritional medicine can administer these intravenous treatments.

Load up on elderberry

Everyone should have a high-quality elderberry extract in the medicine cabinet. The shrub is one of nature's most proven flu fighters. Studies have found it to be quite powerful in treating the flu. For example, one randomized, double-blind, placebo controlled trial involved 60 Norwegian men and women between the ages of 18 and 54 years. All volunteers selected for the study had a fever and at least one respiratory influenza symptom.

The volunteers received 15 mL of standardized elderberry syrup or placebo four times per day for 5 days (starting within 48 hours of their influenza-like symptoms). Symptoms were relieved on average four days earlier and the use of rescue medication was significantly less in those receiving standardized elderberry extract compared with placebo. None of the patients reported any adverse events during the study.[16]

Another noteworthy study, on both children and adults this time, was done by the same team of Israeli researchers. Within just two days a stunning 93.3 percent of the group that got elderberry had significant improvements in their symptoms, including fever. When you compare that to the 91.7 percent of the placebo group who had not shown *any* improvement until day 6, and it's clear to see who the winner is here.

In fact, within just two to three days 90 percent of the elderberry group had kicked *all* of their symptoms to the curb. But it took 90 percent of the placebo group six days to get rid of their symptoms completely.[17] The form of elderberry used in this study is available in a product called Sambucus from Nature's Way. I should mention that elderberry is also very effective for treating coughs.

Final word on flu

Lastly, if you get the flu make sure to eat lightly. You want your body to have to expend as little energy on digestion as it can. You should concentrate on eating broths, herbal teas such as ginger, and soups containing onions and garlic, which are antiviral. In addition, make sure you are drinking plenty of water to keep yourself hydrated and to help to detoxify and move secretions out of the body.

Hot water or tea with honey or cinnamon helps with sore throats and coughing. They also support mucus excretion. Make sure to avoid immune-suppressing foods such as milk products, wheat, fruit juices, and other simple sugars.

Garlic Can Stop the Sniffles

Nothing smells like garlic as it sizzles in a pan… and few natural ingredients have as many health benefits. Hundreds of studies help prove garlic's many health-promoting properties. It is a natural antibiotic and has a big advantage over antibiotic drugs—the body does not become resistant to garlic. Some of garlic's best-known benefits include its power to lower blood pressure, reduce total and LDL (bad) cholesterol and increase HDL (good) cholesterol.

To enhance your health, use garlic liberally in your cooking or take daily supplements—especially if you have high cholesterol or high blood pressure.

Bonus: Research shows that aged garlic extract (AGE), when combined with cholesterol-lowering drugs, can help reduce plaque buildup in the coronary arteries, lowering your risk for heart disease. Garlic is so good for you, I recommend that everyone take it every day.

Dosage: Four milliliters of AGE in liquid form or a total of 1,200 mg in capsule form daily.

AGE has additional special powers, including one that may come in handy this winter—use it to relieve sinus pain and pressure.

How: Tilt your head back and place two drops of liquid AGE into each nostril. Keep your head back for five seconds. You will feel a warm sensation, then your nose will begin to run. The garlic appears to work by acting as an irritant—prompting the sinuses to drain—and an antibacterial, antiviral and antifungal agent, proven in studies to kill the germs that cause sinus infections.

My patients typically report that their sinus pressure and headache are gone within 30 minutes. Administer as needed—typically once a day—and if you're not better in a few days, see your doctor. This treatment is safe for everyone, except perhaps those who get nosebleeds easily—then I wouldn't recommend irritating the nostrils.

Good brands: Kyolic (800-421-2998, www.kyolic.com) and Nature's Answer (800-439-2324, www.naturesanswer.com). AGE is sold in drugstores and health-food stores.

The Hydrogen Peroxide "Miracle Cure" That Your Doctor's Never Even Heard Of

Forty-eight year old Cara had been feeling tired for the past two months. At first she thought it was the stress of family life and her business that were at the root of her fatigue. But those things hadn't changed much for the past few years. She felt as if something else must be going on in her body.

I asked if she was having any signs of menopause such as a changing cycle or hot flashes. If she was in the beginnings of menopause, then her fatigue was likely caused by a drop in hormone levels which could easily be corrected and her energy would come bouncing back. But she didn't have any obvious symptoms of premenopause.

Cara told me that her body would ache at times. She wondered if she might have fibromyalgia. Her muscle aches and fatigue symptoms were certainly similar. I explained that even if she did have fibromyalgia, which I was not convinced she did, if we treated the root cause of the condition her symptoms should go away.

I ordered a battery of blood tests to see what was going on in her body. One of her tests was for Epstein Barr Virus. This virus causes mononucleosis. Between 85 percent to 90 percent of American adults have antibodies to this virus showing past infection. Symptoms commonly include a sore throat, swollen glands in the neck, and extreme fatigue. With rest most people recover from this viral infection in a few weeks, and in more severe cases up to a few months. Of course natural therapies that enhance the immune system can help you recover quicker! In fact a healthy immune system can keep this virus suppressed for the rest of your life.

While experts don't all agree, it appears that some people can have a reactivation of the Epstein Barr virus when their immune system becomes suppressed. Cara's life was causing her a lot of emotional distress and this put her at a higher risk for the virus kicking back in. As you probably already guessed, her test showed that Epstein Barr had once again reared its ugly head.

A powerful weapon against viruses yet virtually unknown

Her treatment will surprise you. It's one of complementary medicine's most powerful weapons against viruses yet virtually unknown except by a minority of doctors—good old hydrogen peroxide, or H_2O_2. Hydrogen

Hydrogen peroxide is naturally produced in your body

Hydrogen peroxide is also created in your digestive tract by friendly Lactobacillus flora. This acts as a fuel source to healthy aerobic (oxygen dependent) bacteria and it eliminates unhealthy anaerobic (do not require oxygen) bacteria. You also find hydrogen peroxide in the breast milk of nursing mothers, presumably for its antimicrobial properties. It's even needed by the body for enzyme reactions involving the production of thyroid and other hormones in the body. H_2O_2 dilates your blood vessels and improves circulation. It's also involved in detoxification pathways to rid the body of harmful toxins.

peroxide was first identified in 1818 and today it is generally used for pulp and paper bleaching, reducing the odor of waste treatment plants, and as a topical antimicrobial agent for the skin or counter surfaces.

Hydrogen peroxide is an oxidative agent. Oxidizing agents are able to destroy microbes like viruses or bacteria. As a matter of fact your white blood cells naturally use H_2O_2 to destroy foreign invaders as part of your immune response. Since the human body naturally uses H_2O_2 it's well tolerated when it is used correctly.

With Cara, I used a special highly diluted medical grade hydrogen peroxide delivered by an IV into her veins. My goal was to enhance what her body would naturally do, by introducing a small amount of H_2O_2 right into her blood stream reducing the viral load of the Epstein Barr Virus. This same effect actually occurs with intravenous vitamin C as well—it naturally increases the level of hydrogen peroxide in the blood stream for an all out assault on harmful intruders. H_2O_2 has an added bonus of significantly increasing the activity of immune cells known as T and B lymphocytes, which are critical for destroying viruses.

H_2O_2 had the potential to help millions

After three treatments Cara was feeling much better and by five treatments her energy had soared. She had her health back! Currently intravenous hydrogen peroxide is used by thousands of holistic doctors around the world, and very successfully I would add. But it's not being used nearly as much as it should be. If the practice was more widely known and used in local doctor's offices and hospitals it has the potential to help millions. Some suspect it hasn't ever been chosen as a conventional therapy because it's not patentable. And most doctors don't know that it's even possible to use it as a treatment.

Side effects with intravenous H_2O_2 are uncommon. But, obviously you should never use hydrogen peroxide internally without medical supervision. As with any intravenous procedure it could cause irritation of the vein, rashes, headache, and anxiety. I rarely see any adverse effects with its use. When used at the right concentration and dose and given over a long enough period of time (about 90 minutes) it rarely causes problems. It should not be given to anyone who is pregnant or anyone with anemia, thalassemia, sarcoidosis, or tuberculosis.[1]

To find a doctor trained in intravenous hydrogen peroxide see the practitioner listing at the American College for the Advancement of Medicine at www.acam.org.

How to Conquer America's Growing Super-Infection Threat—Naturally

Imagine you go to the hospital to get some stitches for a cut, antibiotics for an infection, or God forbid something more serious like a heart attack or a surgery. You receive excellent treatment and you're on the way to recovery… but then you notice your abdomen starting to swell like a balloon. Soon severe abdominal pain causes you to writhe in pain and you have a fever and diarrhea accompanied by blood or pus in your stool.

You've just become yet another victim of a growing health problem that kills almost as many people as car accidents each year in the US. And while it kills approximately 30,000 people a year the problem actually affects 500,000 people a year.[1] I'm talking about *Clostridium difficile*, often referred to as *C. difficile*.

Are you at risk for this super infection?

C. difficile bacteria can cause a variety of digestive symptoms ranging from diarrhea to life-threatening inflammation of the colon known as colitis. Rates of infection from this nasty bug have been increasing at an alarming rate the past decade. If you don't know someone who has had this problem you will.

The fact is *everyone* is susceptible to this infection, but you're even more at risk if you fall into any of the following groups:

- You have cancer or another immune-compromising condition

- You are hospital bound or in a long-term care facilities

- You are taking antibiotics

- You have recently had abdominal surgery or a gastrointestinal procedure

- You have a colon disease such as inflammatory bowel disease or colorectal cancer

- You have had a previous C. difficile infection

Seniors are even more susceptible to the bug than other adults with 25 percent of frail elderly people who get a C. difficile infection dying from it.[2] And, frighteningly, the number of kids getting these infections is skyrocketing. A recent study found a 12-fold increase in C. difficile among children with a stunning three out of four of the infections contracted *outside* of hospital settings![3]

Incredibly, about 20 percent of people who are hospitalized acquire C. difficile during hospitalization. More than 30 percent of those infected go on to develop diarrhea.[4] If you have diarrhea within two months of receiving antibiotics, or if you experience diarrhea within 72 hours after

---

Mainstream medicine goes natural

One "natural," and perhaps cringe-worthy, solution that's been accepted by conventional medicine is a "stool transplant." A healthy donor's stool (and of course the friendly bacteria it contains) is placed in your colon by a gastroenterologist with a scope or special tube that goes down the nose. This increasingly popular procedure increases the good bacteria locally within the colon allowing them to overtake the C. difficile.

being hospitalized, you should be tested for C. difficile infection.

Bacteria... the good, the bad, and the ugly

These bacteria exist throughout the environment in soil, water, and animal and human feces. C. difficile is present in two to three percent of healthy adults and in as many as 70 percent of healthy infants who never develop symptoms and do not require treatment.[5] This red flag tells me that the *balance* of our good bacteria (flora) plays an important role in protecting us against this opportunistic villain.

When levels of good bacteria in our gut get too low, C. difficile thrives and produces toxins that inflame the colon. This is why consuming cultured foods rich in good bacteria known as probiotics (yogurt, miso, tempeh, kefir, sauerkraut) as well as prebiotics that feed your good bacteria (Jerusalem artichoke, onions, leeks, peas, beans, garlic) are so important in preventing intestinal infections.

As conventional medicine has learned the hard way, when you over-use antibiotics bacteria can literally become resistant to the drugs. This is one of the biggest challenges we face with C. difficile. The bug has become resistant to most of our common antibiotics making it much more difficult to treat. And that's not the only harm antibiotics cause. These drugs also alter your gut flora by wiping out the protective good bacteria. This turns your gut into the perfect, breeding ground for C. difficile to thrive. You should always avoid antibiotics unless they're absolutely required!

How the creeping crud spreads

As disturbing as it is to think about, C. difficile is spread through fecal contamination. When someone doesn't wash their hands well enough after using the bathroom they can quickly contaminate surfaces such as telephones, remote controls, medical equipment, bathroom fixtures, light switches, chairs, tables, door knobs, and other frequently touched items. The spores from the bacteria are hearty and can survive for months on these types of surfaces. If you happen to touch a contaminated surface and then later touch your mouth the bugs can end up in the intestines where the damage occurs. This is why frequent hand washing with soap and lots of scrubbing is so important and why the surfaces of hospitals, clinics, nursing homes, and other frequented centers should be cleansed regularly.

The best test to find out if you're infected with C. difficile is a stool culture. If you are infected speedy treatment is required. First, if you're taking an antibiotic that has caused this problem it should be stopped. For mild cases of diarrhea without a fever, abdominal pain, and no increase of white blood cells (determined by blood test) this alone can sometimes resolve the symptoms. (I of course would add probiotic supplementation into the picture, but more on that later.) If your symptoms are more than mild, one of two antibiotics that still work against C. difficile are generally used: Metronidazole (oral or intravenous) or vancomycin (oral) for 10 days.

Unfortunately, about one-third of people treated with antibiotics have a relapse within three to 21 days after the treatment is discontinued. One desperate patient who came to see me had been having relapses on and off for almost an entire year! Repeated rounds of antibiotics could not clear her infection. Fortunately my natural treatment eradicated the problem within just a couple of weeks.

Probiotics to the rescue

In my experience using probiotics during and after antibiotic therapy will *dramatically* decrease the relapse rate. It's a shame that it's not standard protocol. Without changing the environment of the gut and populating it with "intestinal soldiers" you are often fighting a losing battle.

If you have a current infection or a history of infection I can't stress how important it is for you to supplement with the probiotic *Saccharomyces boulardii* (S. boulardii). This non-harmful yeast has been shown in studies to prevent antibiotic-associated diarrhea. A review of studies published in the highly respected *American Journal of Gastroenterology* found that yeast was effective in preventing antibiotic-associated diarrhea found in C. difficile infection.[6]

The probiotic has also been shown to reduce the risk of recurrence of C. difficile when taken in combination with the antibiotics metronidazole or vancomycin.[7,8,9] Research even suggests that S. boulardii helps decrease the toxicity of C. difficile by producing a protein-digesting enzyme that neutralizes the toxins produced by the C. difficile.[10]

But, unfortunately, despite all the research that clearly shows how beneficial S. boulardii is in these super infection cases it's rarely ever used by conventional doctors. That's a real shame since this inexpensive probiotic could greatly reduce the suffering of many and may even save lives.

To prevent C. difficile infection… especially if you're taking antibiotics in an environment such as a hospital or nursing home or if you've had a previous C. difficile infection… I recommend taking five billion S. boulardii organisms twice a day. If you have an active C. difficile infection you should take five to 10 billion organisms twice a day a few hours apart from your antibiotics.

More effective natural solutions

C. difficile is a serious matter. Don't settle for antibiotic therapy alone to treat this super infection. In addition to S. boulardii I also recommend taking a broad spectrum probiotic to boost the levels of immune-enhancing probiotics in your gut. A good choice is one containing the well-studied *Bifidobacterium longum* BB536 strain.

Another natural compound that has helped my patients eradicate C. difficile is colloidal silver. It has a broad-spectrum antimicrobial effect that doesn't seem to damage the good intestinal bacteria like antibiotics do. A good choice is Sovereign Silver. Take one teaspoon three to four times a day.

I have also found certain homeopathic remedies can help get symptoms such as diarrhea and abdominal pain under control quickly.

Three of the more common ones are:

- Arsenicum album—for symptoms of diarrhea accompanied by blood, fever, and chills

- Mercurius—for burning and spasming of the digestive tract.

- Sulphur—for explosive, burning diarrhea that has a very foul odor.

A local naturopathic doctor or practitioner schooled in homeopathy can help you make the choices that are best for you.

Lastly, millions of Americans take acid-suppressing medications known as proton pump inhibitors (PPIs) for acid reflux. Common examples include Aciphex, Dexilant, Nexium, Prevacid, and Prilosec. The FDA issued a statement in February of this year warning that their use may be linked to an increased risk of C. difficile diarrhea.[11]

The reason for the link between C. difficile and PPIs is not entirely clear. It's possible that stomach acid acts as a natural barrier to bacteria like C. difficile preventing them from easily entering the digestive tract. Remember, the infection normally makes its way in through the mouth and down through the stomach and intestines. When you suppress your stomach acid you have removed an important barrier to intestinal infections. If you're taking these medications and have diarrhea see your doctor immediately. And, of course, since most people can resolve their acid reflux with diet changes and weight loss I recommend working with a holistic doctor to resolve your acid reflux naturally.

Part X

Men and Women's Health

Natural Ways to Fight Prostate Enlargement

If you are a man approaching age 45, you have a nearly 50 percent chance of having an enlarged prostate. By age 70, the chances are almost nine in 10 that you'll have it. Called *benign prostatic hyperplasia* (BPH), the condition involves an enlarged prostate that compresses the urethra and partially blocks flow of urine. BPH is the most common prostate problem for men. While it's not life-threatening—it is not, for example, related to the development of prostate cancer—symptoms can be troublesome. Fortunately, there are natural ways to prevent and treat it.

The prostate pressure point

The job of the prostate is to produce fluid that nourishes and transports sperm. This walnut- sized gland weighs approximately 20 g, about as much as two Fig Newtons. Located in front of the rectum and below the bladder, the prostate surrounds the urethra, the passageway that carries urine away from the bladder and into the penis.

A swollen prostate can compress the urethra like a clamp on a garden hose, restricting urine flow. It also may press upward, irritating the outer wall of the bladder. This irritation makes the bladder wall thicker and even more easily irritated. A man with BPH might start having bladder contractions, making him feel the need to urinate frequently even when there's not much urine. Over time, the bladder may lose the ability to completely empty, increasing discomfort.

Possible causes

There remains a lot to be answered when it comes to the causes of BPH. One thing researchers can agree on is that hormonal factors play the largest role.

Research has focused on the hormone *testosterone* and a related substance called *dihydrotestosterone* (DHT). Some researchers believe that testosterone, an anabolic (growth-promoting) hormone, is the main culprit. Others disagree because prostate growth tends to be a problem later in a man's life, while the amount of testosterone is at its highest when males are in their late teens or early 20s.

The conversion of testosterone to DHT increases as men grow older—and DHT is very potent. It stimulates the proliferation of new prostate cells and slows the death of older ones. But if DHT is a cause, why do some men with prostate enlargement have normal DHT levels? Could another hormone be involved?

Now researchers are looking at the effect of the hormone *estrogen* (especially the kind called *estradiol*) on prostate growth. Estrogen isn't just a "female" hormone. Men have it as well, and as they age, estrogen levels increase. High estrogen-to-testosterone ratios could increase the effects of DHT on prostate cells.

Looking for trouble

The most common test to diagnose BPH and other prostate-related problems is a *digital rectal exam*. Your physician inserts a gloved finger into the rectum and feels the part of the prostate next to the rectum for any enlargement or hardness. All men over age 40 should have this test once a year.

A variety of pharmaceuticals can help relieve BPH symptoms, but each has potential side effects. Many physicians prescribe alpha-blockers, such as *terazosin* (Hytrin) or *doxazosin* (Cardura), which relax the neck of the bladder, making urination easier—but these can cause fatigue, weakness, headaches and dizziness. Another prescription drug, *finasteride* (Proscar), relieves symptoms by shrinking the prostate gland, but it can cause impotence and reduced sexual desire.

For men who have serious BPH problems that are interfering with their lifestyle, some doctors recommend surgical procedures—but surgery can lead to impotence or incontinence.

I find that drugs and surgery usually are unnecessary. As long as a man is getting his prostate checked at least once a year and there are no signs of tumor growth or urinary blockage, BPH can be treated with natural therapies. These include improved diet and supplements. Also, 30 minutes of daily exercise has been shown to reduce BPH symptoms quite significantly.

Healing foods

• **Avocados** contain *beta sitosterol*, a *phytonutrient* that protects against prostate enlargement by inhibiting growth factors that cause prostate swelling. Avocados also are a good source of *oleic acid*, a mono-unsaturated fatty acid that is thought to reduce inflammation, which can contribute to BPH. Have at least two weekly servings (one-fifth of a medium avocado per serving). If you do not like avocados, you can have three half-cup servings a week of peanuts, rice bran or wheat germ.

• **Fish** is a good source of *eicosapentaenoic acid* (EPA), a powerful omega-3 fatty acid that helps reduce swelling and inflammation. Eat at least two three-ounce servings of trout, salmon or sardines each week.

• **Ground flaxseed** has been shown to reduce estrogen levels, and it contains anti-inflammatory *omega-3 fatty acids*. I advise men to take one or two tablespoons daily along with 10 oz of water (to prevent constipation). As I have noted on several occasions, ground flaxseed has a mild, nutty flavor and can be added to salads, cereals, yogurt, smoothies and protein shakes or just eaten plain.

• **Pumpkin seeds** are natural sources of zinc. This mineral helps keep your prostate healthy by reducing the activity of the enzyme *5-alpha- reductase*, which produces DHT. Sprinkle a tablespoon or two of pumpkin seeds—raw or roasted, with or without the hulls—on salad, yogurt, cereal, etc. four times weekly.

• **Soy** contains a number of *phytoestrogens* (plant chemicals that balance estrogen), including *genistein*, which can help control prostate enlargement. I prefer fermented soy foods, such as miso, tempeh and fermented soy protein powder, which provide a form of genistein that can be readily absorbed by the body. Have at least one-half cup serving daily.

• **Tomatoes** are rich in the disease-fighting antioxidants known as *carotenoids*. Preliminary scientific research has suggested that tomatoes and tomato products help prevent prostate cancer. They also may have a beneficial effect on prostate enlargement. Consume two servings of fresh tomatoes and two servings of cooked tomatoes (e.g., tomato paste/sauce) weekly (one serving equals one-half to one cup of tomatoes and/or tomato sauce). If you don't like tomatoes, eat watermelon or cantaloupe.

Foods to avoid: Men with BPH should avoid caffeinated beverages and alcohol—they irritate and inflame the prostate. Also reduce your intake of foods that contain harmful fats, such as *hydrogenated* or *partially hydrogenated oils*, that promote inflammation. Stay away from packaged foods that are high in sugar, which also can worsen inflammation.

Natural supplements

The following supplements are listed in order of importance—start with the first and move down the list until you find what works best for you. Many formulas contain a blend of two or three of the ones listed.

• **Saw palmetto berry extract** is a mainstay in the natural treatment of BPH and alleviates most symptoms. It was first used medicinally by Native Americans for prostate and urinary tract problems. Recently, researchers have found that saw palmetto can help the prostate by reducing activity of the DHT-producing enzyme 5-alpha-reductase. A review of

18 randomized, controlled trials involving 2,939 men found saw palmetto to be as effective as the BPH drug finasteride.

It can take six to eight weeks before this natural prostate protector begins to fully take effect. I recommend a product that is standardized to contain 80 percent to 95 percent fatty acids (check the label) and a total daily dosage of 320 mg, which can be taken all at once. Two brands I recommend are Nature's Way Standardized Saw Palmetto Extract and Enzymatic Therapy Super Saw Palmetto, which are widely available at health-food stores. It is best to take it on an empty stomach. A small percentage of men get stomach upset from saw palmetto. If this occurs, try taking it with meals.

• **Pygeum africanum,** an extract that comes from the bark of the African plum tree, decreases the need to urinate at night and improves urine flow during the day. I prefer a formula that combines pygeum with saw palmetto, such as Ultra Saw Palmetto + Pygeum from Jarrow Formulas (www.jarrow.com, or call 310-204-2520 to locate a store near you). The daily pygeum dosage is 100 mg.

• **Nettle root** can provide you modest benefits. The nettle-containing product from Nutrilite, Saw Palmetto with Nettle Root, produced good results in a UCLA study. Over six months, the 44 men in the study showed modest improvements in BPH symptoms. The Nutrilite supplement includes saw palmetto, nettle root, beta-carotene, pumpkin seed oil and lemon bioflavonoid concentrate (Nutrilite, 714-562-6200, www.nutrilite.com). Take one softgel three times daily.

• **Pollen extracts** seem to relax the muscles of the urethra and improve the ability of the bladder to contract. The extract most widely tested is PollenAid (877-472-6469, www.graminex.com). Take three capsules daily before meals with a glass of water.

• **Fish oil** can help reduce prostate swelling and inflammation. Take 3,000 mg to 5,000 mg daily in addition to two weekly servings of fish. If you prefer a vegetarian source of omega-3 fatty acids, use one to two tablespoons of flaxseed oil.

Caution: Fish oil should not be used by anyone who takes blood-thinning medications such as *warfarin* (Coumadin).

Common symptoms of BPH

• A need to urinate frequently.

• Urination that is hard to start or stop.

• Weak urination or "dribbling."

• Sensation of an incompletely emptied bladder.

• Increased need to urinate at night.

• Burning pain accompanying urination.

• Recurring bladder infections.

Fight Osteoporosis the Natural Way—Simple Steps... For Women and Men

Misconceptions abound when it comes to osteoporosis, a dreaded disease that's marked by porous, brittle bones and hunched backs. Most people think of osteoporosis as a women's disease, but it's more than that. While eight million American women have been diagnosed with osteoporosis, more than two million men also are affected by it.

Osteoporosis: A silent problem

Osteoporosis can develop because, starting at about age 35, our bone cells do not make new bone as fast as it is broken down. Our bones become more frail and fracture more easily. Fractures, especially of the hip, spine and wrist, are more likely to occur, even without trauma. Osteoporosis has no symptoms until a bone is fractured. Many people go for decades without a diagnosis of osteoporosis—until they fall and an X-ray reveals porous bones.

Bone density can be measured with a *dual-energy X-ray absorptiometry* (DEXA) scan, but many people don't get this test. I recommend a baseline DEXA scan by age 50, and if results are normal, follow-ups every three to five years.

The most worrisome risk for a person with osteoporosis is a hip fracture. According to the National Osteoporosis Foundation (at www.nof. org), an average of 24 percent of hip-fracture patients age 50 or older die in the year following their fractures, often as a result of long-term immobilization that leads to blood clots or infection. Six months after a hip fracture, only 15 percent of patients can walk unaided across a room.

Virtually every person with osteoporosis who has come to my clinic is confused about the best way to promote bone health. Conventional doctors typically prescribe osteoporosis medication, such as *alendronate* (Fosamax) and *ibandronate* (Boniva). However, these drugs can cause side effects, such as digestive upset and blood clots, and they have been linked to thigh fracture risk. Plus, they don't address the underlying nutritional deficiencies that promote bone loss.

The natural protocol I recommend includes a healthful diet (rich with vegetables, fruit and fish and low in refined-sugar products and red meat)… weight-bearing exercise (such as walking and stair-climbing)… and good hormone balance (deficiencies of some hormones, including testosterone, accelerate bone loss). I also suggest certain bone-protecting supplements.

Caution: People with kidney disease should not take supplements without consulting a doctor. With kidney disease, the kidneys cannot process high doses of nutrients.

My recommendations for women and men: To help prevent osteoporosis, take the first three supplements listed below. If you have osteoporosis or *osteopenia* (a mild bone loss that can be diagnosed with a DEXA scan), take the first three supplements listed and as many of the others as you're willing to try, in the dosages recommended…

Super trio prevents and treats osteoporosis

• **Calcium is the most prevalent mineral in bone tissue**. Taking supplements helps prevent a deficiency. Most studies have found that calcium slows bone loss but does not increase bone density when used alone. Women with osteoporosis should take 500 mg of calcium twice daily with meals. It should be a well-absorbed form, such as citrate, citrate-malate, amino acid chelate or hydroxyapatite. To boost absorption, take no more than 500 mg per dose. Calcium carbonate, which is widely used, is not well-absorbed. For osteoporosis prevention, men and women, as well as boys and girls starting at age 13, should take 500 mg daily.

Calcium supplementation for men who have osteoporosis is more complicated. Some recent research has identified a link between high calcium intake (from dairy products) and increased risk for prostate cancer. A meta-analysis in the *Journal of the National Cancer Institute* that reviewed 12 studies on this association concluded, "High intake of dairy products and calcium may be associated with an increased risk for prostate cancer, although the increase appears to be small." A recent study found that calcium intake exceeding 1,500 mg a day (from food and supplements) may be associated with a higher risk of advanced, and potentially fatal, prostate cancer. The saturated fat in dairy products may raise prostate cancer risk.

Until there is more definitive information, I recommend that men who have osteoporosis, regardless of whether they have eliminated calcium-rich foods from their diets, take no more than a 500-mg calcium supplement daily. Men with prostate cancer should consult their doctors before using calcium supplements.

• **Vitamin D** promotes absorption of calcium. Deficiencies of this vitamin are more common in Americans over age 50 than in younger adults. Sun exposure prompts the body to produce vitamin D, and the kidneys help convert it to its active form. As we age, our skin cannot synthesize vitamin D as effectively from sunlight, and our kidneys become less efficient. People with darker skin, those with digestive problems (due to malabsorption conditions, such as Crohn's disease) and those with limited exposure to sunlight are also at greater risk for vitamin D deficiency. Preliminary studies indicate that an inadequate intake of vitamin D is associated with an increased risk of fractures.

For the prevention of osteoporosis, I recommend 600 IU to 800 IU of vitamin D daily. People with osteoporosis should take 800 IU to 1,200 IU daily. Vitamin D is fat soluble, meaning it is better absorbed when taken with meals (containing small amounts of fat).

For many patients with low vitamin D levels, I recommend 2,000 IU of vitamin D daily. To ensure that vitamin D levels are optimal, I monitor blood levels once or twice a year. Overdosing can lead to heart arrhythmia, anorexia, nausea and other ill effects.

• **Magnesium**, one important constituent of bone crystals, is crucial for the proper metabolism of calcium. A deficiency of magnesium impairs bone-building cells known as *osteoblasts*. Like calcium, magnesium requires vitamin D for absorption.

Researchers from Tel Aviv University in Israel looked at the effect of magnesium supplementation on bone density in 31 postmenopausal women with osteoporosis. This two-year, open, controlled trial (both the researchers and patients knew who was receiving the placebo or the supplement) involved giving the participants 250 mg to 750 mg of magnesium daily for six months and 250 mg for another 18 months. Twenty-two patients (71 percent) experienced a one percent to eight percent increase in bone density. The mean bone density of all treated patients increased significantly after one year and remained at that level after two years. Among an additional 23 postmenopausal women not receiving magnesium, mean bone density *decreased* significantly.

For osteoporosis prevention, take 400 mg to 500 mg of magnesium daily… for osteoporosis, take 500 mg to 750 mg daily. In both cases, take in divided doses.

If you have bone-loss disease

• **Vitamin K** has received attention in recent years for its role in treating osteoporosis. It activates *osteocalcin*, a bone protein that regulates calcium metabolism in the bones and helps calcium bind to the tissues that make up the bone. It also has been shown to inhibit inflammatory chemicals that cause bone breakdown.

Studies have shown that low vitamin K intake and blood levels are associated with reduced bone density and fractures in people who have osteoporosis. A recent meta-analysis published in the American Medical Association's *Archives of Internal Medicine* found that vitamin K supplements were associated with a consistent reduction in all types of fractures. Leafy, green vegetables, such as spinach, kale, collard greens and broccoli, are the best sources of vitamin K, yet many people do not consume these vitamin K–rich foods on a regular basis. High-dose vitamin K (above two milligrams) should be used only under the supervision of a doctor, because excess vitamin K may increase blood clotting. Vitamin K supplements should not be used by people who take blood-thinning medication, such as *warfarin* (Coumadin) or *heparin*, or by pregnant women or nursing mothers. I typically recommend two milligrams to 10 mg daily of vitamin K for people who have osteoporosis to help increase their bone density.

• **Essential fatty acids (EFAs)** have been shown to improve bone density in older women and are believed also to promote bone health in men. Many researchers theorize that osteoporosis develops because of chronic inflammation of bone tissue (due to stress, toxins, poor diet and infection). EFAs, especially those found in fish oil, reduce inflammation. Some studies show that EFAs also improve calcium absorption. I recommend that people with osteoporosis take fish oil daily (containing about 480 mg of EPA and 320 mg of DHA), along with 3,000 mg of evening primrose oil, which contains inflammation-fighting *gamma-linolenic acid* (GLA). Because EFAs have a blood-thinning effect, check with your doctor if you are taking a blood thinner.

• **Strontium** is a mineral that does not get too much attention, because it's not regarded as essential for the human body. However, 99 percent of the total amount of strontium found in the body is located in the teeth and bones. Supplemental strontium is not the radioactive type that you may have heard about in relation to nuclear facilities. Strontium is a valuable mineral for people with osteoporosis, and I often recommend it.

A clinical trial in the *New England Journal of Medicine* found that strontium prevents vertebral fractures and increases bone density. The most common supplemental forms are strontium chloride and strontium citrate. I suggest a supplement that contains 680 mg of elemental strontium daily (similar to the dose used in most studies). Because calcium inhibits strontium absorption, strontium should be taken at least four hours before or after calcium is taken. Strontium should not be taken by pregnant women and nursing mothers. It is not available at most health-food stores, but you can buy it from Vitacost (800-381-0759, www.vitacost.com).

• **Soy**, as a supplement and/or food, has been shown in several studies to improve bone density. Soy contains *isoflavones*, estrogen-like constituents that support bone mass and relieve menopausal symptoms in women. Women and men with osteoporosis or osteopenia need to take 125 mg of soy isoflavones daily in soy protein powder or supplement form and consume three to five servings of soy foods weekly. (One serving equals one-half cup of tofu… one-half cup of soy beans… or one cup of soy milk.)

Caution: Soy supplements are not well studied in women who have had breast cancer, so they should avoid supplements and nonfermented soy products.

• **Vitamin C** is required for the production of the protein *collagen*, a component of bone tissue. I recommend that people with osteoporosis take 1,000 mg twice daily. Reduce the dosage if loose stools develop.

• **Silicon** is a trace mineral required for bone formation. I recommend two to five milligrams daily.

Best osteoporosis formulas

These products contain all the vitamins and minerals described in this article, in the therapeutic doses used for osteoporosis treatment…

• **Bone-Up by Jarrow**. To find an online retailer, call 310-204-6936 or go to www.jarrow.com.

• **Osteoprime from Enzymatic Therapy**. To find a local retailer, call 800-783-2286 or go to www.enzymatictherapy.com.

• **Pro Bono** from Ortho Molecular Products is available from health-care professionals, including naturopaths, holistic MDs, chiropractors, nutritionists and acupuncturists.

Don't Let a Dip in This Critical Hormone Doom You to Fuzzy Thinking, Ho-Hum Sex, and an Early Grave

"I haven't felt this much energy and mental sharpness in years, and I've only been on the testosterone you prescribed for a few days. Is that even possible?" asked Grant, a 56-year old patient I was treating at my clinic.

"The truth is I hear this kind of thing all the time from the guys I'm treating. Men who come in to see me complaining of everything from a lack of energy to trouble getting an erection are astonished at the difference testosterone replacement makes in their lives. And although testosterone *is* certainly a superstar in recharging a man's sexual desire and performance its benefits go far beyond the bedroom.

When a woman's hormones, like estrogen, drop during menopause her doctor will prescribe hormones for her. But most doctors ignore the fact that middle-aged men are experiencing their own rapid decline in hormones. Sadly, many doctors are unaware of how common testosterone deficiency is in men. One study from the New England Research Institutes in Watertown, Massachusetts, looked at testosterone levels in 1,500 men and discovered that 24 percent of them had low total testosterone! That translates to millions of American men suffering needlessly because their bodies are not making enough of this critical hormone.

The reality is if left untreated testosterone deficiency is a major risk to your health. In fact, there's even a medical term for testosterone deficiency... *hypogonadism*. And *andropause* is the name used for the decline of testosterone and other hormones in middle-aged men. Now you don't need to remember either of those terms. All you really need to know about them is that for a guy not having enough testosterone on board can lead to everything from muscle shrinkage (hello old man arms) to growing a set of man boobs.

Research has shown that after we reach age 40, serum testosterone levels start falling between 0.4 percent and 2.6 percent per year. And it's no coincidence that there's a similar drop in bone density, muscle strength, physical function, and sexual function at the same time.[1]

Yet, all too often patients tell me their previous doctor refused to test them for deficiency because they haven't officially reached their golden years. This is negligence in my opinion, and why I include testing of this vital hormone (along with others) in yearly blood work in all my male patients starting at age forty. When men are deficient and they begin testosterone replacement, obvious improvements in their symptoms can often be seen within days to weeks.

Revitalize your sex life

There's no doubt that low testosterone can lead to low libido and erectile dysfunction (ED). It's largely responsible for making a man— well, a man! In fact if you're forty or older and you've had any problems in the bedroom you should be tested for testosterone deficiency.

Testing is even more important if you suffer from diabetes. Research has shown that low testosterone in men with type 2 diabetes is associated with more severe ED, low sexual desire, and low intercourse frequency.[2]

But balancing your levels can quickly make the bedroom your favorite

The tell tale signs of low testosterone[3]

- Incomplete or delayed sexual development

- Reduced sexual desire (libido) and activity

- Decreased spontaneous erections

- Breast discomfort, gynecomastia (enlarged breasts)

- Loss of body (axillary and pubic) hair, reduced shaving

- Very small (especially < five milliliters) or shrinking testes

- Inability to father children, low or zero sperm counts

- Height loss, low trauma fracture, low bone mineral density

- Hot flushes, sweats

- Decreased energy, motivation, initiative, and self-confidence

- Feeling sad or blue, depressed mood

- Poor concentration and memory

- Sleep disturbance, increased sleepiness

- Mild anemia

- Reduced muscle bulk and strength

- Increased body fat and body mass index

- Diminished physical or work performance

room in the house once again.

Head off heart problems

Now, as I've already mentioned, your muscles need enough testosterone to work properly. When our levels are too low we start to get flabby and weak. You know… that dreaded middle-aged spread.

Well, your heart is basically a big muscle. So, naturally, it stands to reason that we need to have enough testosterone to keep our heart muscles healthy. And that's exactly what a growing amount of research is showing us.

We know, for example, that <u>low</u> testosterone is linked to a higher risk of dying from congestive heart failure.[4] And heart doctors have few tools for helping the heart beat with better force—which is the key to reversing heart failure. That's where testosterone comes in. Studies show that the hormone may help with heart failure.

Low testosterone levels could be putting your heart at risk for other problems as well. Not having enough of the hormone could send your total and LDL ("bad") cholesterol numbers soaring. And low levels increase your risks for inflammation, insulin resistance, and blood vessel wall dysfunction to boot.

Not only that. You're much more likely to build plaque in you arteries. In one Dutch study researchers found that men who had the lowest levels of free testosterone also had ten times the thickening of the carotid artery wall, as did the men with higher testosterone levels.[5] And, of course, thickening of your artery walls puts you at a higher risk for having a heart attack or stroke.

Testosterone is, in fact, so important to heart health that studies now report that men with low levels are more likely to die from heart disease. In one of the studies, published in the British journal *Heart*, researchers found that men with both heart disease and low testosterone were almost <u>twice as likely to die</u> over a seven-year period than those with heart disease but normal levels of the hormone.[6] Just one more reason to insist that your doc check your testosterone levels!

Drive away diabetes

Testosterone plays an important role in blood sugar regulation. Metabolic syndrome—the term for a group of factors, including abdominal weight gain and elevated blood sugar levels that increase your risk for diabetes, heart disease, and stroke—is affected by testosterone levels.

Having low levels of the hormone is a known risk factor for type 2 diabetes in men. In fact, up to one-third of men with type 2 diabetes are deficient in testosterone.[7] And testosterone replacement can reduce blood glucose levels by approximately 15 percent.[8]

I have found in my own practice that testosterone replacement combined with dietary changes and targeted nutritional supplements can make a significant difference in blood glucose control.

Reclaim the lean muscles of your youth

Testosterone increases muscle size and strength. (This is why bodybuilders love the stuff and why men tend to naturally be more muscular than woman.) But as we age and our testosterone drops our muscles tend to shrink and lose strength right along with it. If you're getting proper nutrition and exercise but notice a big decrease in your muscle strength or size go see your doctor to have your levels checked.

Restoring your hormone levels to normal can stop and even reverse the decline helping you regain the muscles of your youth.

Keep your brain firing on all cylinders

Your brain has receptors for testosterone, which is why it affects cognitive ability. Preliminary research has shown that a low level of the hormone is associated with an increased risk of Alzheimer's disease later in life. And, testosterone has been found in recent studies to benefit those with depression.[9]

Maintain your bones with testosterone

Studies show that men deficient in testosterone are at higher risk for osteoporosis, with about one in eight men experiencing an osteoporosis-related fracture.[10] If you've been diagnosed with osteoporosis, testosterone is, in my opinion, a better therapy than drugs that carry a whole host of nasty side effects. Of course weight-bearing exercise, a pH-balanced diet, and an assortment of vitamins and minerals are essential also.

Taking your testosterone

There are a variety of ways to administer testosterone. These include weekly or biweekly injections (100 mg weekly or 200 mg bi-weekly), daily application of topical creams or gels (50 to 100 mg each morning), patches (one to two five milligram patches applied nightly), sublingual pellets (varies), lozenges (30 mg twice daily), and pellet implants (varies).

I prefer the topical creams or gels because they're easy to apply and you can easily change the dosage with them. Another good option is the once a week injection which helps you to maintain the most consistent levels of the hormone.

Avoid the commercial brands you see marketed on television. They're very low potency and expensive. Instead, have your doctor prescribe a custom formulation, specific to your body's requirements, through a compounding pharmacy.

Proceed with a bit of caution

There are certain situations when testosterone supplementation should be avoided. If you have breast or prostate cancer you should not start taking testosterone. If you start supplementing with testosterone and your PSA continues to rise over time or your prostate enlarges, then therapy is normally stopped.

While some doctors argue that testosterone therapy causes prostate cancer, the reality is that studies show there is not a statistically significant difference compared to men on placebo.[12] The truth is testosterone does not cause prostate cancer or we'd have a whole lot of young men in their late teens and early 20s being diagnosed with it. And, of course, we don't.

The nutrition connection

You may be able to help balance your testosterone levels simply by making a few changes in your eating habits.

If you have low testosterone it often means you need to get more protein. Just eating 25 more grams of protein a day can help boost your levels. I also recommend that all men include pumpkin seeds in their diet to increase their zinc and omega-3 levels.

Be sure to eat plenty of cruciferous vegetables such as broccoli, kale, cauliflower, and Brussels sprouts because they will help your liver metabolize estrogen. And I also recommend taking two tablespoons of ground flaxseeds a day with 10 oz of water to help your body with estrogen metabolism.

Supplements... the final piece of the puzzle

When I put one of my male patients on a testosterone replacement I also always recommend 50 to 75 mg of zinc citrate (twice a day with food), and a few mg of copper, to prevent the conversion of testosterone into estrogen. As an added bonus it also prevents the buildup of dihydrotestosterone, which is associated with prostate enlargement and scalp hair loss.

At the dosages I have recommended there are no long-term side effects for testosterone therapy. Some doctors recommend estrogen-blocking drugs such as anastrazole (Arimidex) to prevent the buildup of estrogen. This is generally not necessary. Besides, this drug is relatively expensive and can have a host of side effects such as joint pain and digestive upset. In my opinion, my nutritional recommendations, along with zinc work just as well. Not to mention they are much safer and less expensive.

If you have reached middle age your testosterone levels are already on the decline. If your levels dip too low it can affect everything from your energy levels to your heart health. If you think your testosterone levels are dropping too fast, you owe it to yourself to get tested.

Discuss your results with your doctor. It may take many more years until the average family physician incorporates this into his or her practice. Don't wait that long. Starting on testosterone replacement could help you live a longer and happier life

Be sure to test for a baseline

Testosterone deficiency can be diagnosed with a blood test. Most labs consider a total testosterone below 300 ng/dL deficient. If possible you should have your sample drawn in the morning. Testosterone can also be tested with saliva or urine samples. And don't forget, for a first-time evaluation your doctor should also include these other important markers to establish your baseline:

- Luteinizing hormone: Pituitary hormone that stimulates testicle production of testosterone

- Follicle stimulating hormone: Pituitary hormone that stimulates testicle production of testosterone

- Prolactin: Pituitary hormone that when elevated may indicate a pituitary tumor causing testosterone deficiency

- Zinc: Mineral required for testicular production of testosterone

- Complete metabolic panel: Assess liver and kidney function

- Complete blood count: Make sure red blood cell count is normal

- Prostate specific antigen: General marker for prostate health

- Digital exam of the prostate

- Physical exam

If you're getting testosterone replacement therapy you should be tested again after four to six weeks. If your numbers are normal then you should be retested at least every four to six months after that. I also monitor red blood cell counts (which are rarely elevated in testosterone users), liver and kidney function, prostate, as well as estrogen level because testosterone is converted into estrogen within the body. If your testosterone levels are low you should also have a bone density test.

Progesterone for Hot Flashes

Progesterone may help relieve hot flashes and night sweats, say University of British Columbia researchers. Healthy postmenopausal women suffering from hot flashes and night sweats took either 300 mg of oral progesterone or a placebo. Those who took progesterone experienced a 56 percent reduction in the intensity of hot flashes and night sweats and a 48 percent reduction in the number of hot flashes and night sweats, versus 28 percent and 22 percent, respectively, in those taking a placebo. The progesterone did not cause any side effects. Talk to your doctor about using bioidentical progesterone to control hot flashes.

Avoid Mainstream Medicine's Synthetic Hormone Trap: How to Navigate the Maze of Menopause Naturally with Bio-Identical Hormones

In just a few years from now it's estimated that half of US women will be menopausal. And that means with millions of women going through menopause by the year 2015 you, or someone you care about, will likely be managing the maze of menopause soon. Unfortunately, most doctors offer women solutions that just don't fit the bill. They don't always work very well. And even worse, they come with a laundry list of side effects that, frankly, I wouldn't wish on my worst enemy.

But despite never hearing about them from your own doctor there *are* safe natural solutions for managing your menopause symptoms. I will tell you more about them in a few moments. But first let's take a look at the flawed solutions that mainstream medicine offers.

Mainstream medicine's menopause madness

Not surprisingly, most docs reach for the prescription pad as soon as a woman mentions a single menopausal symptom. After all, the drug companies—which stand to rake in billions in sales from this growing segment of society—have trained them well. But what you *may* be surprised to learn is that many of those "menopause" prescriptions that doctor's are writing aren't even menopause drugs at all. In fact, they have nothing to do with hormones. They're drugs, prescribed off label to treat one of the top complaints that menopausal women have, and that's hot flashes.

Two-thirds of women going through menopause experience hot flashes.[1] And that means that relieving them is BIG business for the drug companies, and they just so happen to have pharmacies full of drugs they can offer you for it.

Turning down the heat with drugs

If you tell your doctor that you're having hot flashes he's likely to hand you a prescription for an antidepressant. Serotonin reuptake inhibitors or SRIs—including Prozac, Zoloft, Paxil, and Effexor—manipulate the body's serotonin levels and, as a result, they can reduce hot flashes.[2] But of course that drop in hot flashes can come at a pretty hefty price. Potential side effects of these heavy-duty drugs include agitation, suicidal thoughts, nausea, diarrhea, insomnia, decreased sexual desire, and delayed orgasm or inability to have an orgasm. They have even been linked to bone loss and increased risk of breast cancer. For some women the side effects are as bad as, or worse than, the hot flashes they were trying to get rid of in the first place.

But I'm not done yet. SRIs aren't the only surprising drugs you could find your doctor pushing... uh I mean prescribing... to relieve your hot flashes. The blood pressure drug Clonidine—sold under the brand name Catapres—may help control hot flashes.[3] Clonidine alters blood flow slowing down the activity of your nervous system and, ultimately, reducing the number of hot flashes you have. However, like all drugs, Clonidine can come with a boatload full of potential side effects including dry mouth, constipation, drowsiness, and difficulty sleeping.[4]

And the final item on the list of strange-but-true prescriptions for hot flashes is the common anti-seizure and pain medication gabapentin. You might be more familiar with its brand name Neurontin. This drug, which resembles the natural neurotransmitter GABA, *can* reduce hot flashes for some women. But you may be trading those hot flashes for dizziness, drowsiness, fluid retention, nausea, vomiting, and hostility.[5]

Phew… if you're a woman suffering through hotflashes the *choices* that mainstream medicine offers don't seem much like choices at all. Well, that is of course unless you're willing to sacrifice your health and safety and just live with the consequences.

But the truth is you *can* find drug-free relief with these…

Natural hot flash busters

I've been in this doctoring business for quite a few years now and I'm sorry to say that I've found that many of my colleagues *say* they support natural therapies for menopause symptoms, but they don't. In reality, they share very few details on natural therapies with their patients and they downplay how well they can work despite the evidence.

UN-natural Premarin

Some doctors still claim that the currently out of vogue Premarin… that contains estrogens from pregnant female horse urine… is "natural" because it comes from nature. But don't be fooled! That's nothing more than a word game. Equilins, or horse estrogens, are found only in horses.[6] And the fact is the estrogen found in female horses is just not the same kind you'll find in human women.

In vitro research has shown that Premarin metabolites damage cell DNA.[7] The Women's Health Initiative Trial of 2002 exposed the serious side effects that can come along with dosing up on horse hormones. Heck, the Premarin website itself lists a number of those startling side effects including heart attacks, strokes, breast cancer, and blood clots.[8]

For example, your doctor's probably never told you that you don't have to down a heavy-duty drug like Paxil to find cooling relief from your hot flashes. Our Creator has given us natural compounds that work on those *same* serotonin levels in your brain, but *without* all those nasty side effects. If I have a patient who needs extra relief from hot flashes I skip the harsh drugs and prescribe natural 5 hydroxytryptophan to tweak her serotonin levels instead.

And, few doctors will tell you that both ground flaxseeds and fermented soy foods like tempeh and natto have been shown over and over again to be quite effective at reducing hot flashes for many women. In fact, if your symptoms are mild you may even be able to control them with just food and supplements.

However, for many women diet and supplements alone are not quite enough. If you find that you need a little more help to drive your own symptoms away the best way to deal with the hot flashes, and other common menopause complaints—including night sweats and vaginal dryness—is to balance your hormones.

And despite what your mainstream doctor may tell you, resorting to synthetic hormone therapy (HT) isn't your only—or even your best—option. But you may be wondering…

Does natural really matter?
You bet!

Many doctors… and obviously their patients… are confused about what the difference between natural bio-identical hormones and synthetic hormones actually is. It really all boils down to a couple of important points.

Bio-identical hormones—as the name implies—are identical in structure and function to the hormones your body naturally produces on its own. This means your body recognizes and uses them in the *same* way as nature intended. Unlike synthetic hormones they are not patentable.

Synthetic hormones—as the name implies—are <u>not</u> natural. They're created in a lab and aren't identical in structure or function to the hormones that your body makes. Your body may not recognize them or use them in quite the same way as nature intended. Synthetic hormones are, however, patentable. This means that they usually cost more than bio-identical hormones and they are a huge cash cow for the drug companies.

The bottom line is a simple one. If you're going to take a hormone it should be exactly the same as what you *already* find in your body.

The cells in your body are *designed* to interact with the specific chemical structures of the hormones that your body makes. So, it only makes sense to duplicate this chemical structure. Yet, way too many doctors have swallowed Big Pharma's propaganda and are still clinging to the outdated idea that there's no difference between synthetic and bio-identical hormones. And countless women are suffering as a result.

Don't fall for guilt by association

I'm betting that it will not come as much of a surprise to you that Big Pharma, and its friends over at the FDA, are not big fans of bio-identical hormones. And you don't have to look very far for the reason why. You see, you can't obtain a patent for a substance found in nature. So the increasing popularity of bio-identical hormones cuts directly into drug company profits.

As Big Pharma scrambles to keep control of the hormones market one of the tricks up its sleeve is to cause confusion. Mainstream doctors have been led to believe that the risks of synthetic hormones apply to bio-identical hormones as well. But nothing could be further from the truth. As I explained earlier, our cells were *designed* to interact with the hormones our own bodies make. It stands to reason that natural hormones should be safer than man-made hormone-*like* chemicals. More on that in a moment.

The truth is bio-identical hormones shouldn't even be in the same category as synthetics. Instead, they should be evaluated on their individual merits. We can start by taking a look at…

The bio-identical safety record

Contrary to what your doctor may have told you there <u>has</u> been research done on the safety of bio-identical hormones. And, yes, they've proven themselves to be quite safe and reliable.

One long-term study followed over 80,000 French women for over eight years. Researchers looked for any links between both bio-identical and synthetic hormone therapy and breast cancer. What they discovered was that there was <u>no</u> increase in the risk of breast cancer among users of bio-identical estrogen and progesterone. In fact, the researchers even noted that the use of bio-identical progesterone was particularly important in the outcome of the study.[9]

It also brings up a major mistake made in conventional medicine. The standard of care for a woman with a hysterectomy… surgical removal of the uterus… is to recommend estrogen alone. The reasoning is that although progesterone has been shown to prevent uterine cancer in women supplementing with estrogen since there's no uterus there's no need for prevention.

I tell my female patients without a uterus whose gynecologists have put them on estrogen replacement alone, that I recommend they take additional natural progesterone as well. And when they ask me why I explain, "You still have breasts. Your whole life progesterone has been used to keep the cell dividing effect of estrogen in check. It's important to keep that protective effect." Previous research has even shown that bio-identical progesterone reduces the cancerous effects of synthetic estrogen when it comes to uterine health.[10]

Every once in awhile a new patient who is on synthetic progesterone (progestin) will come to see me. I try to get her off of them as quickly as possible because, again, the evidence is clear here. The natural version is just plain safer. In fact, a medical journal confirmed that natural progesterone is just plain good for your brain and heart, but they were <u>not</u>

willing to say the same thing about the synthetic stuff.[11]

Research has also shown that applying estrogens to the skin (what's known as a *transdermal* application) and the use of natural progesterone offer significant benefits and added safety when compared to using synthetic hormones.[12] (I prefer to prescribe topical forms of hormones, which are absorbed through your skin. With capsules or tablets there's always more of a danger that cancerous estrogen metabolites can build up and you do not get the same anti-inflammatory benefits as you do with topical. As well the dose can be adjusted easier with transdermal form.)

And the benefits of bio-identical estrogens don't end there because it just so happens that…

Natural estrogen is better for your brain

Yes, it turns out that bio-identicals are not only safer; they're better for your brain too! A recent study, published in *American Journal of Geriatric Psychiatry*, highlighted the benefits that *natural* estrogen has on the brain.

The lead investigator summarized the study by saying, "We found consistently that [synthetic estrogen—conjugated equine estrogen] may not be good for the brain, at least in women with increased risk of dementia. And 17β-estradiol [bio-identical estrogen] had better effects."

The researchers found that those women who received bio-identical estrogen scored higher on tests of verbal memory performance. And when the researchers controlled for menopause related variables the women, as a group, also performed better on tests that measured executive function (this is the process that helps us connect past experiences with the present), visual memory, and attention.[13]

But natural hormones aren't just better for your brain…

Bio-identicals are also better for your heart

According to a study published in a major medical journal for cardiologists, researchers have *also* acknowledged the heart benefits of natural progesterone and estrogen.[16] The study revealed that progesterone has positive effects on lipids (blood fats) and plaque buildup in the arteries. In other words they can help keep your arteries clear and your blood flowing smoothly.

The authors showed that when you apply estrogen to the skin it helps the heart in several different ways. The topical estrogen causes the blood vessels to relax, it makes the arteries less thick, and it keeps the blood vessels from getting inflamed.

Trying natural testosterone

Let's face it, when you mention the word testosterone most people immediately think "the male hormone." But the truth is women's bodies need testosterone too. And when it comes to reversing some of the most trying symptoms of menopause… such as low libido, fatigue, depression, memory, bone loss, and vaginal dryness and thinning… it's bio-identical testosterone that can really get the job done.

Plus, as an added benefit it turns out that testosterone may help your heart. One study, published in a major cardiology journal, found that bio-identical testosterone therapy fights the waxy plaque that can build up inside your arteries.[14]

Oh, and despite what you may have been told about the supposed dangers of testosterone the research clearly shows that properly administered testosterone therapy is quite safe. In fact, one review that crunched the data from a number of testosterone studies confirmed this quite clearly. The reviewers noted that there's, "Little evidence of risk for [liver] toxicity, endometrial hyperplasia, behavioral hostility… or adverse cardiovascular effects" in women receiving testosterone replacement therapy.[15]

So you've weighed all the evidence, the arguments for going the natural root just make sense, and you've made the decision to try natural bio-identical hormones. But now what?

Committing to going natural

Remember, you *do* have natural, safe, and effective choices for dealing with your menopause symptoms. Making the commitment to go natural with hormone replacement therapy is one of the best gifts you can give yourself. If your doctor has told you that you're only option is synthetic hormones… well… it's simply time to find yourself a new doc and get a second opinion.

Your best bet is to seek out a doctor who's trained in the safe and proper use of bio-identical hormones and who will work with a compounding pharmacy that can tailor your hormone regimen to your body's exact needs. You can get a referral from the American College for advancement in medicine at www.acam.org or the American Association for Naturopathic Physicians at www.naturopathic.org.

In addition, I see women (and men) who need to have their hormones balanced daily at the Stengler Center for Integrative Medicine in California. You'll find the information to contact my office on the inside front cover of this issue. Or, if you're in the Portland, Oregon, area I recommend *A Woman's Time*, the clinic of noted naturopathic gynecology expert Tori Hudson, ND.

PART XI

Dr. Stengler's Urgent Health Warnings

Put Away Those Dangerous Drugs... And Try These Natural Alternatives

Isn't it strange when some wholesome-looking actor appears on a TV commercial to promote a pharmaceutical? The ad tells you how great the drug is, then proceeds with a long, rapid-fire listing of potential side effects. What a contradiction!

It's difficult to believe, but Americans spend close to $200 billion each year on prescription drugs. Now, many people are concerned about the side effects of these medications—and with good reason. Each year, 2.9 percent to 3.7 percent of hospitalizations in the US are due to adverse reactions to medications.

The solution is to get healthy—and to stay healthy—using natural methods. Many nutritional supplements can be used safely and effectively in place of prescription medications. Whether you're treating heartburn, high blood pressure, elevated cholesterol, depression or any number of other common ailments, there are excellent natural alternatives to be considered.

Caution: Do not stop taking a prescription drug or begin using a supplement unless you are being monitored by a health professional. These natural alternatives work best when combined with diet and life-style improvements, particularly regular exercise, stress-reduction techniques and adequate sleep.

Stomach medications

Up to 18 percent of Americans experience heartburn at least once weekly. Heartburn that occurs more than twice per week may be *gastro-esophageal reflux disease* (or GERD), a condition in which stomach contents back up into the esophagus. The most commonly prescribed drugs for heartburn and GERD are *esomeprazole* (Nexium), *lansoprazole* (Prevacid), *rabeprazole* (Aciphex), *omeprazole* (Prilosec), *pantoprazole* (Protonix). Known as *proton pump inhibitors* (PPIs), all of these drugs block the production of stomach acid. And they carry a hefty price tag—about four dollars per dose. Potential side effects include diarrhea, vomiting, headache, rash, dizziness, abnormal heartbeat, muscle pain, leg cramps and water retention.

Natural alternatives: Try them in this order —each one alone—for two weeks at a time until you find what works effectively for you. You can take more than one at a time.

• **Licorice root** (in chewable wafers or powder form) reduces heartburn and irritation of the digestive tract lining. Take 500 mg to 1,000 mg three times daily 30 minutes before meals. A special type of licorice root, known as *deglycyrrhizinated licorice* (DGL), does not elevate blood pressure, as do some varieties of the herb. DGL is widely available at health-food stores and pharmacies. It should relieve your symptoms within two weeks. Take as needed if symptoms recur.

• **Nux vomica**, a homeopathic remedy derived from the seeds of the poison nut tree, has helped many of my patients reduce or eliminate heartburn. It soothes irritation of the digestive lining and is believed to help the upper esophageal valve close more efficiently, thereby preventing reflux. Take two 30C potency pellets three times daily until your symptoms are eliminated. Improvement should occur within two weeks. Resume treatment if symptoms return. Because nux vomica is also used to treat asthma, it is good for asthmatics who suffer from heartburn.

• **Aloe vera**, a cactuslike member of the lily family, soothes and promotes healing of the lining of the digestive tract. Some individuals who don't respond to DGL get relief from aloe vera. Drink one-quarter cup of aloe vera juice or take a 500-mg capsule three times daily.

Antidepressants

Sertaline (Zoloft), *escitalopram* (Lexapro) and *fluoxetine* (Prozac) are the most popular prescription antidepressants sold in the US. They belong to a class of drugs called *selective serotonin reuptake inhibitors* (SSRIs). *Serotonin*, a *neurotransmitter* (chemical messenger) produced by nerve cells in the brain, plays an important role in balancing mood. SSRIs temporarily block serotonin from returning to the neuron that released it, boosting the amount of available serotonin.

Potential side effects of SSRIs include drowsiness, nervousness, insomnia, dizziness, nausea, tremors, loss of appetite, headache, diarrhea, dry mouth, irregular heartbeat, skin rash, weight loss or weight gain and activation of mania in patients with *bipolar disorder* (also known as manic-depressive illness). These drugs also can cause sexual side effects, including loss of libido and decrease in the intensity of orgasms. In July 2005, the FDA warned that children and adults taking antidepressants should be monitored for signs of worsening depression or suicidal thoughts.

Natural alternatives: Try them in this order for six to eight weeks. If effective, continue indefinitely. You can take more than one at a time.

• **S-adenosylmethionine** (SAMe), the nutritional supplement derived from the amino acid *methionine*, is excellent for mild to moderate depression. SAMe is thought to work by increasing the production of mood-boosting neurotransmitters. Some studies have shown SAMe to be as effective as pharmaceutical antidepressants—or, in some cases, even more so. Take 400 mg two or three times daily on an empty stomach. Do not use this supplement if you are taking an antidepressant or antianxiety medication—or if you have bipolar disorder. Like SSRIs, SAMe may activate a manic phase in bipolar patients.

• **5-hydroxytryptophan (5-HTP)** is a quick-acting, mood-enhancing amino acid that I recommend for my patients with mild to moderate depression. In the body, 5-HTP is converted into serotonin, helping to raise levels of this mood-balancing neurotransmitter. Take 100 mg two to three times daily on an empty stomach. Do not take 5-HTP in combination with pharmaceutical antidepressant or antianxiety medication.

• **St. John's wort** is an herb that is widely used in Europe to treat depression. In a review of 23 studies, it was found to be as effective as pharmaceutical therapy for mild to moderate depression. I recommend taking 600 mg of a 0.3 percent *hypericin extract* in the morning and 300 mg in the afternoon or evening. St. John's wort should not be used by women who take birth control pills or by anyone taking HIV medication or immune-suppressing drugs. Do not take St. John's wort with antidepressant or antianxiety medication.

• **Fish oil** has been shown to help mild to moderate depression. Take a formula that contains 1,000 mg of combined *docosahexaenoic acid* (DHA) and *eicosapentaenoic acid* (EPA) daily. Nordic Naturals and Carlson's both make good formulas that are available at health-food stores. Fish oil can be taken indefinitely.

• **B vitamins** improve the efficiency of many functions, including the conversion of glucose to fuel and the synthesis of neurotransmitters. Deficiencies of B vitamins (notably B-3) can lead to anxiety and agitation. Take a 50-mg B complex daily for as long as you like.

Cholesterol-lowering drugs

An estimated 11 million Americans take the cholesterol-lowering medications called *statins. Atorvastatin* (Lipitor), *simvastatin* (Zocor) and *rosuvastatin* (Crestor) are the most commonly prescribed in the US. One month's supply of one of these drugs costs $80 to more than $120.

These drugs work by inhibiting a liver enzyme that helps produce the "bad" cholesterol, known as *low-density lipoprotein* (LDL) cholesterol. These drugs also decrease fats in the blood known as triglycerides and increase "good" *high- density lipoprotein* (HDL) cholesterol levels. The possible side effects include abdominal pain and digestive upset, joint pain, and muscle weakness and pain. One of the most frightening side effects is *rhabdomyolysis*. This condition affects only one in 100,000 people taking statins each year, but it results in severe pain and may cause kidney failure.

Natural alternatives: Try red yeast rice extract, then retest cholesterol levels in three months. Continue if effective. If not, try policosanol.

• **Red yeast rice extract** is a supplement that has been shown to reduce total and LDL cholesterol levels by 11 percent to 32 percent and triglyceride levels by 12 percent to 19 percent. It has been shown to raise HDL by 15 percent to 30 percent. Take 2,400 mg of red yeast rice extract (containing 9.6 mg to 13.5 mg total *monacolins*) daily. Side effects, such as mild gastrointestinal discomfort, are rare. As with many products, red yeast rice extract should be avoided by people with liver disease.

• **Policosanol**, a derivative of sugarcane, is another well-researched cholesterol-lowering supplement. The *American Heart Journal* published a review of placebo-controlled studies, which found that taking 10 mg to 20 mg of policosanol daily lowered total cholesterol by 17 percent to 21 percent and LDL cholesterol by 21 percent to 29 percent. The supplement raised HDL cholesterol by eight percent to 15 percent. Policosanol does not effectively lower triglyceride levels, so I do not recommend it for people who need to reduce these blood fats. Anyone else with high cholesterol should consider taking 10 mg to 20 mg daily.

Important: If your cholesterol levels are significantly elevated (in the mid-300s or higher), you may need to take a statin before trying these natural alternatives. Statins also may be prescribed to help reduce inflammation following a heart attack.

Blood pressure medication

High blood pressure (hypertension) is estimated to affect one of every four adult Americans. *Atenolol* (Tenormin), *lisinopril* (Zestril) and *furosemide* (Lasix) are the most popular prescription drugs for high blood pressure. These drugs are relatively inexpensive—ranging from $11 to $36 per month.

Tenormin (a so-called beta-blocker) works by blocking off nerve impulses of the sympathetic nervous system, the portion of the involuntary nervous system that helps control the body's response to stress (the "fight or flight" reaction). Blood pressure is then lowered by reducing the heart rate and the force of the heart muscle contraction. Possible side effects include digestive upset, fatigue, insomnia, impotence, light-headedness, slow heart rate, low blood pressure (a dangerous condition that can lead to fainting and fatigue), numbness, tingling, sore throat and shortness of breath.

Lisinopril is an *angiotensin-converting enzyme* (ACE) inhibitor. It triggers the relaxation of blood vessels. Relaxed blood vessels help lower blood pressure. Side effects of lisinopril could include chest pain, cough, diarrhea as well as low blood pressure.

Furosemide is a diuretic that causes water excretion. By blocking absorption of salt and fluid in the kidneys, the drug causes an increase in urine output. Water excretion helps reduce blood volume, which means less work for your arteries and veins. Potential side effects include irregular heartbeat, dizziness, abdominal pain or diarrhea, low blood pressure and an imbalance of electrolytes (key minerals that are needed for vital body functions), leading to muscle cramps or weakness.

Important: If you have moderate to severe high blood pressure (160/100 and above), you may need prescription medication. You may be able to limit your need for prescription blood pressure drugs if you work with your doctor to incorporate natural therapies.

Natural alternatives: Try the first two extracts below for 30 days. If your blood pressure doesn't improve, try using all of the natural treatments together. You should see improvement within four weeks—and can continue the regimen indefinitely.

• **Hawthorn extract**, derived from the berry of a thorny shrub with white or pink flowers, dilates artery walls, decreasing *systolic* (top number) and *diastolic* (bottom number) blood pressure by about 10 points each. Take 250 mg to 500 mg three times daily. Hawthorn extract can have a mild blood-thinning effect, so check with your doctor first if you are taking a blood thinner, such as *warfarin* (Coumadin).

• **Bonito fish extract**, a protein from the muscle tissue of the bonito fish, acts like a natural ACE inhibitor. I recommend a daily dose of 1,500 mg.

• **Coenzyme Q10**, an enzyme found in the energy-producing mitochondria of all cells, has been shown to reduce both systolic and diastolic blood pressure by five to 10 points. You may need to take 200 mg to 300 mg daily for a blood pressure–lowering effect.

• **Calcium and magnesium** relax the nervous system and arteries, lowering blood pressure. I suggest 500 mg of calcium and 250 mg of magnesium twice daily.

Cholesterol Mania—
Stop Taking Drugs You Don't Need

Cholesterol-lowering "statin" drugs are big business now. *Atorvastatin* (Lipitor), one of the most popular drugs in this class, is among the most commonly prescribed medications in the US. With approximately 12 million Americans using it, US sales of Lipitor totaled nearly six billion dollars in 2008.

Why are so many people taking these drugs? It's long been known that elevated cholesterol levels are associated with an increased risk of heart disease, but now consumers are being given an additional incentive to use these drugs. The National Institutes of Health's National Cholesterol Education Program (NCEP) Adult Treatment Panel III recently released updated guidelines for cholesterol drug therapy. According to these guidelines, 37 million Americans—that's one in five adults—are eligible for cholesterol-lowering medication. Previous guidelines recommended these drugs for 13 million Americans. I find the new guidelines very suspect. Read on, and you will understand why.

The updated recommendations are based on a review of five clinical trials using statins. One of the key changes in the new guidelines involved lowering the optimal range for LDL "bad" cholesterol in the blood in all adults to less than 100 mg/dL. Individuals with cardiovascular disease or other risk factors, such as diabetes, smoking or hypertension, are told to aim for the same level—with an "optional target" of less than 70 mg/dL. It is rare for any of the patients I test—whether they are healthy or not—to have LDL levels below 100 mg/dL. I encourage my patients to strive for an LDL level of 100 mg/dL to 130 mg/dL with an HDL "good" cholesterol level of 50 mg/dL or higher.

The evidence for the recent NCEP guidelines was challenged in a letter from the Center for Science in the Public Interest (CSPI), a nonprofit consumer advocacy organization that conducts research in health and nutrition.

The CSPI letter, which was signed by more than three dozen physicians, epidemiologists and other scientists, urged the NIH to convene an independent panel to conduct a second review of the studies. They wrote, "There is strong evidence to suggest that an objective, independent reevaluation of the scientific evidence from the five new studies of statin therapy would lead to different conclusions than those presented by the current NCEP. The studies cited do not demonstrate that statins benefit women of any age or men over 70 who do not already have heart disease."

The letter also cited concerns that were raised after one study showed that statin therapy significantly *increases* the risk of some types of cancer in the elderly. (Research has, indeed, shown that statins can increase risk of nonmelanoma skin cancer and breast cancer. Other research, however, has linked statin use to a decreased risk for some types of cancer, such as colon and prostate malignancies.)

There was another alarming discovery. Eight of the nine authors of the new LDL recommendations had financial ties to statin drug manufacturers, including Pfizer, Merck, Bristol-Myers Squibb and AstraZeneca. In response to the CSPI letter, the NIH declared that the scientific basis for the new guidelines was adequate and there was no conflict of interest for panel members.

No conflict? Is it pure coincidence that most of the authors of the guidelines had financial ties to statin manufacturers? Now millions of Americans are following these misguided recommendations for statin therapy instead of using natural treatments.

Understanding the dangers of statins

Statins first became available in the US during the late 1980s, when they were marketed as a unique treatment for elevated cholesterol—they inhibit an enzyme called *3-hydroxymethylglutaryl-coenzyme* A (HMG-CoA) reductase, which is involved in the production of cholesterol in the liver. In addition to Lipitor, other statins include *rosuvastatin* (Crestor), *lovastatin* (Mevacor), *pravastatin* (Pravachol) and *simvastatin* (Zocor).

The most common side effects of statins are headache, nausea, vomiting, constipation, diarrhea, rashes, weakness, muscle and joint pain and increased liver enzymes. The most serious, but rare, side effects are liver failure and *rhabdomyolysis*, a life-threatening condition that causes extensive damage to muscles.

In addition, statins deplete the body of *coenzyme Q10* (CoQ10), a naturally occurring substance that your body needs to create energy in cells, particularly heart cells. In one study, the CoQ10 blood levels of Lipitor users were reduced by 50 percent after 30 days of statin use. To prevent a deficiency of CoQ10, I recommend that my patients who use statins take 100 mg to 200 mg daily of CoQ10.

Cholesterol-lowering the natural way

The general medical community pays lip service to diet and lifestyle changes as a first line of therapy for abnormal cholesterol levels—but many patients are pressured to begin drug therapy right away, while diet and lifestyle changes are only an afterthought. Conventional doctors often tell patients that they have a genetic cholesterol problem and that cholesterol-lowering medication is their only option because diet and lifestyle changes would not be sufficient. Some people, such as those who have acute cardiovascular issues or extremely high total cholesterol levels (above 350 mg/dL) and/or significantly elevated LDL levels (above 200 mg/dL), are usually not able to control their cholesterol levels through diet and lifestyle changes alone. However, many people can bring their cholesterol and lipid levels into normal range by watching what they eat, exercising and reducing their stress levels. Nutritional supplements also are an option.

If your cholesterol is mildly or moderately elevated (total cholesterol 200 mg/dL to 239 mg/dL… and/or LDL above 70 mg/dL), get a baseline cholesterol test if your levels haven't been tested in the last six months. Then try the diet and lifestyle changes described in this article for eight to 12 weeks.

People who are unable to reduce their cholesterol levels through diet and exercise and/or who have family members with high cholesterol *are* likely to be genetically predisposed to the condition. Such people should *not* rely on lifestyle changes alone.

Better: They should combine the healthful practices described here with regular supplement use.

Important: There are times when I recommend statin treatment—immediately after a heart attack to reduce inflammation and when there is extreme elevation in total cholesterol (400 mg/dL or higher) and/or LDL cholesterol (210 mg/dL or higher), usually due to genetics.

Diet and lifestyle changes

My top suggestions for improving cholesterol levels…

1. Reduce saturated fat in your diet to less than seven percent of daily calories. Saturated fat is found mainly in beef, veal, pork and poultry (especially in dark meat and the skin of any meat). Saturated fat is plentiful in most dairy products, except nonfat yogurt, reduced-fat cheese and skimmed milk. Small amounts are found in coconut and palm oils, so consume these sparingly. To monitor your saturated fat intake, keep a daily record based on food label information.

Avoid products that contain trans fatty acids, which often are found in deep-fried foods, bakery products, packaged snack foods, margarines (except products with cholesterol-reducing plant stanols or plant sterols), crackers and vegetable shortening. If a product contains more than 0.5 grams of trans fat per serving, the label will list the trans fat content. Avoid foods that "hide" trans fats by using the term "partially hydrogenated" on their labels and claiming zero grams of trans fat. Common offenders include baked goods, crackers and packaged mixes. Cardiovascular disease is linked to trans fat intake because this unhealthful fat raises levels of LDL cholesterol and blood fats known as triglycerides, while lowering beneficial HDL cholesterol. Cook with organic olive or canola oil. Macadamia nut oil also is healthful.

2. Consume two weekly servings of foods rich in heart-healthy omega-3 fatty acids. Sources include some types of fish—anchovies, Atlantic herring, sardines, tilapia and wild or canned salmon. For a list of the fish not contaminated with mercury or *polychlorinated biphenyls* (PCBs), check www.oceansalive.org, the Internet site of the Environmental Defense Fund, a Washington, DC–based, nonprofit group dedicated to solving environmental problems.

3. Eat five to seven daily servings of fruits and vegetables. Produce contains antioxidants that prevent oxidation (cell damage from negatively charged molecules known as free radicals) of cholesterol, as well as fiber that helps lower cholesterol.

4. Consume foods that contain soluble (dissolves in liquid) fiber, such as beans, barley, oats, peas, apples, oranges and pears. Soluble fiber reduces the absorption of cholesterol from the intestines into the bloodstream. For example, a daily bowl of oatmeal can reduce total cholesterol by as much as 23 percent. Oatmeal also has been shown to curb LDL cholesterol levels without lowering beneficial HDL cholesterol.

5. Eat nuts, such as walnuts and almonds, which are rich with healthful monounsaturated fatty acids. One study conducted in Barcelona, Spain, showed that a walnut-rich diet reduces total cholesterol by

4.4 percent and LDL cholesterol by 6.4 percent. Macadamia nuts, pistachios, almonds, hazelnuts and pecans also have been shown to reduce cholesterol levels. Eat a handful of walnuts or any of the nuts listed above daily.

6. Add ground flaxseed (up to one-quarter cup daily, taken in two doses) to protein shakes, cereal and/or salads. Flaxseed has been shown to reduce total and LDL cholesterol. Drink 10 oz of water for every two tablespoons of flaxseed consumed, to avoid intestinal blockage.

7. Consume 20 g to 30 g of soy protein every day (in food or protein powder form). Some studies suggest that soy protein may lower cholesterol levels in some people with high cholesterol. Because soy protein can have a potential estrogen-like effect, it should be avoided by women who have breast cancer or a family history of the disease.

8. Reduce daily intake of simple sugars, such as those in crackers, cookies and soda. Found in abundance in processed packaged foods and many baked goods, they have been shown to decrease HDL cholesterol. By cutting back, you also reduce risk of elevated insulin levels, which lead to increased production of cholesterol by the liver.

9. Exercise regularly. Thirty minutes of exercise, such as brisk walking, swimming, biking or tennis, three to five times a week is effective for lowering elevated cholesterol.

10. Lose weight and body fat. Weight loss by people who are overweight reduces cholesterol levels and prevents insulin resistance, a blood sugar problem that can lead to high cholesterol.

11. Don't smoke. Smokers have lower levels of HDL cholesterol and an increased risk of heart attacks.

12. Practice stress-reduction techniques, such as deep breathing and biofeedback. Stress has been shown to elevate cholesterol in most individuals.

Harmful Heartburn Drugs

Let's take the bad news first. Popping a pill to alleviate heartburn can raise your risk for breaking a bone, getting an ulcer and perhaps even developing cancer. Since heartburn affects more than 60 million Americans at least once a month, the potential for harm is huge.

Heartburn (which has nothing to do with the heart) is not a disease, but a symptom—a burning sensation behind the breastbone. Most people have occasional heartburn (also called indigestion), typically brought on by a large or spicy meal.

Chronic heartburn usually signals *gastroesophageal reflux disease* (GERD). Basically a mechanical malfunction, GERD occurs when the valve between the stomach and esophagus, called the *lower esophageal sphincter* (LES), fails to close properly, permitting stomach acid to back up. The esophagus doesn't have the stomach's strong protective lining, so acid damages esophageal tissues and causes pain.

Symptoms of GERD include persistent heartburn, acid regurgitation, chest pain, dry cough, bad breath and hoarseness in the morning. Untreated, GERD can scar the esophagus, making it hard to swallow… and may damage esophageal cell DNA, raising the risk of esophageal cancer.

Now for the good news: Natural treatments can safely heal GERD.

Get the facts here—then work with your doctor to discontinue danger-ous drugs as you incorporate natural therapies.

Banish the burn, weaken the bone?

Each year, GERD patients in the US are given about 100 million prescriptions for *proton pump inhibitors* (PPIs), which suppress the stom-ach's production of *hydrochloric acid*. PPIs include *rabeprazole* (Aciphex), *esomeprazole* (Nexium), *lansoprazole* (Prevacid), *omeprazole* (Prilosec) and *pantoprazole* (Protonix).

The Journal of the American Medical Association published an analysis of 16 years of medical records from 13,556 patients with hip fractures and 135,386 patients without fractures (all over age 50).

Conclusions: Patients who took PPIs at average doses for more than a year had a 44 percent increased risk of breaking a hip. Those who took higher-than-average doses more than doubled their risk of hip fracture.

Ironically, PPIs are frequently advised when GERD develops as a side effect of the osteoporosis drug *alendronate* (Fosamax). In other words, patients with brittle bones are given a drug to improve bone density… but the drug causes reflux, so patients are then given PPIs, which make bones even weaker!

Other GERD drugs that impede acid production include *histamine-2 receptor antagonists* (H2 blockers). Over-the-counter (OTC) H2 blockers include *cimetidine* (Tagamet HB), *famotidine* (Pepcid AC) and *ranitidine* (Zantac 75)—each of which also comes in prescription strengths. OTC *antacids*, which neutralize acids, have a similar effect. Antacids include Alka-Seltzer, Maalox, Mylanta, Pepto-Bismol, Rolaids and Tums.

What is the connection between the acid-suppressing drugs and frac-tures? Hydrochloric acid promotes absorption of calcium and other min-erals necessary for proper bone formation. When stomach acid is sup-pressed, the body cannot effectively absorb minerals—setting the stage for osteoporosis.

More reflux drug dangers

Stomach acid helps to break down protein into *amino acids*, which the body uses for tissue healing and immune response. When stomach acid is suppressed, protein is not properly digested. The resulting amino acids that are absorbed can trigger an *autoimmune reaction* (in which the immune system attacks the body's own tissues), causing pain and swelling of muscles, joints and digestive organs.

Heartburn drugs can decrease absorption of other drugs, too. These include some antibiotics, antifungals and the heart medication *digoxin* (Lanoxin).

When acid is low, *Helicobacter pylori*—a bacterium that causes stomach ulcers and increases the risk of stomach cancer—can flourish. So can fungi and bacteria that target the intestines, leading to bloating, diarrhea, constipation, gas and itchy rectum.

Paradoxically, drugs that reduce stomach acid can actually *increase* heartburn. When acid does not fully break down foods, the body may develop food sensitivities that further irritate the LES and stomach.

My view: GERD medications should not be utilized—especially for more than a few weeks—unless natural treatments have been tried for four to six weeks and failed to alleviate heartburn and other symptoms.

Anti-indigestion diet

Recently, a commentary in *Archives of Internal Medicine* reviewed 16 studies on the effects of changes in diet on heartburn symptoms. The report concluded that dietary restrictions did not help.

I adamantly disagree. All the studies reviewed looked only at whether a particular food either increased acidity in the stomach or decreased pressure exerted by the LES—but not at the real-world issue of whether avoiding that food alleviated symptoms. As hundreds of my patients can attest, heartburn may disappear with appropriate dietary changes. Avoid carbonated beverages, alcohol, coffee, nonherbal tea, cow's milk, citrus, chocolate, peppermint and spicy foods. If symptoms improve, reintroduce these foods one at a time to see which specific ones trigger your heartburn—and then avoid those foods in the future. If problems persist, a holistic doctor can test your sensitivity to different foods (using blood tests and other methods) to identify the culprits.

Trusted trio of safe soothers

For additional relief, I recommend the three natural GERD-combating supplements *par excellence*. All are sold at health-food stores and are safe for everyone (but not recommended for pregnant women).

Start with *aloe vera*, an anti-inflammatory plant that soothes the digestive tract lining. Three times daily, 20 minutes before meals, swallow 600 mg in capsule form… or use four tablespoons of extract… or two teaspoons in powder form, mixed in water.

If heartburn persists after one week, add the homeopathic remedy *Nux vomica* to your regimen. Though no formal studies have been done, I believe that it strengthens the nerve impulses to the LES and helps it to close properly. Take two tablets of 30C potency twice daily until symptoms are gone. Thereafter, use as needed for occasional symptoms.

If symptoms remain after three weeks, also take *deglycyrrhizinated licorice root* (DGL). This stimulates the protective mucus of the stomach, soothing the LES and esophagus. Chew two 400-mg tablets three times daily, 20 minutes before meals.

Helpful: If heartburn makes it hard to sleep, avoid eating within two hours of bedtime. Also, raise the head of your bed six inches by placing wooden blocks beneath the bed frame's head two legs. Gravity helps keep stomach acid down, so heartburn is less likely to keep you up.

Toxic Toilet Paper: Revealed… How Your Toilet Paper May Be Making You Sick!

B y now you probably *already* know that the hormone-like compounds hidden in plastic products like water bottles may be bad for your health. In fact, these compounds… like BPA, PCBs, and phthalates… have been linked with everything from autism to cancer.

But I bet you never considered that some of those *same* toxins could be invading your bathroom time too!

Researchers, from the Department of Waste Management at Dresden University of Technology in Germany, tested toilet paper (and other paper products) for various estrogen mimics known as xenoestrogens. They wanted to find out what the levels of those xenoestrogens are in the papers, and if they were finding their way into wastewater.

Shockingly, they found that all but one of the hormone pretenders were in the toilet paper… and at very high concentrations.[1] Meaning, of course, you're exposed to those <u>same</u> levels when you visit the bathroom!

The scientists also found that the xenoestrogens in the toilet papers do pass through to the wastewater. They warned that toilet paper "should not be mixed with biological waste e.g. for co-composting or co-fermentation in order to derive organic fertilisers."

I did some research but didn't find any American toilet paper brands that were *guaranteed* free of these nasty toxins. However, knowing the American spirit I'm sure a xenoestrogen-free toliet paper will be coming along soon. I'll be sure to let you know if I discover any.

Your Prostate Drug Could Be Killing You! Common Prostate Drugs Given to Millions Linked to Aggressive Prostate Cancer

There are lots of good things about getting older. With age comes wisdom, which means as we pack more birthdays under our belt we're much more confident in ourselves and our decisions. Plus studies show that contrary to the grumpy old person stereotype, as we get older we're actually much more content and satisfied with our lives. And with kids grown-up and moving out of the house you might suddenly find yourself with the extra time you always wanted to pursue hobbies and just relax.

But if you're a guy there's one thing that often comes with age that's anything but welcome. I'm talking about prostate problems. In fact, having an enlarged prostate… a condition known as benign prostatic hyperplasia (BPH)… is so common that there are currently millions of men taking prescription drugs to treat the problem. Doctors prescribe these drugs to shrink the prostate and help improve bothersome symptoms including night-time urination, weak stream, urgency to urinate, leaking, and incomplete bladder emptying.

The shocking link between prostate drugs and prostate cancer

Unfortunately, it turns out that those millions of men may be unknowingly trading their bothersome prostate symptoms for something much, much worse. Shockingly, research has now revealed that BPH drugs increase your risk of developing an *aggressive* form of prostate cancer! Most men develop some form of prostate cancer if they live long enough. Fortunately most are slow growing and do not kill. The concern is that the aggressive forms can spread quickly to vital organs of the body and become fatal.

In two large trials the link between 5-alpha reductase inhibitors (5-ARIs) and this form of prostate cancer was so strong that, in a rare move, the FDA actually mandated a change to the drug labels. Specifically, the labels must now carry a warning about the increased risk of being diagnosed with a more serious form of prostate cancer.[1] These medications include Proscar (finasteride), Avodart (dutasteride), and Jalyn (dutasteride and tamsulosin). This warning also extends to the popular medication Propecia used for male pattern hair loss, because it contains a low dose of finasteride.

5-ARIs inhibit the enzyme that converts the male hormone into dihydrotestosterone (DHT). DHT is one of the hormones thought to stimulate prostate enlargement. And the drugs have been shown to reduce the overall risk of prostate cancer. Sounds good so far, right? But the paradox of these medications is that at the same time they *increase* the risk of more serious, aggressive prostate cancers. No doubt this is a scary trade-off.

As a reader of *Health Revelations* you're probably already aware that PSA is not a great test for identifying prostate cancer. But, unfortunately many doctors still mistakenly rely on this number alone as an indicator. In these cases a diagnosis may be delayed because 5-alpha reductase inhibitors could be masking the cancer since they can reduce prostate specific antigen (PSA) blood values by approximately 50 percent.[2] So, in other words, a man taking these drugs could have a normal PSA level

The PSA coin toss

PSA is not a great test for prostate cancer screening. In fact, in 2010 Richard Ablin, PhD, the researcher who discovered PSA in 1970, has stated that the PSA test is a "hugely expensive public health disaster" and "hardly more effective than a coin toss."[3] Indeed two large studies recently published in the *New England Journal of Medicine* demonstrated that "PSA screening had either no or little effect on the death rate from prostate cancer."[4] To be fair there is some usefulness for the PSA test. Ablin confirms that the PSA test can be useful in monitoring men who had treatment for prostate cancer.[5] Also, consistent increases in PSA levels (known as PSA velocity) may indicate prostate cancer, although the research in this area is inconclusive.

despite having an aggressive prostate cancer forming.

If you're taking one of these drugs and want to continue with them I recommend that you request prostate ultrasound testing in addition to blood work and a yearly digital prostate exam. This combination of approaches can help your doctor catch any potentially aggressive forms of cancer earlier. The better long-term choice, of course, is working with a doctor skilled in natural medicine who can help you take advantage of nature's nontoxic remedies to relieve your troubling BPH symptoms. My patients find they work well.

Reduce PSA levels and heal your prostate naturally

Recent research published in the *British Journal of Nutrition* found that omega-3 fatty acids and coenzyme Q10 significantly lowered PSA levels in healthy men. The study involved 504 men who were randomly assigned to receive 400 mg of coenzyme Q10, omega-3 (4.48 grams of EPA and 2.88 grams of DHA), 2,400 mg of gamma-linolenic acid (GLA), or a placebo daily for 12 weeks. Those taking the omega-3 and coenzyme Q10 supplements had a 30 percent and 33 percent reduction in their PSA levels, respectively. Those taking GLA had an increased level of PSA by about 15 percent.[6]

I regularly recommend omega-3 supplements and omega-3 rich foods to my male patients because they reduce prostate inflammation and swelling. Diets that are rich in omega-3s, such as the Mediterranean diet, have a protective effect against a variety of different cancers, including cancer of the prostate. And of course omega-3 fatty acids benefit many other parts of the body—including the brain, joints, skin, heart and arteries, and immune system to name just a few. Good food sources of omega-3 are flaxseed and fish including salmon, sardines, and trout.

In the same *BJN* study GLA was shown to *increase* PSA levels. GLA is a type of fatty acid that comes from the omega-6 family of fatty acids. When you get too many omega-6 fats in your diet it encourages inflammation and it's believed to increase your risk for a variety of inflammatory health conditions including cancer. Another study, published in the journal *Nutrition Research*, concluded that "a high dietary ratio of (omega-6 to omega-3) fatty acids may increase the risk of overall prostate cancer among white men and possibly increase the risk of high-grade prostate cancer among all men."[7] Americans typically get way too many omega-6 fatty acids in their diet in the form of vegetable oils, processed packaged food, and restaurant meals. Reducing the omega-6s in your diet could help reduce your cancer risks.

Make your diet prostate-friendly

Prostate health is greatly influenced by what you put in your mouth. Red meat, dairy products, and animal fat are all associated with prostate cancer.[8] I believe refined sugar products—which includes most bread—should be added to that list as well.

The prostate is very sensitive to hormones. These foods can increase the levels of male hormones and growth hormones in the body leading to prostate enlargement and even cancer. So for a healthy prostate it's best to cut back on *all* of them. And when you do choose to eat them make sure you're picking hormone-free organic products.

Better yet, just slash animal-derived proteins from your diet entirely if you can manage it… except for organic eggs and cold water fish such as salmon, sardines, or trout. Instead focus on protein-rich plant sources such as beans, lentils, pumpkin seeds, and quinoa. This will help reduce inflammation and growth of the prostate.

The truth about soy and prostates

I'm often asked what I think about soy foods and their effect on the prostate. Many clinicians tell patients that soy is "bad" for the prostate because it contains phytoestrogens—naturally occurring chemicals in plants that mimic the hormone estrogen. The reality is that there are a stack of studies showing just the opposite. Soy consumption by men is associated with a *reduction* in prostate cancer![9]

It turns out that phytoestrogens can inhibit the growth of various cancers. One well-studied compound found in soy is genistein. Genistein has been shown to reduce prostate cancer cell activity. According to the National Cancer Institute, "Several laboratory studies have found that treating human prostate cancer cells with isoflavones (such as genistein or daidzein) interferes with pathways in prostate cancer cells related to inflammation and cancer growth and spread."[10]

Unfortunately, most of the soy available in the US has been highly processed with solvents to remove soy oil from the bean. And even worse, most of it has been genetically modified so the chemicals they provide are different from what our bodies were designed for. In the Far East soy is consumed as a whole food no matter whether it's cooked, roasted, fermented, or sprouted. Eating just two ounces of fermented soy foods a couple of times a week can have a protective effect. Fermented soy products include tempeh, tofu, natto, and soy miso.

Prostate-cancer fighters from the produce aisle

Men who eat lots of vegetables have a lower risk of prostate enlargement and prostate cancer. But fitting in the five to seven servings of vegetables a day you need to protect yourself against cancer can be quite a challenge. An easy way to sneak more veggies into your diet… and a trick I use myself… is to drop an assortment of vegetables into the blender each morning with a protein drink mix and some unsweetened coconut or almond milk. I like to include carrots, beets, zucchini, and romaine lettuce along with several cancer-crushing cruciferous veggies like broccoli, cauliflower, Brussels sprouts, cabbage, bok choy, collard greens, and kale.

Vegetables are naturally rich in immune-enhancing nutrients, including carotenoids and vitamins C, E, and K. They also contain compounds known as glucosinolates, which are converted into the anti-cancer compounds indole 3, carbinol, and sulforaphane in the body. These nutrients help the liver break down estrogen, a hormone that stimulates prostate growth when levels are too high (which is often the case in overweight men).

Prostate healer from the Middle East

Pomegranate trees are a common sight in the Middle East, Israel, and Iran. But it wasn't until the late 1700's that the fruit tree made it to North America. Today the pomegranate has become quite popular and you can get it in most grocery stores. But the benefits of the fruit go well beyond its snacking potential. It turns out that the delicious pomegranate may also be a cancer fighter.

Test tube studies show that pomegranate causes cancer cell death and inhibits blood flow to tumors.[11,12] An interesting study out of UCLA looked at the effect of pomegranate in men who had radiation or surgery for prostate cancer. Researchers found that when these men were given eight ounces of pomegranate juice daily the time it took their PSA levels to double (a common measurement that doctors use to judge how a prostate problem is progressing) became *significantly* longer. In addition, there was a drop in the growth of cancer cells and a spike in cancer cells dying off.[13]

As a side benefit, pomegranate juice has been shown to improve erectile dysfunction by improving penile blood flow.[14] Aim to drink two to eight ounces of the juice a day or to eat a fresh pomegranate several times a week to promote prostate health.

Protect your prostate with ketchup

Hidden inside tomatoes and some other pink and red fruits is a powerful prostate-friendly nutrient called lycopene. Lycopene is a type of carotenoid or pigment that provides tomatoes with their deep red color. It's also found in watermelon, pink grapefruit, and guava.

German researchers found elderly men with benign prostatic hyperplasia who were given 15 mg lycopene supplements had their PSA levels drop. Along with that drop the men's prostates stopped growing. The PSA levels of the men who were given a placebo, however, didn't budge and their prostates continued to grow.[15]

Several studies have linked lycopene-rich foods to a reduction in prostate cancer risk. In fact, just one serving a day has been shown to have a protective effect. Your body is able to use more lycopene from the foods you eat if the cell walls of the food are broken down. So choose foods like tomato juice, ketchup, and tomato sauces (organic, of course) to make sure you're getting the most benefit.

Kill cancer cells and suppress inflammation with common spices

You may already have a bottle of this cancer-fighter in your kitchen cabinet. I'm talking about the delicious golden yellow spice turmeric. Several studies show that eating turmeric lowers the risk of a variety of cancers, including prostate. Turmeric has a unique ability to suppress inflammation and keep cancer cells from multiplying. Make it a goal to use a teaspoonful with meals a couple times a week. It's also available as a supplement.

Turmeric isn't the only spice-rack staple that could play a role in keeping your prostate healthy. If you're a fan of spicy foods you're sure to be familiar with fiery cayenne. You may even be familiar with the spice's medicinal use a topical pain reliever and as a circulation-booster when eaten. But you probably never realized that it may also play an important role in prostate health.

Research has shown that cayenne induces prostate cancer cell death.[16] Researchers from Nottingham University found it destroys the mito-chondria (energy producing factory) of cancer cells.[17] You can add a pinch of cayenne to your dishes to spice up meal time and protect your prostate at the same time. And if your taste buds lean towards the mild side you can pick up the spice as a supplement instead. Cayenne has a blood-thinning effect so be sure to check with your doctor before using large amounts of the spice.

Top it all off with the right tea

Tea is a known cancer fighter. But too much caffeine can be irritating to the prostate and bladder, which means for some men tea can make urinating more difficult. Your best bet is to pick a green tea, which will have significantly less caffeine but is still loaded with the anti-cancer and anti-inflammatory compounds you want.

There are many studies that show that regularly drinking green tea—generally three to five cups or more a day—has a protective effect against prostate cancer. Green tea is rich in powerful antioxidants known as polyphenols. The most important is EGCG. These antioxidants protect against damage to cell DNA (genetic material that controls cell repli-cation), cause cancer cells to stop replicating, improve immunity, and support the liver's ability to rid the body of cancer-causing compounds. I recommend picking an *organic* green tea, which is readily available in most supermarkets and health food stores.

The Common Household Poison That's Making You and Your Children Dumber

You do your best to take care of your family. You eat the right foods, you exercise, and you try to avoid chemicals that can damage your health. But what if I told you that there was a dangerous chemical lurking in your home that was nearly impossible to avoid? And what if I revealed that the chemical was "hidden" in plain sight on virtually every bathroom countertop and in approximately 70 percent of Americans' tap water? And what if your friendly neighborhood dentist insisted it's a necessity to prevent cavities?

You may have guessed by now that I'm talking about fluoride, which interestingly the FDA regards as a drug.

The truth is we've been deceived. We've been sold a bill of goods since we were children. The party line is that we need fluoride to prevent cavities. Only a negligent parent or crazy person would refuse to allow their child to use toothpaste with fluoride or get fluoride treatments when they go to the dentist, right?

At every turn picture perfect models beam their bright white fluoridated smiles at us from TV commercials while they tell us how great their fluoride-laced toothpaste is for us and our families. But there's a much darker side to fluoride that overshadows those shiny smiles. And since our government thinks it knows what's best for our health they're literally dumping this toxin into the majority of our water supply!

The REAL cause of the dumbing down of America

Although studies have shown for decades that ingesting fluoride has a boatload of detrimental health effects, one recent study has caught even mainstream medicine's sluggish attention. Researchers from the Harvard School of Public Health and China Medical University in Shenyang analyzed 27 studies and found that fluoride harms intelligence, lowers IQ, and has a distinct negative effect on overall cognition of children.[1]

Sadly, the researchers had to rely on data from Chinese studies since little research on the toxicity of fluoride has been completed in the US. (Yes, we're practically shoving this poison down our kid's throats and yet its effects have gone virtually un-researched here in this country.)

Overall, researchers determined that 26 of the 27 studies found that a high fluoride level in water negatively affected brain function in children. In a Harvard University press release discussing the results one author compared this toxin to heavy metal poisoning when he commented: "Fluoride seems to fit in with lead, mercury, and other poisons that cause chemical brain drain. The effect of each toxicant may seem small, but the combined damage on a population scale can be serious, especially because the brain power of the next generation is crucial to all of us."[2]

The Environmental Protection Agency and American Dental Association will no doubt put their own spin on these frightening findings. They will likely try to discredit the research pointing out that these were studies in China and don't apply to citizens of the US. Don't listen to them. The fact is we're not talking about one or two studies here, but 27! And the last time I checked both the government *and* mainstream medicine considered Harvard to be a very credible research organization.

The authors of the study commented that they were forced to use

Chinese studies since there is very little in the way of American research on the safety of fluoride ingestion through the water supply. You would think that *before* dumping fluoride in the American water supply, and loading up our toothpaste tubes with the stuff, there would be at least *some* long-term safety data. But nope, you'd be wrong. Instead we have to rely on Chinese research.

Let's go back to 2008 and a systematic review published in *Biological Trace Element Research*. Those researchers found that children in China who live in an area with fluoridated water have five times greater risk for a lower IQ than children who live in a nonfluoridated or slightly fluoridated area.[3] And since researchers compared the toxicity of fluoride to that of lead and mercury, both known toxins that adversely affect brain function, there's no reason to believe that fluoride won't also negatively affect the adult brain.

But it's not just the brain we need to be concerned about. According to some toxicology experts, fluoride ingestion has a poisoning effect on other parts of the body too.

The toxin that targets everything from your teeth to your ticker

Fifty percent of fluoride is metabolized by your kidneys (where it can also cause damage) and is excreted through the urine. The rest gets stored in your bones and teeth where—paradoxically—it causes damage. According to the Centers for Disease Control and Prevention, almost half of American adolescents have fluorosis.[4] This is a disfigurement of tooth enamel that is a result of exposure to excessive fluoride and that appears as white patches to brown mottling. Also, a 1995 *Journal of Dental Research* study found that bone strength in animals decreases with an *increased* level of fluoride in bones.[5] There are also data suggesting that excess fluoride may increase the risk of bone fractures, joint pain, and bone cancer.[6]

But fluoride's ravaging rampage doesn't end with your teeth and bones. Frighteningly, emerging research that suggests your ticker may be in trouble too. Research from the Netherlands found that excessive fluoride can lead to abnormal calcification of heart tissue and impaired function in animals. And remember that fluorosis I just mentioned? It turns out that in one study kids with the condition were found to have heart rhythm abnormalities.[7]

Fluoride's damaging effects may run even deeper

And fluoride doesn't just target brains, teeth, bones, and hearts. (As if that wasn't enough!) It turns out that the damaging effects of this toxin may run even deeper than that, effecting entire body systems.

Research in 2010 points to chronic fluoride exposure as a possible cause of inflammation *throughout* the body. The researchers also found that fluoride exposure reduces energy production by the cells.[8] (Since fluoride's toxicity is similar to lead and mercury this finding didn't surprise me.)

Excessive fluoride is also associated with hormone disruption, with hormones produced by the thyroid particularly affected. In fact, fluoride was once used for the treatment of hyperthyroidism, where the thyroid gland is producing too much thyroid hormone. So it stands to reason that large doses of it can suppress thyroid function.

The tooth untruth

Fluoride supporters will often point out that there has been a dramatic decline in cavities and tooth decay in the US during the past half century. But this is simply a case of misdirection. You must keep in mind there is also much better dental hygiene being practiced today. And, in addition, many European countries—where fluoride water enrichment was stopped in the 1970s—show a similar decline in cavities due to better oral hygiene.

Following fluoride to the source

While it's true that fluoride exists naturally in water, soil, and some plants, the reality is that it enters our bodies from many manmade sources. It's a by-product of phosphate fertilizer production and an industrial waste product of the aluminum smelting industry. And of course it's added too much of the nation's water supply.

Even the government has had to begrudgingly admit that excessive fluoride exposure is a problem. In 2011, the US Department of Health and Human Services announced there was too much fluoride in the nation's water supply. They recommended reducing the amount of fluoride added to water to 0.7 ppm everywhere. Previously the limit had been 0.7 ppm in warm climates where people drink a lot of water to 1.2 ppm in cooler climates where people typically consume less water.

And of course any product where water has been involved in the manufacturing process exposes people to fluoride. This includes baby formula, cereals, soda, juice, tea, wine, and beer. In addition, nonorganic foods may be laced with additional fluoride because certain pesticides can contain the toxin. To reduce your fluoride load make sure to use a reverse osmosis filtering system or drink spring water, which is usually low in fluoride.

You should work with a holistic dentist to avoid toothpaste enriched with fluoride. An average tube contains enough fluoride to kill a child, hence the warning to call poison control if your child has been ingesting toothpaste containing fluoride. Fluoride-containing toothpaste contains a fluoride concentration between 1,000 ppm to 1,500 ppm.

And remember, even if you don't swallow the toothpaste there could be fluoride absorption through the cheek and veins under the tongue directly into the blood stream. There are plenty of toothpastes, chewing gums, and mouthwashes available that are fluoride-free. Take a look at your local health food store.

Make the switch to dental products containing xylitol. Several studies have demonstrated that this natural product derived from plant fiber is effective in reducing cavities. A recent Italian study in schoolchildren at high risk for cavities found that six months of using high-dose xylitol chewing gum was effective in controlling cavities, a result that was still seen two years later.[9]

The battle has begun

The Centers for Disease Control and Prevention proclaimed the fluoridation of water "one of 10 great public health achievements of the 20th century."[10] I believe that history will show us instead, that it was one of the biggest medical blunders of all time, ranking up there with the use of drinks containing mercury to treat fevers and other illnesses. We have made great strides with the mercury fillings fiasco. However, we've been losing the battle when it comes to fluoride. For the sake of our health and that of our children, please support national and local networks fighting against water fluoridation.

WARNING:
These Common Medications Could Be Destroying Your Hearing!

Most people agree that next to vision hearing is our most important sense. Unfortunately it tends to decline for all of us as we age. And noise damage earlier in life can put you risk for hearing loss as well. But there's one major cause of hearing loss you won't hear about from your doctor (no pun intended). In fact, approximately 40 million Americans have hearing loss because of the medications they take!

Men need to be careful with erectile dysfunction medications known as PDE-5 inhibitors. Common examples are Viagra, Cialis, and Levitra. These drugs may do wonders for your love life, but could cost you your hearing. A 2011 study, which reviewed reports of hearing loss found in men who took Viagra or other drugs for erectile dysfunction, showed an association between the drugs and hearing loss. And shockingly 66.7 percent of the group studied had their hearing decline… a condition the researchers referred to as "Viagra deafness"… within 24 hours of starting the medication.[1]

But if you're not a guy, or aren't on an E.D. medication, you certainly aren't off the hook. There are plenty of other medications that can be toxic to the sensitive hearing components of your ear. (Known in medical circles as "ototoxic.") For example, common antidepressants or anti-anxiety medications such as Xanax can have an effect on your hearing as well. And one of the many reasons I advise my patients to limit their use of antibiotics is a potential for hearing loss. Antibiotics such as tetracycline or erythromycin can have this side effect.

Next are the chemotherapy drugs including the commonly prescribed carboplatin and cisplatin. And millions of Americans on blood pressure medications may be putting their hearing at risk when they take their prescribed diuretics (some folks call them "water pills"). The commonly prescribed class of drugs known as loop diuretics… including the drug Lasix… increases your risk for hearing loss.

But it's the last class of drugs I want to warn you about that might surprise you most of all. In fact, these drugs are *so* common that you might not even think of them as drugs at all. I'm talking about nonsteroidal anti-inflammatory drugs. Yes, despite their image of being gentle and safe NSAIDs—which include ibuprofen, naproxen, and aspirin—do indeed increase your risk of hearing loss.

Now I, of course, realize that there are times you might need to be on a medication. But if you're taking one of these potential hearing destroyers the good news is that you don't have to sit idly by hoping that you don't start to lose your hearing.

Instead you can be proactive by…

Protecting your hearing with super nutrients

Coenzyme Q10 is often referred to as the heart nutrient, but it turns out it's tops for ears too. CoQ10 has been shown in various animal and human studies to protect against hearing loss and actually improve hearing![2,3] I recommend 100 to 200 mg daily.

You've heard before that fish is brain food right? Well it turns out that that nutrients in seafood are great for the ears too. Research shows that there's a relationship between higher intakes of the nutrients found in seafood and decreased incidence of hearing loss. Having fish in your diet can reduce inflammation and is important for keeping the nerves involved in hearing in good health. Be sure to eat cold-water verities… like salmon or sardines… two to three times a week.

Lastly, vitamins A and E have been shown to be critical nutrients in preventing hearing loss.[4] A study in the *Journal of Nutrition, Health, and Aging* found that getting enough vitamin A and E in your diet can significantly reduce your risk of hearing loss.

Emerging research is suggesting that free radical damage to the hearing apparatus of the ear is a significant cause of hearing loss. Antioxidants like vitamins A, E, and CoQ10 are critical to reducing the nerve damaging effect of the free radicals that we're exposed to in everyday life.

Is Cancer on Tap in YOUR Kitchen?

If you're a guy I want you to put down that glass. Back slowly away from the sink. And whatever you do don't drink another sip of water until you answer one simple question for me.

Have you taken your birth control pills today?

Yes, I'm aware that it's an outrageous question. No man has ever *willingly* swallowed a birth control pill. But that's why what I'm about to tell you is so disgraceful.

You may be shocked to learn that…

Your tap water may be laced with hormones

The fact is you could be swallowing birth control hormones with every sip you take of tap water. And with every swallow, those hormones could be sending your risk of prostate cancer climbing right through the roof.

It's not pleasant to think about, but it's reality. Leftovers from birth control pills, including synthetic estrogen and progestin, are *literally* being flushed down our toilets and contaminating our water supply. And unfortunately, those of us with a prostate gland are suffering the consequences since our prostates are particularly sensitive to hormones.

A recent study in the *British Medical Journal* (BMJ) took a deep look at the data we have available on prostate cancer. But, ironically, they didn't initially set out to learn anything about prostates at all. However, they just couldn't ignore the unintentional findings that their research was turning up.

Originally the team was researching how many women were using contraception, including birth control pills, intrauterine devices, condoms, or vaginal barriers. But they accidentally also uncovered a strong link between birth control pill use and cases of prostate cancer worldwide.

Making a rePEEt performance in your drinking glass

Birth control pills are in a class of chemicals known as endocrine disturbing compounds. Other examples of endocrine disruptors include detergents, pesticides, cosmetics, and building materials. When a woman is on birth control pills, whenever she pees she literally releases hormone residues into the sewage system. And unfortunately water treatment facilities do not filter out these compounds, or even test to see if they are there. So they end up in our drinking water.

To be honest I've never been a fan of birth control pills as a form of contraception. They cause an imbalance in a woman's hormones and come with inherent risks such as breast cancer (yes, even the highly touted low-dose versions), weight gain, and blood clots. Now emerging evidence is showing the health hazards of these drugs extend to men as well. And I can only imagine what they're doing to our children.

Studies have already shown that contamination from these synthetic estrogens is causing infertility and deformities in animals. It only stands to reason that this should set off alarm bells about what they may be doing to humans as well. And this study in *BMJ* is not the first one to link them with health problems in humans. However, because the link was so significant, and seen worldwide, it <u>has</u> finally made more researchers sit up and take notice of the potential health hazards of these pills.

Protect yourself from prostate cancer

Prostate cancer is the most common male malignancy in the Western world. To lower your risks of becoming a victim you need to start protecting yourself against estrogen overload today. First, make sure you're drinking purified water. Water that's been run through a reverse-osmosis filter or distilled are both good options. And if you use a water bottle make sure it's bisphenol A free.

Next, eat one to two servings of cruciferous vegetables a day to help your body metabolize estrogen. Also be sure to get plenty of fiber into your diet. Regular bowel movements will help your body literally expel harmful estrogens. And you should start using natural skin care products that are free of estrogenic parabens.

I often test the estrogen level of men. If the level is too high I put them on a detox program. This includes purified water, organic food, and ground flaxseeds. In addition I have them supplement their diet with phytonutrients such as indole 3 carbinol, diindolylmethane, and glutathione, which helps their livers rid their bodies of the extra estrogen.

The Bitter Truth About Artificial Sweeteners and Cancer

You probably know aspartame by its brand names NutraSweet and Equal. The popular artificial sweetener is a staple on restaurant tables around the world. It adds the sweet taste to diet soda, instant tea, sugarless candy, and chewing gum. Heck, it's even dumped into over-the-counter cough syrups and liquid pain relievers to make them syrupy sweet.

Aspartame is popular because it tastes similar to sugar but adds no calories to foods. According to the Calorie Control Council the fake sweetener is used in more than 6,000 products and it's eaten by more than 200 million people around the world.[1] And while it's classified by the US Food and Drug Administration (FDA) as a "general purpose sweetener" I prefer to call it "bad news."

Aspartame sounds fine and dandy—until you start looking at its sordid past and the results of a very concerning recent study. Researchers at Brigham and Women's Hospital and Harvard Medical School conducted this recent test. It looked at the relationship between drinking regular and diet soft drinks and risks of lymphoma and leukemia in more than 77,000 women and 47,000 men over 22-years. Researchers found that drinking more than one serving of diet soda a day was associated in certain groups with increased risk of developing leukemia, multiple myeloma, and non-Hodgkin's lymphomas compared with participants who do not drink as much diet soda.[2] More specifically it found that greater intake of diet soda was associated with:

- Higher leukemia risk in men and women (pooled analysis)

- Higher multiple myeloma risk (in men only)

- Higher risk non-Hodgkin's lymphoma risk (in men only)

The type of analysis done in this study doesn't *prove* by itself that aspartame causes cancer. But it's another great reason to avoid the sweetener. Or at least, use it sparingly. Aspartame eventually breaks down into formaldehyde a chemical that can cause cancer. The main source of this potential poison is diet soda.

Your brain on aspartame

Aspartame is made of two amino acids, aspartic acid and phenylalanine *combined* with a methyl ester group. Now you don't need to remember all those 20 cent words. Instead, just remember that according to some reports aspartame may wreak havoc on your brain and nervous system. Some critics of the sweetener believe that it acts as an excitotoxin—a chemical substance that damages neurons by stimulating excess activity. It's also been widely reported that the Food and Drug Administration (FDA) has received more than 10,000 complaints about aspartame. These complaints included headaches, dizziness, and even seizures.

Don't settle for sucralose

Sucralose, known by the retail name Splenda, is a common artificial sweetener in the US. No long-term human studies have been conducted on Splenda. And the studies done on animals aren't reassuring. They reveal links to reduced thymus growth rate… enlargement of the liver and kidneys… decreased packed cell volume… and increased risk of cataracts. Admittedly, the amount of sucralose fed to the study animals was very high—yet there's still a great need for clinical studies on humans.

Saccharin side effects?

Saccharin, sold as Sweet'N Low and Necta Sweet, has been a controversial artificial sweetener since its introduction in the early 1900s. Some users report reactions to saccharin, including itching, hives, headache, and diarrhea. A study done in the late 1970s showed that high doses can cause bladder cancer in male rats. Based on those findings saccharin was banned in Canada (but they're considering lifting the ban). In 1977, Congress required warning labels for products containing saccharin, although this requirement has since been repealed.

Stevia is safe and sweet

Americans have been tricked to believe that artificial sweeteners pose no risk. Here's the truth: In susceptible people, artificial sweeteners may be associated with variety of health problems, from weight gain to headaches to mood changes to possibly cancer. Why take unnecessary risks? There are all-natural alternatives that can satisfy the pickiest sweet tooth, without adding unwanted calories.

Stevia rebaudiana (stevia) has been a popular natural sweetener in the US health food industry for the past 17 years. The plant grows in the rain forests of Brazil and Paraguay, and in Asia. Stevia is up to 300 times sweeter than table sugar and has almost no calories. I have found it has no detrimental effects on blood sugar readings.

In studies, stevia lowered blood pressure in people with mild hypertension and reduced blood glucose levels in patients with type 2 diabetes. Also, an extract from stevia leaves contains antioxidant polyphenol flavonoids which protect against DNA damage, according to a study published in *the Journal of Agricultural and Food Chemistry*.[3]

Stevia is available in liquid, powder, and tablet form. To sweeten an eight-ounce beverage, such as coffee, tea, or lemonade, you generally need to use only one tablet, a pinch of the powder, or three to five drops of the liquid. Follow directions on the label.

You can bake with stevia, substituting one teaspoon of powder or liquid extract for each cup of sugar. Stevia can have a bitter aftertaste, depending on the brand and amount used. Fortunately recent stevia extracts have less of the bitter aftertaste that was once a problem. Even soda pop conglomerates Pepsi and Coca Cola are introducing products sweetened with stevia.

The xylitol option

Xylitol is a white substance that looks and tastes like sugar. You find the natural sweetener in fruits, vegetables, and the bark of some trees. The human body also produces xylitol naturally while breaking down other food sources. In the 1960's it was approved as a food additive by both the World Health Organization and the FDA. Xylitol has 40 to 50 percent fewer calories than sugar. It has no detrimental effects on blood sugar levels and is safe for people with diabetes.

Xylitol has another surprising benefit. The sweetener reduces the formation of cavity-causing plaque. It does this by preventing bacteria from adhering to the mucous membranes of the mouth and sinus and helps to build tooth enamel. Xylitol is used in sugar-free chewing gums, mouthwashes, and toothpastes—products I buy for my own family.

This natural sweetener works very well for beverages. However, xylitol should not be used for baking breads or other foods that contain yeast. In some people, xylitol can trigger diarrhea. To avoid this, start with a small amount and let your digestive tract adjust to it gradually. Xylitol is available in powder form. One popular product is Xylosweet.

The zero calorie fruit extract

Lo han kuo (also spelled luo han guo) is the fruit of *Momordica grossvenori* plant, a member of the cucumber family that grows in southern China. For several centuries, the fruit has been used by practitioners of Chinese medicine to treat dry coughs, sore throats, skin conditions, digestive problems, and to calm the nervous system. People make tea, juice, soup, candy and cake from the dried fruits.

It contains no sugar or calories, and it's safe for people with diabetes and hypoglycemia (low blood sugar). It doesn't lose its sweetness when heated, so it can be used in baking and cooking. The FDA has approved lo han kuo as a "generally regarded as safe" (GRAS) food ingredient. There's no known toxicity associated with this fruit extract. Lo han kuo products I find have a taste similar to maple syrup and leave no aftertaste.

One product that's been popular with my patients is Lo Han Sweet made by the company Jarrow. It's a combination of Lo Han and Xylitol. It can be found online and in health food stores.

Part XII

Dr. Stengler's Top 19 Healing Secrets

Dr. Stengler's Quick Cures

Homeopathy promotes healing by utilizing substances that mobilize the body's natural self-defense processes. For uncomplicated health problems, such as occasional digestive upset or a cold, patients can be helped with simple, common homeopathic or herbal remedies sold in health-food stores. My quick cures…

For nosebleeds

Pinch the nose closed, and keep your head tilted downward (not back, which can cause choking). If you continue to bleed profusely from a nosebleed (or any other small wound), take the homeopathic remedy *Phosphorus* (dissolve two 30C pellets under the tongue) to cut down on bleeding time. Take five minutes after the bleeding begins. If bleeding continues, wait five minutes and take another dose.

For spring allergies

To reduce spring allergy symptoms such as burning, watery eyes, sneezing and runny nose, use the homeopathic remedy *Allium cepa*. Take two pellets of a 30C potency three times daily for one to two days. Symptoms should improve. If symptoms recur during allergy season, you can take the dose again.

For earache

For an earache caused by infection, use Herb Pharm Mullein/Garlic Compound eardrops. A blend of garlic and mullein (an herb), the drops combat infection and reduce inflammation without killing health-promoting bacteria, as antibiotics do. Place two or three warm drops (heat the bottle first) in the affected ear. Repeat three or four times daily or until pain is gone. Do not use if your eardrum is perforated or if your ear contains fluid or pus. Available online as well as at health-food stores.

For motion sickness

If you are prone to nausea and dizziness while riding in a car or on a boat, travel with the homeopathic remedy *Cocculus*, which is available at health-food stores. It works very quickly. Dissolve two pellets of 30C potency under your tongue. Wait five minutes. If you don't feel better, take an additional two pellets of 30C potency. Breathing fresh air also will help you feel better.

For digestive upset

For gastrointestinal complaints, such as belching or upper abdominal bloating, use the homeopathic preparation *Carbo vegetabilis*, available at health-food stores. Take two 30C pellets. If digestive upset continues, take this dose again in 10 minutes. Wait another 10 minutes, then take again, if needed. There are no side effects. If this remedy doesn't help after three doses, stop taking it.

For menstrual cramps

To ease the pain of menstrual cramps, take cramp bark, the dried bark of the cramp bark shrub (*Viburnum opulus*). This herb works as a gentle muscle relaxant. Known to quickly ease menstrual cramps, it can be used to help all types of muscle problems, including leg cramps or a stiff neck. Follow the instructions on the label. There are no reported side effects or interactions.

For constipation

Try the herb senna (*Cassia senna*), which is a natural laxative. Take 500 mg in capsule form (standardized to 20–60 mg *sennosides*). Or drink one cup of senna tea. Do not use senna for long-term relief (more than one week) of constipation or if you are pregnant or have Crohn's disease or ulcerative colitis.

For food poisoning

As your body rids itself of the contaminated food, you can restore the good bacteria in the intestine by taking probiotics, such as *Lactobacillus (L.) acidophilus* and *L. bifidus*. Take five billion colony-forming units four times daily on the first day. That should help your body fight and eliminate the intestinal infection.

For mosquito bites

To reduce the swelling, pain and itch of mosquito and other insect bites, use the homeopathic preparation *Ledum* (Ledum *palustre*). Take one pellet of 30C potency. If the itchiness and discomfort have not subsided in 30 minutes, take another pellet. There are no side effects—and Ledum is safe for everyone. Those who get boil-like bites can also mix two 30C pellets of Ledum in two ounces of water in a spray bottle, then spray bites every hour to reduce discomfort.

For sunburn pain

To ease the pain of sunburn, take the homeopathic preparation *Cantharis*. Use a 30C potency four to six times daily for two days. This remedy helps to prevent or reduce blistering and burn pain. Cantharis is safe for everyone. In addition, you can apply a gel of 90 percent to 99 percent aloe.

For canker sores

For canker sores, those painful, open sores inside the mouth, use *deglycyrrhizinated licorice* (DGL), a preparation of the licorice plant with anti-inflammatory properties that speed the healing of ulcers. Take 1,000 mg to 3,000 mg daily of DGL in a chewable tablet while you have the canker sore. DGL is safe for everyone.

Head-to-Toe Diagnostic Clues Part 1

Stand in front of a mirror and stick out your tongue. Is your tongue's surface smooth or cracked? Stroke your fingers across the back of your upper arm. Do you feel tiny bumps on the skin? You may never have noticed—but to a holistic doctor, such small physical signs provide clues to your health. Close observation gives me a sense of a patient's problem even before I hear about symptoms or see lab test results—giving us a head start on healing.

What your hair and face reveal about your health

In a two-part feature, I'll take you on a top-to-bottom tour of the body, describing subtle signs suggesting health problems and outlining treatments. Unless noted, all products are sold at health-food stores or pharmacies and are safe for everyone (but if you take medication, check with your doctor before using them). In cases where my advice may differ from the instructions on product labels, I have recommended dosages. Here, I will cover the hair and face… in the next article, I'll cover the rest of the body (including the arm and its mysterious bumps).

Hair's health clues

• **Brittle hair**. Hair that breaks easily and has split ends could signal nutritional deficiencies. I suggest taking supplements of the mineral *silicon* at five milligrams daily... the sulfur compound *methylsulfonylmethane* (MSM) at 3,000 mg daily... and a vitamin B complex at 50 mg twice daily. *Essential fatty acids* (EFAs) will also help, so take fish oil supplements with 500 mg to 1,000 mg of combined *eicosapentaenoic acid* (EPA) and docosahexaenoic acid (DHA), or two tablespoons daily of *flaxseed oil, perilla oil* or *hemp seed oil.*

Helpful: Shampoo enriched with vitamin B-7 (biotin), such as Natural Biotin Shampoo (Jason Natural Products at 866-595-8917 or www. jason-natural.com).

• **Hair loss**. It's often blamed on genes, but for some men and most women, hair loss is actually due to excess cortisol (a stress hormone) or testosterone... or deficiencies of *estrogen, progesterone* or *thyroid hormone*. Low thyroid hormone also causes partial loss of the eyebrows. These imbalances are associated with poor diet, stress, exposure to toxins or (for women) pregnancy or menopause. Hormone imbalances can be confirmed with saliva, urine and/or blood testing.

Mild cases of hair loss can be corrected in men and women with natural over-the-counter (OTC) remedies. Try...

• The herbs *saw palmetto* (for men) and *chasteberry* (for women).

• Cream containing progesterone (for women). Use under the supervision of a physician—excessive dosages may cause irregular menstrual cycles.

If hair loss occurs at a time of high stress, also take oral supplements of...

• The herb *ashwagandha* (in extract form).

• An herbal relaxation formula with *passionflower, oat straw* and/or *valerian root.*

If these remedies don't halt hair loss within six weeks, you may have a severe hormone imbalance. Talk to your doctor about bioidentical prescription hormone therapy.

• **Sensitive scalp.** When patients report that it hurts to comb their hair, I suspect a deficiency of nutrients involved with nerve function.

Solution: Daily supplements of vitamin D at 800 IU to 2,000 IU, plus 500 mg of magnesium in divided doses. Scalp pain also can be due to a sensitivity to shampoos or styling products. Switch to more natural hair products, available at health-food stores.

• **Dandruff.** It does not take a doctor to spot telltale flakes, but few people realize that dandruff often stems from nutritional deficiencies. Take a vitamin B complex at 50 mg twice daily... a multivitamin that includes 200 mcg of the mineral selenium... and EFAs, such as fish oil or flaxseed, perilla or hemp seed oil. Dandruff also may be linked to low stomach acid, which impedes nutrient absorption.

Helpful: OTC tablets of *betaine hydrochloride* (which mimics stomach acid), at 500 mg to 700 mg three times daily with meals, plus the herbs *gentian root* and *dandelion root*, which stimulate stomach acid production. (Do not use these if you have an ulcer.)

Secrets seen in the eyes

• **Bloodshot eyes.** Persistent red in the eyes without nasal congestion suggests a food sensitivity, typically to dairy products, soy, sugar, wheat or gluten (a sticky protein found in wheat, rye and barley). To recognize triggers, eliminate suspected foods from your diet, one by one, for several weeks to see if symptoms improve.

An unusual diagnostic tool: Noninvasive *electrodermal testing*, which measures a body's electrical response—from acupuncture points and energy-flow meridians—to the foods being tested. (This test is available from holistic physicians and chiropractors.)

Also, blood testing can measure the body's production of antibodies in response to various foods. Those foods that trigger reactions can be avoided… or a desensitization program that involves exposure to small but steadily increasing amounts of the allergen can "teach" the immune system to stop overreacting.

• **Dark circles**. This classic sign of sleep deprivation also can indicate food allergies. Less often, dark circles suggest that the liver is not effectively removing toxins from the body. To improve liver function, eat carrots and beets or drink their juices… and take daily supplements of *chlorella* (a type of algae), plus the herbs milk thistle, dandelion root and wheatgrass.

• **Pale inner eyelids**. Whenever I gently pull down a patient's lower eyelid, I hope to see a healthy pink-red color. A pale eyelid interior suggests iron-deficiency anemia—especially if the patient has bleeding hemorrhoids… has a heavy menstrual flow… or is a vegan (one who eats no meat, fish, dairy foods, eggs or honey). If blood tests confirm an iron deficiency, I prescribe 100 mg to 200 mg of chelated iron daily, to be taken only until test results return to normal.

Ear exam

• **Earwax**. Excessive buildup often signals a food sensitivity or an EFA deficiency. To remove earwax, place two drops of warm (not hot) olive oil in the affected ear… leave in for one hour (lie on your side, ear up)… then rinse in the shower or bathtub. Repeat as necessary. OTC earwax removal products with peroxide can be used in a similar manner.

• **Popping noises**. Often due to chronic *serous otitis media* (fluid behind the eardrum), these noises may be caused by an EFA deficiency or food sensitivities.

Helpful: A naturopathic or osteopathic doctor or a chiropractor can gently manipulate the head and neck to release trapped fluid.

What i know from a nose

• **Runny nose**. When red eyes accompany a runny nose, I suspect an environmental allergy —to pollen or dust mites, for example. For relief, take supplements of *stinging nettle leaf* and *quercetin* (an anti-inflammatory plant compound)… and rinse eyes twice daily with one ounce of saline solution mixed with five drops of the herb *eyebright* in tincture form.

• **Red nose.** Flushing on the nose and cheeks that's accompanied by red bumps may look like pimples, but it could be due to the inflammatory skin disease *rosacea*. Its cause is unknown, although there may be an underlying vascular problem. A bacterial infection called *Helicobacter pylori* (which also causes stomach ulcers) may be associated with rosacea, too. Such an infection can be diagnosed with a blood test and treated with antibiotics or oral supplements of the amino acid *zinc carnosine*… an herbal preparation of *mastic gum*… and/or *betaine hydrochloride*. Since bacteria on the skin may exacerbate problems, use a topical cream with the compound *alpha lipoic acid.* Too much estrogen and/or too little progesterone also may contribute to rosacea.

Helpful: A hormone-balancing progesterone capsule or cream (for women)… or the herb *burdock root* in capsule form, at 500 mg three times daily (for men and women).

What a mouth tells me

• **Swollen gums**. These usually indicate poor dental hygiene, but they also can suggest a deficiency of vitamin C or *flavonoids* (healthful plant pigments), especially if the patient bruises easily. Try 1,000 mg of vitamin C twice daily… plus 300 mg of *grape seed extract* daily. In a vegetarian or a person who takes cholesterol-lowering statin medicine, swollen gums suggest a deficiency of the naturally occurring nutrient *coenzyme Q10* (CoQ10), needed for basic cell function.

Helpful: 100 mg to 200 mg of CoQ10 daily.

• **Pale or swollen tongue.** A light red tongue is a sign of good health, but a pale pink tongue may indicate iron deficiency. A swollen, smooth, sore tongue suggests a deficiency of B vitamins. Blood tests can confirm deficiencies, and supplements or injections can correct the problem.

• **White tongue coating**. A thin coating is normal, but a thicker white coating suggests a *Candida albicans* yeast infection—either limited to the mouth or reflecting an overgrowth of yeast in the digestive tract. This is common with long-term use of antibiotics. Restrict simple sugars… eat yogurt with live cultures… take antifungal herbs, such as oregano oil… and take probiotics, such as *Lactobacillus acidophilus* and *bifidobacterium*, to restore beneficial bacteria to the digestive tract.

• **Rough tongue**. Grooves in the middle of the tongue plus a sticky coating of mucus are associated with chronic digestive problems, such as *irritable bowel syndrome* (IBS) or *ulcerative colitis*. Scalloped indentations on the sides of the tongue suggest liver or gallbladder problems.

Solutions: A more healthful diet… digestive enzyme supplements, such as Enzymedica Digest Gold (888-918-1118, www.enzymedica. com), taken with meals… herbs to aid digestion, including ginger and gentian root… and/or herbs that support liver and gallbladder function, such as *milk thistle, turmeric, artichoke* and *dandelion*.

• **Splotchy tongue**. Small bumps called *papillae* normally cover the tongue's upper surface. Smooth, sensitive splotches amidst the bumpiness result from the loss of papillae on certain areas, creating a "geographic tongue."

Likely cause: Vitamin B deficiency. Take 50 mg of a vitamin B complex twice daily.

Also try: The homeopathic remedy *Taraxacum* (derived from dandelion root). Take two pellets of a 30C potency twice daily for two weeks.

Cheek checkup

• **Sunken cheeks**. Few American doctors realize that hollow cheeks can indicate a deficiency of *cortisol* or growth hormone. Saliva or blood testing can identify the problem, which then can be treated with hormone therapy, if necessary.

• **Puffy cheeks**. I can tell whether a woman takes birth control pills because her puffy cheeks are a tip-off. Daily supplements of 50 mg of vitamin B-6 and 500 mg of magnesium help the liver to process the estrogen from the pills, reducing water retention.

Now that you know what to watch for, give your head a good look. If you notice any of the signs above, talk to your doctor—who will applaud your diagnostic skills.

Head-to-Toe Diagnostic Clues
Part 2

Did you stroke your fingers across the back of your upper arm? Did you feel tiny bumps on the skin? When I asked this earlier, I left readers wondering—because Part 1 of this two-part feature discussed what the face and hair reveal about health. In Part 2, I'll review the rest of the body—and share the secret behind those tiny bumps, plus many other subtle health clues.

Unless noted, all treatments below are safe for everyone. Supplements are sold at health-food stores.

News from the neck

• **A bowtie-shaped bump**. This distinctive swelling at the base of the throat is a *goiter*, or enlarged thyroid gland, due to a deficiency of iodine. The thyroid gland needs iodine to manufacture thyroid hormone. Deficiencies are common in people who avoid salt.

Solution: Eat iodine-rich sea vegetables, strawberries, eggs and dairy foods (in moderation)… take 150 mcg to 300 mcg of iodine daily in capsule form… and consult an endocrinologist.

• **Stiff neck**. Tight muscles or restriction of the neck vertebrae can result from poor posture or sleeping with a pillow that is too soft or too hard.

Recommended: Massage and/or acupuncture, particularly if you also have headaches or neck pain... a cervical pillow that fits the neck's natural curve... and the muscle-relaxing mineral magnesium (250 mg, or mg, twice daily), taken with calcium (500 mg twice daily) for optimal effect, until stiffness is gone.

Warning: A stiff neck along with a fever and severe headache may indicate *meningitis*, a serious infection that requires emergency care.

What the torso tells me

• **Sagging breasts**. In a woman, sagging breasts may simply be her natural shape—or may indicate a deficiency of the hormones *estrogen* and/or *progesterone*, particularly if accompanied by hot flashes and overall loss of skin elasticity. If saliva and/or blood tests confirm a deficiency, *hormone-replacement therapy* (HRT) may be appropriate.

Flabby breast tissue is not uncommon in overweight men because fat cells produce estrogen, a hormone that contributes to breast enlargement. A diet rich in *cruciferous* vegetables (broccoli, cauliflower, collard greens, cabbage), plus two tablespoons of ground flaxseeds every day (taken with 10 oz of water), help the liver to break down excess estrogen—and also provide a good start on a sensible weight-loss plan.

• **Apple-shaped abdomen**. A person who's as big or bigger around the waist as around the hips may have *insulin resistance*—in which the body's cells don't readily accept the glucose-transporting hormone insulin, so the pancreas produces more insulin to compensate. This leads to an accumulation of fat around the waist. Insulin resistance is a risk factor for diabetes. Excessive insulin also contributes to inflammation—which sets the stage for cardiovascular disease, Alzheimer's disease, arthritis and cancer.

For a rotund patient, I recommend regular exercise and a diet high in fiber and low in refined carbohydrates. Supplements of a fat called *conjugated linoleic acid* (CLA) at 1,000 mg three times daily can aid weight loss and promote the cells' proper use of insulin. *Slimaluma*, a plant extract (taken at 500 mg, one hour before breakfast and dinner), curbs appetite and reduces abdominal fat. I also test levels of *dehydroepiandrosterone* (DHEA), since supplementation of this hormone in people who have low levels can reduce belly fat and improve insulin resistance.

Clues in the skin

• **Hairless skin**. Sparse body hair in men and women suggests a deficiency of the hormones *testosterone* and/or *DHEA*, which can increase the risk for depression, fatigue, poor memory, low libido, osteoporosis and heart disease. If tests confirm the diagnosis, prescription testosterone HRT and/or nonprescription DHEA oral supplements (best used under a doctor's supervision) may be warranted.

• **Skin tags**. These small, soft, protruding bumps are connected to the skin by a narrow stalk of tissue. They are usually benign and painless but can become irritated. Skin tags are most common on the eyelids, neck, armpits, upper chest and groin… tend to appear in middle age… and are more common in women. Growths can be removed surgically, electrically (*cautery*) or by freezing (*cryotherapy*), but they may grow back. The cause of skin tags is unknown, but natural remedies may halt the spread and prevent recurrence. Take daily supplements of *biotin* (300 mcg)… *chromium* (200 mcg to 400 mcg)… *alpha lipoic acid* (300 mg)… and *cinnamon extract* (500 mg). Also try homeopathic *Thuja occidentalis*, at two pellets of a 30C potency twice daily for a month.

Secrets held in the hands and arms

• **Weak pulse at your wrist**. Every doctor checks a patient's pulse, looking for a steady rate of 60 to 80 beats per minute. However, I like to employ some of my Chinese medicine training by evaluating more subtle signs. For example, a very strong pulse can indicate stress, while a weak pulse that is hard to detect suggests that the heart is not contracting as forcefully as it should or that certain organs are not functioning well. A complete pulse diagnosis can be made by a practitioner of Oriental medicine. For a referral, contact the American Association of Acupuncture &

Oriental Medicine (866-455-7999, www.aaaomonline.org).

• **Abnormal fingernails**. Spoon-shaped nails or pale nail beds that do not quickly return to their normal color after being pressed suggest iron-deficiency anemia… ridges can indicate an infection or low thyroid function… white spots mean a zinc deficiency… and brittle nails signal a deficiency of protein, essential fatty acids, calcium and/or silicon. Nail abnormalities also result from reduced stomach acid, which leads to poor nutrient absorption.

Solution: In addition to a daily multivitamin, take two capsules (with every meal) of *betaine hydrochloride*, a beet extract that increases stomach acid… or a full-spectrum digestive enzyme, which improves nutrient absorption.

Lessons from the legs and feet

• **Stiff knees**. A stiff-legged gait and aching knees can signal *osteoarthritis*, a degeneration of cartilage (tough, elastic tissue that allows bones to slide smoothly over one another). Its causes include previous injuries, inflammatory disease and nutritional deficiencies. To lubricate joints and help repair cartilage, take daily *glucosamine* (1,500 mg)… *chondroitin* (1,200 mg)… combination *eicosapentaenoic acid* and *docosahexaenoic acid* (1,000 mg)… and *hyaluronic acid* (200 mg in two divided doses).

• **Inward- or outward-rolling feet**. I watch patients walk, looking for *pronation*—a biomechanical problem common among the flat-footed, in which the feet tilt inward—or *supination*, in which the feet roll outward. Either condition can lead to pain in the feet, knees, hips and lower back. A chiropractor or podiatrist can provide supportive custom-made orthotic shoe inserts to promote proper foot alignment.

Helpful: Exercise the muscles of the arch by picking up marbles with your toes.

The answer you've been waiting for...

Those itty-bitty, not-so-pretty bumps on the back of the arms are *follicular hyperkeratosis* and usually signal a vitamin A deficiency. Take 5,000 IU—the upper limit for pregnant women—to 10,000 IU of vitamin A daily until bumps clear up, typically four to six weeks. Thereafter, to prevent a recurrence, take a daily multivitamin that contains at least 2,500 IU of vitamin A or *beta-carotene* (which the body converts into vitamin A) and eat beta-carotene–rich foods, such as dark green and orange-yellow vegetables.

Beat Bad Breath

About half of Americans have bad breath (*halitosis*). Fortunately, a simple natural approach often eradicates the problem.

So many conditions could contribute to bad breath, including gum disease, degrading silver fillings, chronic dental and/or throat infections and ulcers and other digestive problems. Go to a dentist to find the cause because bad breath may indicate a bigger problem. *If your dentist cannot find a problem, try these suggestions…*

Take one teaspoon of liquid *chlorophyll* (the green pigment in plants) straight or diluted in a glass of water after meals. Chlorophyll (available at most health-food stores) freshens breath and supports detoxification of the digestive tract.

Many people who have bad breath have an overgrowth of bacteria in the mouth, which is typically caused by certain foods, sugar, lack of good bacteria and/or infection. For these cases, I recommend rinsing with *xylitol*, a natural sugar alcohol found in many fruits, berries, vegetables and mushrooms. Xylitol prevents bacteria from adhering to teeth and gums. I have seen good results with a product called Spry Cool Mint Oral Rinse, used twice daily. About $5 a bottle.

The Awesome Healing Power of Silver

You know that silver is a precious metal and an industrial commodity—but did you know that it also is a powerful healing agent? Silver has antimicrobial and antibacterial properties, and it has been used throughout the ages to cure infections and help heal wounds. Now interest in silver is growing in the medical community because new studies have found that it can kill a wide range of bacteria and viruses, including the very dangerous *E. coli* and *Staphylococcus*.

The form of silver generally used as medicine is colloidal silver, which is the suspension of microscopic particles of silver in liquid.

Before the advent of antibiotics, colloidal silver was used to treat infections. Silver utensils and vessels (with silver linings) were known to kill germs better than utensils and vessels made of other materials. But after antibiotics came into vogue, silver went out of favor with conventional doctors except for a few uses—as a salve for burns and wounds... in nitrate eye solutions to prevent blindness in newborn babies... and as an antibacterial coating in the lining of catheters.

Holistic physicians, however, never stopped prescribing colloidal silver to prevent many types of viral, bacterial and fungal infections, with generally excellent results. Now, with various bacteria strains becoming increasingly resistant to the effects of antibiotics, the rest of the medical community is once again becoming interested in colloidal silver. Because silver attacks microbes in several different ways at once, it's more difficult for the microbes to develop protective mechanisms. In a Taiwanese study published in the journal *Colloids and Surfaces B: Biointerfaces*, colloidal silver was found to kill the potentially deadly superbug known as *methicillin-resistant Staphylococcus aureus* (MRSA) and *Pseudomonas aeruginosa*, another dangerous superbug, on surfaces (such as doorknobs and light switches, where it is known to colonize and spread among people). A study in *Current Science* found that colloidal silver can boost the effectiveness of standard antibiotics when used in combination with them. Colloidal silver's effectiveness against a range of viruses, including *hepatitis C*, *herpes* and *HIV*, also has been shown in both laboratory tests and in people.

My approach

I recommend colloidal silver in liquid form, drops or spray to many of my patients with infections of all kinds, including those of the eyes, ears, throat, respiratory tract, digestive tract or urinary tract. To determine how to use each form of colloidal silver, follow the instructions on the label. *For example, it can be...*

• **Ingested** (one teaspoon of the preparation four times daily, up to seven days).

• **Put into a saline solution to treat pinkeye** (two drops in one-half ounce of saline solution, and rinse the eye with the solution three times daily for seven days).

• **Placed directly in the ear** (two drops in the affected ear three times daily for seven days).

• **Sprayed on cuts**.

Other uses: Colloidal silver often is used by holistic physicians to fight infection intravenously. I frequently prescribe colloidal silver to be taken for several months by patients with Lyme disease... or I recommend it instead of antibiotics for infections. For these types of uses, it is best taken under a doctor's supervision (see below for the risks).

Brand to try: Sovereign Silver (888-328-8840, www.natural-immuno genics.com). This high-quality solution contains the smallest particles of any colloidal silver product on the market, with an average diameter of 0.8 nanometers (eight angstroms) per particle. Small particle size is important for several reasons. It enables the particles to penetrate and kill microbe cells more easily... and makes it easier for your body to flush them out of your system once they've done their job.

Safety issues

Colloidal silver is safe for children, but it is not recommended for women who are pregnant or breast-feeding, because it has not been studied in these populations.

Ingesting silver products has, in rare cases, been linked to an irreversible condition called *argyria*, in which the skin turns bluish gray. While this is clearly a side effect that no one wants to encounter, case studies show that this condition occurs only when silver products are consumed for a year or more and/or as a result of ingesting very large amounts—at least one gram, which would require drinking an absurd amount of properly prepared colloidal silver solution (more than 100 quarts daily).

I have never had a case of argyria with the hundreds of patients I have treated with colloidal silver, nor have any of my colleagues witnessed this in their patients. With most commercially made silver products, I consider the risk for argyria to be negligible even with a regimen that lasts for several months (as long as the correct dose is used).

Do not attempt to make a colloidal silver product yourself, and do not ingest someone else's homemade product. A variety of do-it-yourself kits are available. However, these kits create silver particles that are quite large, making them less effective at killing microbes and more difficult for the body's cells to eliminate than smaller particles. Large silver particles are more likely to produce argyria with long-term use.

Healing Outside the Box of Mainstream Medicine

Almost invariably, new patients tell me, "Conventional medicine is not helping me. I'm here to try something different." Patients are now waking up to the fact that most diseases can be helped or healed through natural medicine. Yet success requires that patients and their doctors "think outside the box" of mainstream medicine.

Healing sometimes takes more than an open mind, however. I'm often very impressed by my patients who demonstrate dedication to a new lifestyle... perseverance in spite of setbacks... and courage to combat a discouraging prognosis. Here are the stories of four patients from whom I've learned invaluable lessons. I hope you find them inspiring, too.

Listen to your body

"I've lost track of how many different doctors I've seen in the past three years," said Nancy, 39, a real estate agent and mother of four. "They never agree on what's wrong, other than to imply that my problems are in my head. But my body is telling me something isn't right."

Nancy had a daunting list of two dozen symptoms, including relentless fatigue, widespread muscle pain, dry skin, hair loss, weight gain, *hypoglycemia* (low blood sugar), recurring respiratory infections, dizzy spells, panic attacks and heart palpitations. Her various medical doctors had run numerous blood tests and other laboratory analyses over the years, but the results had always been "normal." Several times Nancy was offered antidepressants, which she refused. "I'm not sick because I'm depressed—I'm depressed because I'm sick," she told me.

Instead of trying to treat Nancy's symptoms one by one, I searched for a connection among her seemingly disparate problems—and recognized that many of them suggested low thyroid function. I ordered a blood test for *free T3*, the most specific marker of thyroid function available. (T3 is one of the thyroid hormones, and the "free" level is the amount not bound to protein and therefore available for use by the body's cells.) This test is not routinely ordered by most doctors, though I think it should be used more often.

The test confirmed that Nancy's free T3 level was low. I prescribed Armour Thyroid, a brand of natural thyroid hormone in tablet form that contains T3 and a blend of other thyroid hormones found in the human body. Most thyroid prescriptions do not contain T3, but instead contain only T4, a less potent and less effective thyroid hormone.

The results were fantastic. Within one week, Nancy's fatigue had eased and her mood had improved. During the next three months, her energy level returned to normal... muscle pain disappeared... respiratory infections cleared up... weight and blood sugar stabilized... skin and hair condition improved... and her mood lifted. Nancy said, "I can hardly believe how well I feel from just one simple type of treatment."

Self-help strategy: Before seeing a dozen different specialists for a dozen different symptoms, consult a holistic physician. He/she will evaluate you as a whole person, rather than as a collection of problematic body parts—and may identify a single root cause behind all your symptoms. A good holistic doctor also will acknowledge that you know your own body best and will take all your concerns seriously.

Help cells to help themselves

A dedicated farmer and proud new grandparent, David was devastated when his oncologist reported that his prostate cancer had spread to his breastbone and that chemotherapy could not help. In an attempt to keep the cancer from spreading further, David underwent radiation treatments. He also received injections of drugs to reduce his body's production of testosterone and estrogen, since these hormones are associated with prostate cancer. Despite these measures, his prognosis was bleak. "Get your affairs in order," his doctor advised. "You've got about 12 months." David was 64 years old.

Though he had never given credence to alternative medicine, David decided that he had nothing to lose. At his son-in-law's urging, he came to see me.

I emphasized the need for David to help his cells detoxify—to release toxins that could be causing the cancer and to minimize the harmful side effects of the radiation treatments. I also recommended that we stimulate his immune system so that it could more effectively combat the disease.

First line of defense: A detoxifying diet.

Although David had been a lifelong beef lover, frequent beer drinker and occasional cake baker, David immediately gave up red meat, alcohol and sugary foods, and greatly increased his intake of nutritious vegetables and fish. He also began taking daily supplements of cancer-fighting vitamin C and selenium... the herbal detoxifiers dandelion root, burdock root and milk thistle... and various natural immune boosters, including *echinacea* and *Oregon grape root.*

The nutrients did their job better than David had dared to hope. He is now cancer-free—16 years after his doctor had predicted his imminent demise. David remains conscientious about his detoxifying diet-and-supplement regimen. "It's the reason I'm here today," he says, "watching my grandson grow up."

Self-help strategy: By detoxifying the body, it's often possible to fight serious diseases at the most basic cellular level. By being open-minded about alternative therapies, you increase treatment options and optimize healing.

Say no to drugs... and yes to nutrition

Victor, 12, was in trouble at school. For years, the boy's behavior had caused problems in the classroom, and recently his restlessness and outbursts had worsened. His grades, never good, had dropped perilously close to failing. After Victor's pediatrician diagnosed *attention deficit hyperactivity disorder* (ADHD), the school psychologist and principal pressured the boy's parents, warning, "If Victor does not go on ADHD medication, he will be asked to leave the school."

But Victor's mother stood firm—"Those drugs can have serious side effects. We need to explore all other options first." That is when the family contacted me.

I shared the family's concerns about ADHD medicine, such as *methylphenidate* (Ritalin) and *amphetamine/dextroamphetamine* (Adderall XR), which can cause nausea, loss of appetite and stunted growth... headaches, dizziness and tics... insomnia and exhaustion... irritability and mood swings... and heart palpitations, blood pressure changes and an increased risk of heart attack. We agreed to try nutritional therapies first and to use drugs only as a last resort.

Fortunately, we had all summer vacation to address Victor's problems. The boy's diet was already good—but nonetheless, I suspected a deficiency of *essential fatty acids* (EFAs), which are vital structural components of cell membranes that affect the health of the brain, nervous system and cardiovascular system.

The clue: Victor's skin was extremely dry. EFA deficiency is a common cause of dry skin, and studies show that EFA supplementation improves mood and focus in some children with ADHD.

To boost Victor's intake of EFAs, I started him on daily supplements of fish oil (Nordic Naturals DHA, 800-662-2544, www.nordicnaturals.com)

and evening primrose oil. In addition, I prescribed the homeopathic remedy *Lycopodium clavatum*, made from club moss, to improve mood and concentration. I also had Victor take daily supplements of *phosphatidylserine*—the nutrient essential for the normal functioning of brain cell membranes and naturally found in soy, rice, fish and leafy green vegetables.

Victor was tested by a child psychologist before starting his treatment with me and again after 10 weeks. To the psychologist's amazement, Victor improved so markedly that he was no longer considered to have ADHD. During the ensuing school year, his teachers reported that Victor's behavior was exemplary. When I asked the boy during a follow-up visit, "How are your grades?" he grinned from ear to ear as he answered, "I made the honor roll!"

Self-help strategy: Many behavioral problems result from biochemical imbalances. Before resorting to drugs, investigate potential side effects—and explore natural alternatives that can safely restore the body's proper balance.

Perseverance pays off

Turning 40, Joanne laughed at the idea of a midlife crisis. She was happily married and had a busy, successful medical practice as a doctor of chiropractic. Life was good, and the future looked bright.

But then Joanne began to experience recurring pain in her bladder and the surrounding pelvic area, plus a frequent and urgent need to urinate. Her doctor diagnosed *interstitial cystitis* (IC), a condition that affects more than 700,000 people in the US (primarily women), yet is still not well understood. Joanne tried every treatment her doctors could suggest—including the prescription drug *pentosan polysulfate* (Elmiron), which is intended to repair the bladder lining, and a surgical procedure called bladder distension, which stretches the bladder by filling it with gas or water to increase its capacity—but nothing brought relief.

After five years, Joanne was in such severe and incessant pain that she could no longer see patients, take care of her two-year-old or find any pleasure from sex. Compounding her problems, she also experienced an early menopause, with symptoms that included dozens of hot flashes a day, frequent insomnia and severe fatigue, heart palpitations, anxiety, mood swings and trouble concentrating.

As I took her medical history, I noticed that her IC symptoms had eased during her pregnancy. This suggested that her IC was connected to her hormone balance and that menopause was aggravating the condition. Blood and saliva tests confirmed that she had a deficiency of *estrogen*, *progesterone* and *thyroid hormones*.

Finding the root of Joanne's problem was easier than treating it. For seven months, we used a trial-and-error approach, looking for a precise mix of hormone-replacement therapies to alleviate her IC and menopausal symptoms. Finally, we hit upon the perfect solution—a mix of an *estriol* (estrogen) vaginal cream… an estrogen/progesterone combination transdermal (or skin) cream… and oral thyroid hormone tablets. Two months later, Joanne's pelvic pain and urinary urgency were gone, her menopausal symptoms had abated, and her sex life was back on track. "I'm enjoying being a mom," she reported, "and I may reopen my chiropractic practice. I've got my life back!"

Self-help strategy: Joanne deserves credit for her patience as we worked to figure out the best treatment for her individual needs. Too many people give up if they don't find a quick fix. For health problems— as with most of life's challenges—perseverance is the key to finding a solution.

Having Trouble Sleeping? These Solutions Can Help

Consistently getting a good night's sleep is not just a luxury—it's essential to your health. Insufficient sleep not only leaves you feeling tired and irritable but also weakens your immune system and puts you at risk for depression, weight gain and chronic headaches. To get the full health benefits of sleep, most adults should aim for at least seven hours of uninterrupted sleep a night.

Many of my patients have trouble sleeping. I often help them determine the nature of their sleep problem—and what might help.

See below for some of my natural remedies. Don't try three solutions at once. Once you find the remedies that work for you, you can use them indefinitely. Before starting, check to make sure that your sleep problem is not caused by any prescription medication you might be taking.

Trouble falling asleep

If you have trouble falling asleep for any reason when you first go to bed, try…

• **Sublingual melatonin.** *Melatonin*, the hormone produced in the pineal gland in the brain, helps to control both sleep and wake cycles. Sublingual melatonin supplements (lozenges placed under the tongue) generally work better than either the capsules or tablets. Start with 1.5 mg of sublingual melatonin, 30 to 45 minutes before bedtime. (If this doesn't help within three nights, try three mg.) Do not take melatonin if you are pregnant, breast-feeding or taking oral contraceptives.

If you have feelings of anxiety, depression or stress, start with…

• **5-Hydroxytryptophan (5-HTP)**. The body uses this amino acid to manufacture the "good mood" neurotransmitter serotonin. Taking a 5-HTP supplement increases the body's *serotonin* production, promoting the sense of well-being and better resistance to stress. Start with 100 mg one hour before bedtime. (If symptoms don't improve within three nights, try 200 mg.) Don't take 5-HTP if you are pregnant, breast-feeding or taking an antidepressant or antianxiety medication.

If 5-HTP (above) doesn't help and you need a more aggressive approach to anxiety and depression, add…

• **SedaLin**. This supplement, manufactured by Xymogen (healthcare professionals can order it at 800-647-6100, www.xymogen.com), can help relax the nervous system. It contains *Magnolia officinalis extract*, from the bark of a type of magnolia tree, to relieve anxiety… and *Ziziphus spinosa extract* from a shrub to treat irritability and insomnia. Take one capsule at bedtime for a minimum of two weeks to allow your hormone levels to adjust. (SedaLin also can be used on its own to relieve anxiety and nervousness during waking hours. Since its main role is to calm the nervous system, it won't make you drowsy.) It is not recommended for women who are pregnant or breast-feeding.

If you are over age 60, try…

• **Calcium and/or magnesium**. These supplements can help seniors, who are most likely to be deficient in these minerals, fall asleep by relaxing the nervous system. Take 500 mg of calcium with 250 mg of magnesium one hour before bedtime. Some people are helped by taking either the calcium or the magnesium alone. Find what works best for you.

If you are menopausal, try…

• **Natural progesterone**. This *bioidentical* hormone (not to be confused with the pharmaceutical *progestin*) has a natural sedating effect for women with sleep problems related to insufficient progesterone.

Best: Have your hormone levels tested. If progesterone is low, apply a total of one-quarter to one-half teaspoon of progesterone cream to the inner forearm and wrist or the inner thighs 30 minutes before bedtime.

One over-the-counter brand to try: Emerita Pro-Gest (800-888-6041, www.emerita.com).

For a stronger effect, take a progesterone capsule (100 mg to 150 mg), available by prescription.

If you have trouble getting back to sleep…

• **Eat a light snack before bedtime**. Some people wake up in the night because their blood sugar dips, triggering the adrenal glands to produce *adrenaline*—exactly what you don't want while sleeping.

Solution: Eat a small snack before bedtime, such as six ounces of organic yogurt.

If you consistently wake up between midnight and two am, try…

• **Balancing stress hormones**. Many people wake up in the wee hours and are unable to fall back to sleep quickly because of an imbalance in stress hormones. Melatonin can help. *In addition, try…*

• **Walking after dinner**. Exercise of any kind decreases the production of stress hormones. Exercise as early as possible during the evening, at least three hours before bedtime.

• **Listening to relaxing music**. One study showed that listening to relaxing music (such as classical) for 45 minutes before bedtime resulted in better-quality and longer sleep.

If you consistently wake up between 2 am and 4 am, try…

• **Balancing other hormones**. Waking between two am and four am can be related to hormone imbalances, including an *estrogen* deficiency in menopausal women (note that this is a different sleep problem than that caused by *progesterone* deficiency described above)... *testosterone* deficiency in males age 50 and older... and/or *growth hormone* deficiency in people age 60 or older. Have your hormone levels tested—and if they are low, obtain a prescription for a bioidentical hormone.

New Nasal Device for Sleep Apnea

I see many patients with obstructive sleep apnea, a disorder in which breathing stops during sleep because soft tissue at the back of the throat collapses and closes the airway. These patients often snore loudly and wake up dozens—even hundreds—of times per night. One of the most common treatments for sleep apnea is a therapy called continuous positive airway pressure (CPAP), in which an air pump blows air into a hose connected to a mask worn on the face. The air pressure created by CPAP keeps the airway open.

Although CPAP can be very effective, the mask can feel cumbersome and the machine can be noisy, so many patients stop using it. Now there is a new FDA-approved treatment called Provent that features a less cumbersome way to keep the airway open. Many of my patients have switched from CPAP to Provent and report that it is more comfortable. *Here's why Provent is worth trying for this condition…*

How it works: Patients place a small, disposable adhesive patch over the opening of each nostril. Each patch contains a small valve. When you inhale, the valves open, allowing you to breathe freely. During exhalation, the valves partially close, increasing air pressure in the nasal passages, which keeps the tissue pushed away so that breathing is easier.

In a study conducted by the makers of Provent and other researchers and published in *Journal of Clinical Sleep Medicine*, 34 study participants used Provent all night on 94 percent of nights during a month.

While Provent was not tested head-to-head against CPAP, if it is used consistently, it will certainly have a greater impact on sleep apnea than CPAP, which is used inconsistently by patients.

My advice: If you have sleep apnea, try Provent, especially if you do not use your CPAP regularly. Available by prescription only and covered by some insurance, Provent costs $50 for a 30-night supply. CPAP machines cost between $200 and $800.

Side effects of Provent include mouth-breathing–related nasal, sinus or middle-ear discomfort. People with severe respiratory disorders, heart failure or very low blood pressure should not use Provent.

For details about Provent, call 888-757-9355 or visit www.provent therapy.com.

Breakthrough Treatments for Hair Loss

Why do some men go bald in their 30s while others have a full head of hair until their final days? Why do some women have everthinning hair, while others never seem to lose a single strand?

Blame your genes, first of all. If your mom, dad or a grandparent had hair loss, chances are greater that you will, too. Even so, there are ways to slow hair loss and stimulate growth.

The hormone factor

You grow and shed hair all the time. Of the 100,000-plus strands of hair on your head, it is perfectly normal to lose 50 to 100 every day. Once a hair is shed, a new hair grows from the same follicle. Hair grows at a rate of nearly one-half inch per month (faster in warm weather, slower when frost is on the vine). Baldness results when the rate of shedding exceeds the rate of regrowth.

Hair loss usually accelerates when you are beyond age 50. One hormone, *dihydrotestosterone* (DHT), seems to be the chief culprit. DHT is a derivative of testosterone (the sex-determining hormone that is more abundant in men than women). In both men and women, DHT increases in the presence of the enzyme 5-alpha reductase, which is produced in the prostate, adrenal glands and the scalp. *5-alpha reductase* is more likely to proliferate after age 50. When DHT is overproduced, hair follicles are damaged. Some follicles die, but most shrink and produce thinner, weaker hairs—and the weak hairs are the ones that fall out.

An oily skin substance called *sebum*—produced by the *sebaceous glands*—makes matters worse. Excess sebum clogs follicles and contributes to high 5-alpha reductase activity, which stimulates production of DHT.

Stress

Among my own patients, stress is a factor for both men and women. I have found that highly stressed women, in particular, have higher-than-normal levels of *cortisol*, a stress hormone that can contribute to hair loss.

A study published in the *Journal of Clinical Biochemistry* confirms that cortisol is indeed elevated in some women who suffer hair loss—and that when they learn to cope better with stress, hair growth improves.

For stress relief, I recommend daily exercise, such as brisk walking, as well as relaxation techniques, including deep breathing and meditation. B vitamins and *ashwagandha* (a stress-reducing herb from India) also can help counteract the effects of cortisol.

A regular daily dose of 100 mg of a B-vitamin complex and 250 mg to 500 mg of ashwagandha can help control cortisol levels. Look for Sensoril Ashwagandha, a patented extract formula by Jarrow Formulas, available at many health-food stores or by calling 310-204-6936 or at www.jarrow.com.

A promising formula

Taking a daily multivitamin and mineral supplement as well as the herbal remedy saw palmetto also can help slow hair loss. A daily scalp massage with essential oils is beneficial, too.

• **Saw palmetto** helps block the effects of DHT on hair follicles, strengthening hair. In a study in the *Journal of Alternative and Comple-*

mentary Medicine, researchers used a product containing *saw palmetto* and a plant compound called *beta-sitosterol* that is found in saw palmetto and other plants. The study included 19 men between ages 23 and 64 who had mild-to-moderate hair loss. Men in one group were given a placebo daily… and men in the other group received the saw palmetto/beta-sitosterol combination (none of the participants knew which group they were in). After five months, researchers found that 60 percent of the men who received their saw palmetto/beta-sitosterol combination showed improvement, while only 11 percent of the men receiving a placebo had more hair growth.

In my clinical experience, saw palmetto is helpful for both men and women. I recommend 320 mg to 400 mg daily of an 85 percent *liposterolic extract*. It is safe to use long term but should not be taken if you are pregnant or nursing.

For a more aggressive approach, you should also take beta-sitosterol. Source Naturals (800-815-2333, www.sourcenaturals.com) offers a 113 mg tablet that can be taken daily. It is available at health-food stores and at www.iherb.com.

• **The essential oils of rosemary and lavender** have been shown to improve hair growth when applied to the scalp. My own belief is that they improve blood flow to the scalp, ensuring that nutrients get to the sites where they're needed.

You can purchase these essential oils in separate containers. Pour some of your regular shampoo into the lid of the shampoo bottle, then add five to 10 drops of each essential oil. Massage into the scalp and leave on three to five minutes before rinsing thoroughly.

Other supplements

If you have tried these approaches for two to three months and still aren't satisfied with the growth of your locks, here are some other supplements that can help both men and women…

• **Biotin**, a nutrient that is required for hair growth, is particularly good for brittle hair. Food sources of biotin include brewer's yeast, soybeans, eggs, mushrooms and whole wheat. For supplementation, take 3,000 mcg daily for at least two months or use a biotin-enriched shampoo daily.

• **MSM (methylsulfonylmethane)** is a great source of sulfur, an integral component of the amino acids that are the building blocks of hair protein. MSM improves the strength, sheen and health of hair. In one study, 21 adults (16 men and five women) who were assessed by a certified cosmetologist under the direction of a medical doctor were given MSM or a placebo and then were reassessed at the end of six weeks. The participants did not know who was given MSM and who was given a placebo.

People given MSM showed significant improvement in hair health, while those taking a placebo showed few or no changes. I recommend a 3,000 mg daily dose of MSM. Look for Opti-MSM or Lignisul MSM, available from many manufacturers and at health-food stores.

• **Essential fatty acids** keep hair from becoming dry and lifeless by decreasing inflammation. Inflammation worsens the quality of hair follicles, and essential fatty acids are needed for the proper development of hair. Food sources include walnuts, eggs, fish, olive oil, flaxseed and hempseed and flax oils. Or you can take a formula like Udo's 3-6-9 Oil Blend, produced by Flora (800-446-2110, www.florahealth.com). Follow directions on the label. The formula contains both *omega-3 fatty acids* (from flax oil or fish oil) and *omega-6 fatty acids* from evening primrose oil or borage oil. Don't expect immediate results, however. It can take four to six weeks to see improvement.

Organic Foods... Worth the Cost?

O*rganic* is the buzzword these days, not just in natural-food stores but even in conventional supermarkets. But what does the term mean? Are organic foods really important for your health?

Under USDA guidelines, organic means the food hasn't been contaminated with man-made chemicals. Organic crops also are produced by farmers whose growing methods conserve soil and water. This helps ensure sustainable and nutritious produce for future generations.

Foods from all major food groups are available in organic form. Organic meat, poultry, eggs and dairy products come from animals that have not been given antibiotics or growth hormones. Animal feed also must be organic. Organic fruits, vegetables and grains come from fields that have been free of synthetic fertilizers and pesticides for at least three years. The foods must be grown without treated sewage sludge, which is commonly used as fertilizer. Organic farmers use animal manure, composted plant material, etc.

Organic farmers also avoid *ionizing radiation*—the process of applying radiation to raw meat, poultry and produce. In meats, the process kills pathogenic bacteria and other microorganisms. In produce, it kills spoilage-causing bacteria and lengthens shelf life. Instead of radiation, organic farmers follow strict hygiene and sanitation practices and climate control—such as that provided by refrigeration.

There are various classifications for organic foods, and the rules can be tricky. A food that is 100 percent organic can be labeled "USDA organic" or "100 percent organic." Any mixed ingredient foods that are at least 95 percent organic also can have this seal. Foods in which at least 70 percent of the ingredients are organic (excluding salt and water) can highlight organic ingredients on the front of the package. If a product contains less than 70 percent organic ingredients, they may be called out on the side of the box, but the term "organic" can't appear on the front.

Organic produce prices vary but usually are only slightly higher than those of conventional fruits and vegetables. Organic dairy products are typically 15 percent to 20 percent more expensive than conventional dairy products, and organic meats and poultry cost two to three times as much as their traditional counterparts.

A richer source of minerals

One study published in the *Journal of Applied Nutrition* compared the amount of healthful minerals and toxic metals in organically and conventionally grown produce—apples, potatoes, pears and sweet corn—as well as wheat. Over a two-year period, average levels of essential minerals were much higher in organic foods than in conventional foods. In addition, organic foods, on average, contained 25 percent less mercury and 29 percent less lead than conventional foods—both metals are toxic to the nervous and immune systems.

Pesticides, which are known hormone disrupters and suspected toxins to the nervous and immune systems, are a concern of mine. More than 1 billion pounds of pesticides and herbicides are sprayed on US crops each year. I believe that pesticides may contribute to the development of cancers of the breast, bone marrow and prostate.

Research has shown that people who live in agricultural areas where pesticides are used have an increased mortality rate from Parkinson's disease, a degenerative disorder of the nervous system. I am especially concerned about children who consume pesticides and other toxins in food. Of course, the absence of hormones and antibiotics in organic dairy and meat makes these foods more healthful than nonorganic varieties.

While organic foods cost more, they are worth the extra expense. However, it's still better for children and adults to eat nonorganic produce than to avoid it altogether.

Best: Incorporate organic foods—particularly dairy and produce— into your diet as much as possible.

Nontoxic Cleaning

Do you suffer from unexplained headaches, breathing problems (asthma or burning of the airway), mood swings and/or skin rashes? These and other chronic problems may be related to the cleansers you use in your home. Common ingredients include ammonia and chlorine (both skin and lung irritants), *formaldehyde* (an irritant to the nervous system and a suspected carcinogen) and *trisodium nitrilotriacetate* (a suspected carcinogen).

You should be particularly concerned if there are infants or young children in your home—developing bodies are more susceptible to injury from toxic substances than those of adults. In my home, we use nontoxic, biodegradable cleansers, from laundry detergents to disinfectants. Much of household cleaning and laundry can be done using inexpensive, safe and natural ingredients—baking soda, lemon juice, vinegar, borax and vegetable soaps, such as coconut, Castile or beeswax soap.

Look for products that are biodegradable, nontoxic, recyclable and nonpetroleum-derived with a phosphate concentration of 0.5 percent or less by weight. This information should appear on the manufacturers' Internet sites. Seventh Generation provides a complete line of nontoxic household products (to find a retailer, call 800-456-1191, www.seventhgeneration.com) as does Earth Friendly Products (800-335-3267, www.ecos.com). Both brands work very well.

Plundering the Pineapple for Bromelain

Bromelain is actually a group of protein enzymes derived from the pineapple plant, whose healing powers were described in medical literature as far back as 1876. Though the active enzymes are found in the fruit as well as the stem, commercial products are made exclusively from the stem.

Bromelain is utilized for many purposes—as a digestive aid, anti-inflammatory, natural blood thinner, mucus-thinning agent, immune-system enhancer and for skin healing. It also helps improve the absorption of particular supplements (such as *glucosamine*) and medications such as antibiotics.

One of bromelain's unique actions is to reduce inflammation in people who have conditions such as arthritis or heart disease. It can also help control the inflammatory process after an injury. It breaks down blood clots at the site of an injury, so swelling is reduced and, at the same time, there is increased circulation to the site of injury or inflammation. Bromelain also helps control some of the body's naturally produced chemicals that tend to increase an inflammatory reaction after an injury.

Maxing your antibiotics

Bromelain is used in many countries to increase the absorption and utilization of antibiotics.

In one study, 53 hospitalized patients were given bromelain in various combinations with appropriate antibiotic medications. Their conditions included a wide range of health problems, including pneumonia, bronchitis, skin *staphylococcus* infection, *thrombophlebitis, cellulitis, pyelonephritis* (kidney infection) and abscesses of the rectum. Twenty-three of the patients had been on antibiotic therapy without success. Bromelain was administered four times a day along with antibiotics or by itself.

To compare, a control group of 56 patients was treated with antibiotics alone.

Of the 23 patients who had been unsuccessfully treated with antibiotics, 22 responded favorably to the combined treatment. The rate of improvement was across-the-board, for every type of disease, when patients were given the combination of bromelain and antibiotics.

For doctors involved in the study, it was an eye-opener. Many had not realized that bromelain was able to potentiate the effects of antibiotics in this way.

I hope we'll see larger-scale studies in the near future. Such promising results suggest that people may be able to take lower doses of antibiotics if they simultaneously take bromelain. (Many doctors are eager to reduce the rampant overuse of antibiotics, which is leading to ominous new strains of resistant bacteria.)

Those with weak or compromised immune systems could be the greatest beneficiaries of combination treatments with bromelain and antibiotics. Infants, seniors and AIDS patients are particularly good candidates for the combined therapies.

Dosage: The dosage of bromelain is designated in two different ways with regard to supplements. One is *milk-clotting units* (M.C.U.) and the other is *gelatin-dissolving units* (G.D.U.). Look for products that are standardized to 2,000 M.C.U. per 1,000 mg, or to 1,200 G.D.U. per

1,000 mg. Most people require a dosage of 500 mg three times daily between meals.

What are the side effects? Side effects are rare with bromelain. However, allergic reactions can happen in sensitive individuals. Increased heart rate and palpitations have been observed in some people at dosages near 2,000 mg. Those on blood-thinning medications need to check with their doctor first before using bromelain.

Recommendations for...

• **Arthritis**. Bromelain is a popular component of natural arthritis formulas. It is helpful for both osteoarthritis and rheumatoid arthritis.

One study found that the supplementation of bromelain enabled people with rheumatoid arthritis to decrease their corticosteroid medications. In addition, patients noticed significant improvements in joint mobility and also noticed less swelling. This study is encouraging because many people suffer side effects from corticosteroid therapy—and the less medicine they have to use, the better. If bromelain supplementation can reduce the amount of steroids needed, the risk of serious side effects decreases as well.

My experience is that most people with arthritis can maintain a good quality of life if they take the opportunity to try bromelain and other natural treatments.

• **Burns**. A bromelain cream has been shown to eliminate burn debris and speed up the healing of burned skin.

• **Cancer**. Various studies have looked at a link between bromelain treatments and cancer deterrence or recovery. In one study, 12 patients with ovarian and breast tumors were given 600 mg of bromelain daily for at least six months. (Some treatments continued for several years.) Resolution of cancerous masses and a decrease in metastasis was reported.

Bromelain in doses of over 1,000 mg daily have been given in combination with chemotherapy drugs such as 5-FU and *vincristine,* with some reports of tumor regression.

Although I do not rate bromelain as one of the more potent anticancer herbs, it is worthy of more study. For those who are using chemotherapy to fight cancer, the addition of bromelain offers the promise of making the therapy more effective.

• **Cardiovascular disease**. Holistic practitioners have expressed a great deal of interest in using bromelain for treatment and prevention of cardiovascular disease. We know that bromelain helps break down *fibrinous plaques* in the arteries, allowing for more efficient circulation. In theory, at least, this is a sure way to help prevent strokes.

When we prescribe routine tests to determine whether individuals are at risk for cardiovascular disease, fibrin is one of the markers that we're beginning to look at routinely. (In other words, a lot of fibrin in the blood is one indicator that stroke could be somewhere on the horizon.) The fact that bromelain can help "break down" this fibrin is significant. In one study, bromelain administered at a dosage of 400 to 1,000 mg per day to 14 patients with *angina* (chest pain) resulted in the disappearance of symptoms in all patients within four to 90 days.

Bromelain also offers the potential to break down plaque, those fatty deposits that impair blood flow through the arteries. The enzyme has been shown to dissolve arteriosclerotic plaque in rabbit heart arteries. While more studies need to be done, I've talked to many practitioners who notice that their patients with heart problems do better on bromelain.

• **Digestive problems**. Bromelain has long been used as a digestive aid in the breakdown of protein, and there are now many "digestive-enzyme formulas" that routinely include bromelain as one of the primary ingredients. Either bromelain alone or the enzyme formulas can be helpful for people who have digestive conditions such as colitis or *irritable bowel syndrome* (IBS). In addition, we now know that incomplete protein breakdown is implicated in immune reactions that lead to inflammatory conditions like arthritis.

• **Injuries**. Bromelain's most well-known use is in the treatment of injuries, and it definitely helps to reduce pain and swelling if you have bruises. In one early clinical trial, doctors gave bromelain to 74 boxers who regularly suffered bruising on the face, lips, ears, chest and arms. When bromelain was given four times a day, all signs of bruising disappeared by the fourth day among 58 of the boxers.

A control group, comprised of 72 boxers, was given placebos—a look-alike capsule made from inert substances. In that group, 62 of the boxers needed seven to 14 days before the bruises cleared up. (Only 10 were free from signs of bruising after four days.)

• **Respiratory mucus**. Bromelain thins mucus. If you have bronchitis and another kind of respiratory-tract condition, you'll probably discover that dosing with bromelain will help you expel the mucus more easily. For similar reasons, taking bromelain has been shown to improve cases of sinusitis.

• **Surgery recovery**. Bromelain is a valuable supplement in helping people to recover more quickly from surgery.

In one study, patients who were given bromelain supplements two to four days prior to surgery were able to recover from pain and inflammation more quickly than those who didn't take the enzyme. The bromelain-takers took an average of 1.5 days to be pain free, compared with an average of 3.5 days for those who went without it. Without bromelain, it took an average of 6.9 days for inflammation to go down, but only about two days for those who had bromelain supplements.

In my opinion, supplements such as bromelain should be routinely given to those recovering from surgery. Just think of all the days of suffering patients could avoid!

• **Thrombophlebitis**. In studies, bromelain has been proven very effective in the treatment of vein clots, as thrombophlebitis is commonly called.

• **Varicose veins**. Bromelain has value in the treatment of varicose veins. I do not rate it so effective as horse chestnut and some of the other herbs, but it certainly helps.

Fish Oil for Heart Disease and More

Gary's father had died at the age of 54. "It was a heart attack," Gary told me.

Now 44 himself, Gary almost felt as if he were living on borrowed time. He could hear the clock ticking.

I assured him that most cases of heart attacks can be prevented. I also let him know he was doing the right thing—showing some concern about his heart health before anything happened. Most people, sad to say, wait until they've had a heart attack before taking the measures that they could and should have taken years before.

True, there are inherited factors that make some individuals more susceptible than others to heart attack—specifically, *homocysteine* and *cholesterol* levels just seem to be higher in some people than in others. But most heart attacks are due to diet and lifestyle factors.

Gary had done enough reading to be aware of that. It was one reason he wanted to get started on an aggressive program to keep his heart as healthy as possible.

Among the strategies we discussed were stress reduction, exercise, a series of lab tests, and, of course, diet and supplements. I emphasized the importance of *omega-3 fatty acids* found in fish, especially cold-water fish such as salmon, mackerel, herring and sardines. Above all, I recommended fish-oil supplements, such as salmon oil, to optimize the amount of these heart-healthy fatty acids. As part of a total strategy for heart health, the steady intake of fish oil could, potentially, add decades to his life expectancy.

Oil well

Among the essential fatty acids that we need to live, omega-3s are very important. These are fats that your body cannot manufacture on its own, so they need to come from food sources or supplements.

While omega-3 is also found in flaxseed and flaxseed oil, the kind that you get from fish and fish oil has some unique properties that are not present in these other foods. The fish and fish oils are a direct source of two long-chain fatty acids known as EPA (*eicosapentanoic acid*) and DHA (*docosahexanoic acid*), and both are very important for heart health.

Another reason doctors are confident about the benefits of fish oil is pragmatic. The vast majority of studies on essential fatty acids have been done on fish oils. There are sound reasons to believe that oils such as flaxseed oil may be nearly as effective, but to date, they haven't been studied so much. It is the fish oils that have been studied and shown to be effective.

Fish became more popular as a "healthy heart" food when researchers studied the "Mediterranean diet"—that is, the diet of many cultures around the Mediterranean during the 1960s in Crete, parts of Greece and southern Italy. (There, as in many other cultures, the "American diet" has crept in, raising the rate of heart disease and other chronic diseases.) In the classic Mediterranean diet, people had many plant foods (vegetables, legumes, fruit, bread, pasta, nuts), lots of olive oil, and low to moderate amounts of fish, poultry, meat, dairy, eggs and wine.

Nutritionists believe the consumption of fish was one of the key benefits of this diet, which resulted in a much lower incidence of obesity, heart disease, diabetes, and cancer. A four-year study of the Mediterranean diet found that people could reduce their risk of heart attack by as much as 70 percent.

Sea rations

In a more direct study of fish consumption, a team of researchers who looked at mortality data from 36 countries confirmed that life expectancy is longer in those countries where people get a lot of fish in their daily diet. Men and women who eat more fish have a lower risk of early death from all kinds of illnesses, particularly stroke and heart disease.

Essential fatty acids form a group of hormone-like messengers known as *prostaglandins*. The omega-3 fatty acids as found in fish oil—helped along by the EPA and DHA in the fish—tend to decrease inflammation, thin the blood and balance the immune system.

In the immune system, EPA appears to be particularly important for its anti-inflammatory effects, so it's helpful to people who have arthritis. DHA is critical for the proper development and function of the brain because your brain cells need it to transmit electrical impulses efficiently. It's not surprising, therefore, that a DHA deficiency can lead to memory, behavior and learning problems.

Some studies have also indicated that supplementing infant formula with DHA can improve children's IQ. Interestingly, it's also important for mood regulation, and studies have shown that a deficiency can contribute to depression.

The DHA found in fish oil also appears to calm down hyperactive children. It's also required for proper retinal development for infants.

Dosage

Fish oil capsules generally are available in 500 to 1,000 mg doses. When purchasing the capsules, pay particular attention to the amounts of EPA and DHA stated on the labels. You want fish oils that contain about 18 percent EPA and 12 percent DHA: In other words, totalling about 30 percent of the omega-3 fatty acids found in these fish oils.

(Some of the newly developed, high-potency fish oils now contain even higher concentrations of EPA and DHA.)

For preventative purposes, I recommend that people eat foods high in DHA and EPA such as cold-water fish. (Eggs also contain DHA.)

If your health is generally good, I'd advise taking 2,000 mg of a daily fish-oil supplement such as salmon oil. But if you're susceptible to specific diseases such as arthritis, high blood pressure and other conditions, I'd advise getting a higher dose—as much as 6,000 to 10,000 mg per day. However, you'll probably want to check with your health practitioner to find an optimal dose for your condition, since the supplement can be costly.

If you're taking the concentrated fish-oil capsules that provide higher concentrations of EPA and DHA, I recommend salmon oil or tuna oil capsules that have been tested for heavy metal contamination and rancidity. I am also a big fan of the oil blends that contain a combination of essential fatty acids such as DHA, EPA, and GLA. An ideal formula also has vitamin E in it. If not, take vitamin E *with* the fish oil to prevent the oil from going rancid.

Fish-oil capsules should be stored in the refrigerator once they are opened. Don't leave the container standing in bright light or keep it in a warm room.

What are the side effects?

Some people who take fish oil experience digestive upset including burping—which can be disconcerting because you may burp a "fishy" smell. But you probably won't have that problem if you take the capsules with meals.

Also, some companies produce specially designed capsules that ensure the oil makes it into the small intestine before breaking down. Such claims are advertised so you might want to try their capsules to see whether their product alleviates the problem of burping or "fish breath."

Since fish oils also have a blood-thinning effect, check with your doctor if you are taking any blood-thinning medications.

You may have an increase in LDL cholesterol while supplementing fish oil. If a blood test shows your cholesterol count is on the rise, you can take a garlic supplement to help neutralize this potential effect of the fish oil.

Although people have relatively few and minor problems with the side effects of fish oil, there's a risk that the capsules can contain rancid oil. It's easy to check, however. Just cut open the end of a capsule. If the fish oil has gone rancid, you can easily smell the strong odor. You're better off getting a fresh bottle with new capsules.

Finally, check the label of any brand you buy to make sure the product was tested for contaminants such as heavy metals.

Here are my fish oil recommendations for various conditions...

ADD and ADHD

Many school-age children have been diagnosed with *attention deficit disorder* (ADD) or *attention deficit hyperactivity disorder* (ADHD), and their problems are sometimes related to nutritional imbalances. (Excess sugars and some additives in junk food have been blamed.)

Essential fatty acids such as DHA are critically important for proper brain function, but—well, how many children do you know who eat fresh cold-water fish three times a week? When children aren't getting enough DHA and they're loading up on saturated fat, trans fatty acids and omega-6 fatty acids from fast-foods, the inevitable result is a fatty-acid imbalance.

DHA supplementation has been shown to decrease aggression while a child is under stress. The DHA in fish oil helps to improve the chemical balance in the brain while giving the general benefits of omega-3 fatty acid supplementation.

I recommend that bottle-fed infants receive omega-3 supplementation, especially DHA, for proper brain and retina development. Breast-fed infants receive these critical essential fatty acids in the breast milk. I suspect that, before long, DHA supplementation will be required in all commercial baby formulas.

Arthritis

Numerous studies with fish oil have been done on people with rheumatoid arthritis and the results have been very positive. For aggressive treatment using fish oil, take 6,000 mg daily. Some people need doses that are even higher, so talk to your health practitioner about the optimum dose if you have severe rheumatoid arthritis.

If the fish oil is helpful in reducing stiffness and pain, there's a good chance you'll be able to reduce the dosages of pharmaceuticals. Drug therapy for rheumatoid arthritis focuses on *prednisone, methotrexate* (also used for chemotherapy) and anti-inflammatory medications—all of which can have serious toxicity when used on a long-term basis. With fish oil, on the other hand, there is no toxicity, so it is a far more benign treatment than the classic pharmaceuticals. One study found that many patients were able to go off their anti-inflammatory drugs while supplementing fish oil and experienced no relapse in their rheumatoid arthritis. Researchers found that the fish oil had a balancing effect on the entire immune system.

It is recommended, as the result of studies, that a minimum daily dose of 3,000 mg EPA and DHA is necessary to derive the expected benefits, although I find not all my patients need this high a dosage. Once you start taking fish oil, you can expect to stay on it for at least 12 weeks before it begins to yield benefits. But after that, you can stay on it indefinitely.

Despite the many improvements you can get from fish oil, I do have to say it should be part of a total program when you're treating rheumatoid arthritis. It's also important to improve your diet and take steps to reduce the toxins in your body. I've seen the quickest results with detoxification programs when they also involved homeopathic remedies. But fish oil is a good long-term therapy for some people, and it can definitely help keep inflammatory conditions under control.

Although not so well studied, essential fatty acids found in fish oil are helpful to decrease the stiffness associated with osteoarthritis, the most common form of arthritis, where the cartilage has degenerated.

Asthma

The rate of asthma keeps skyrocketing. Sadly, children's asthma is continuing to increase at an alarming rate. Environmental pollution and poor dietary habits are largely to blame.

Essential fatty acids in fish and fish oil help to suppress the inflammatory chemicals involved in this disease. Studies show that children who eat oily fish more than once a week have one-third the risk of getting asthma as children who do not eat fish or eat lean fish on a regular basis.

Fish-oil supplements are helpful for both children and adults with asthma. Again, the benefits of fish oil take months before the natural antiinflammatory benefits begin to take hold.

Cancer

Omega-3 fatty acids are important for a healthy, well-functioning immune system. If you can get more omega-3 fatty acids in your diet and also take supplements, there's a good chance you can help protect yourself from certain types of cancers.

Animal studies have shown that fish oil can augment certain types of chemotherapy to fight cancer more effectively. Fish oil has also been shown to help treat *cachexia*, which is the loss of muscle mass and weight in cancer patients.

Cardiovascular disease

With many studies to back up its benefits, fish oil is often recommended as a preventative for heart and circulation problems. Along with the population studies showing that consumption of fish oil slashes the rate of cardiovascular disease are literally hundreds of studies that support these observations. Fish oils reduce cholesterol and triglyceride levels and also act as a natural blood thinner, which results in the lowering of blood pressure.

Chronic obstructive pulmonary disease

Over 17 million Americans suffer from this group of serious breathing disorders that includes asthma, bronchitis, and emphysema. Smoking, as you might expect, is the factor that multiplies your chances of getting any of these diseases. But for smokers as well as nonsmokers, there are some benefits in eating fish as often as possible.

Crohn's disease and ulcerative colitis

Inflammatory bowel diseases such as Crohn's disease and *ulcerative colitis* can be helped by fish-oil supplementation.

In one study of ulcerative colitis, people who took fish-oil supplements (high in omega-3s) were able to cut their steroid medications in half. Again, I see fish oil as one component of a total natural-therapy program to address and alleviate these digestive conditions. Other measures include stress reduction, improving digestive capacity and maintaining a healthful diet.

Herbal medicines as well as homeopathy are excellent therapies to help turn these conditions around without relying on pharmaceutical drugs that may have many damaging side effects.

Depression

The brain is 60 percent fat and needs essential fatty acids, especially DHA, to function properly. It has been shown that people with deficiency in DHA are much more likely to suffer from depression.

Consuming fish on a regular basis is a good way to prevent depression. I recommend concentrated DHA supplements for those already battling depression.

As a side note, I believe it's time that more research is done on nutritional deficiencies to find out how they can cause mental diseases such as depression. I see an increasing number of people using pharmaceutical antidepressants on a long-term basis, without exploring other preventives. As we learn more about genetic susceptibility to depression, we will also discover what nutrients and other therapies can help correct what people have come to call *genetic depression*. To date, fish oil is certainly one of the most important of the nutrients we have been able to identify as necessary for healthy brain functioning.

Eczema

I have found that *flaxseeds* and *flaxseed oil* in combination with *GLA* work well for eczema. It also makes sense to consume cold-water fish rich in omega-3 fatty acids. Fish oil is also another option to treat eczema.

High blood pressure

High blood pressure is one of the biggest risk factors for heart disease and stroke. Numerous studies have shown that fish oil reduces blood pressure. I find fish oil works best as part of a natural program—combined with stress-reduction techniques and a regimen that includes herbs such as hawthorn, minerals such as magnesium and calcium, along with the natural supplement *CoQ10*.

High triglycerides

With fish oil, you can lower high triglyceride levels, which are an independent risk factor for heart disease. As I've mentioned, fish oil can increase LDL cholesterol, so you'll want to supplement with garlic to help balance out its effects.

Insulin resistance

The inability to metabolize carbohydrates effectively leads to high blood-sugar levels and a corresponding spike of the hormone insulin (the component that helps get the blood sugar into the cells). As a result, many different biochemical reactions can occur, one of which is weight gain.

Clinical studies have shown that omega-3 fatty acids, such as those in fish oil, help improve the body's utilization of insulin. (It's interesting that an essential fatty acid can help *decrease* body fat!) This insulin-balancing effect is also important in relation to diabetes.

Kidney protection

People who receive organ transplants require extensive immune-suppressing drugs. These are needed to keep the body from rejecting the donated organ, but some of the drugs (such as *cyclosporine*) are so powerful that they can have life-threatening side effects.

In the case of patients who have had kidney transplants, however, it's been shown that they resume normal kidney function more quickly when omega-3–rich fish oil is supplemented. It appears that the fish oil actually protects the kidneys from the damaging effects of the immune-suppressing drugs.

Lupus

Two pilot studies have shown fish oil to benefit people with *lupus*, an autoimmune condition where the immune system attacks its own tissue. For patients with lupus, I recommend eating cold-water fish regularly and supplementing with fish oil. It may take six months to a year before there's any improvement, but sometimes the benefits can be dramatic.

Multiple Sclerosis

Dr. Roy Swank, the doctor who developed a natural protocol for multiple sclerosis (MS), recommended fish oil as well as flaxseed oil. In fact, Dr. Swank advocated that patients who have MS should eat fish three times a week or more. He was also a proponent of cod liver oil— one of the popular fish oils—as a daily supplement.

Psoriasis

Several studies have indicated that 10 to 12 g of fish oil daily can improve psoriasis. I routinely recommend fish oil and dietary fish as well as other natural therapies to improve this inflammatory condition.

Schizophrenia

Some preliminary studies are showing that EPA and DHA may be helpful in the treatment of schizophrenia. More research needs to be done, but I would not be surprised to see these essential fatty acids become accepted as part of the routine treatment for schizophrenia. Dr. Abraham Hoffer of Victoria, British Columbia has already demonstrated that a knowledgeable practitioner can provide a full-scale treatment of schizophrenia with nutritional therapies.

The Truth About Vitamin E

For more than 30 years, vitamin E has been one of the most widely used supplements. It has been touted as a key antioxidant, helping to prevent heart disease, particular cancers and other serious illnesses. But several years ago, vitamin E became quite controversial, because a few studies showed that it could be harmful. So it left many people wondering, *Is vitamin E safe? Is it effective? For what conditions? And what type of vitamin E should one use?*

Vitamin E is found naturally in wheat germ, nuts, seeds, whole grains, egg yolks and leafy, green vegetables. Animal products are a poor source of vitamin E. The recommended dietary allowance for vitamin E is 15 mg, or approximately 22 IU, per day. Serious vitamin E deficiency is rare, although many Americans don't get enough of the vitamin. People on low-fat diets are susceptible to low vitamin E levels, because fat is needed for absorption of vitamin E. And people with the genetic condition cystic fibrosis have trouble absorbing vitamin E.

Vitamin E has been shown to be important as a supplement for people with specific diseases, such as Alzheimer's and diabetes, and those with a high susceptibility to certain conditions, such as bladder cancer and eye disease. Vitamin E prevents LDL "bad" cholesterol from becoming *oxidized* (damaged), thereby helping to guard against plaque formation in the arteries, known as atherosclerosis. Also, low vitamin E levels are associated with an increased risk of major depression, rheumatoid arthritis and *preeclampsia* (a condition during pregnancy characterized by high blood pressure and swelling of the hands and face).

Controversial studies

Two well-publicized studies have raised questions about vitamin E. The first was a meta-analysis (a study of other studies) led by researchers from the Johns Hopkins School of Medicine in 2004. The researchers reviewed 19 vitamin E studies that followed almost 136,000 patients. Most of these studies targeted populations at high risk for a chronic disease, usually coronary heart disease. Nine of the 19 studies focused on vitamin E alone, while the other 10 studies combined vitamin E with other vitamins or minerals. These studies ranged from 1.4 to 8.2 years in length. Vitamin E dosage varied from 16.5 IU to 2,000 IU per day, with a median dosage of 400 IU per day. The meta-analysis found that those taking 400 IU or more of vitamin E daily for at least one year were 10 percent more likely to die from all causes than those who took a smaller dose.

There are several problems with this analysis. First, researchers combined data that used both natural supplements (which provide the same type of vitamin E as that found in food) and synthetic forms of supplemental vitamin E. Previous research has shown that natural forms of vitamin E are better utilized by the body than cheaper, synthetic forms. The 1996 Cambridge Heart Antioxidant Study used only a natural form of vitamin E and found that a dose of at least 400 IU daily substantially reduced the rate of nonfatal heart attacks after one year of use.

The biggest criticism of the meta-analysis was that most of the studies included elderly people who had existing health problems such as cancer, Alzheimer's disease, heart disease and other potentially fatal illnesses. Even the authors of the research stated, "The generalizability of the findings to healthy adults is uncertain. Precise estimation of the threshold at which risk increases is difficult."

Another study, which was published in the March 16, 2005, issue of the *Journal of the American Medical Association*, focused on patients age 55 or older with vascular disease or diabetes. The study concluded that for people with vascular disease or diabetes, long-term supplementation with natural vitamin E does not prevent cancer or cardiovascular events and may increase risk for heart failure. This study provides no evidence that vitamin E is unsafe for people who are healthy.

Positive findings

Many studies exist that demonstrate both the safety and effectiveness of vitamin E (in natural and synthetic forms). *A few examples…*

• **A Harvard study of more than 80,000 healthy, female nurses** ages 34 to 59 found a 41 percent reduction in the risk of heart disease in those who had taken daily vitamin E sup- plements of 100 IU or more for at least two years.

• **A study of almost 40,000 male health professionals** ages 40 to 75 found that those who took daily vitamin E supplements of at least 100 IU for more than two years experienced a 37 percent lower risk of heart disease.

• **A National Institute of Aging study focusing on 11,000 people between the ages of 67 and 105** found that those who used vitamins C and E supplements in various dosages had a 53 percent reduction in mortality from heart disease and a 42 percent reduction in death from all causes, compared with nonusers.

• **One study of moderate-severity Alzheimer's patients** conducted at Columbia University in New York City showed that a very high daily dose of vitamin E (2,000 IU) delayed the progression of Alzheimer's disease.

Different types

Vitamin E really refers to a family of compounds. There are more than 12 vitamin E compounds found in nature (currently eight forms are available in a supplement form). There are two primary groups of compounds—*tocopherols* (found in foods such as corn, soy and peanuts) and *tocotrienols* (found in rice, barley, rye and wheat). Many foods contain a blend of these two groups. Both have subgroups called *alpha, beta, gamma* and *delta*.

The most commonly used natural supplement form is *alpha-tocopherol*, and most studies have researched this form. But if you take just alpha-tocopherol you can reduce blood levels of gamma- and delta-tocopherols, which is not a good thing. Epidemiological (population) studies indicate that higher blood gamma-tocopherol levels correspond to the reduction of prostate cancer and coronary heart disease. Also, delta- and gamma-tocotrienols reduce the liver's production of cholesterol. One of the positive aspects of the negative vitamin E studies I mentioned earlier is that they have pushed researchers to look deeper into what vitamin E supplements should really contain.

I spoke with Barrie Tan, PhD, president of American River Nutrition, Inc., and adjunct professor of food science at the University of Massachusetts, Amherst, who's a leading specialist in the production and supplementation of vitamin E. He explains that 70 percent of (dietary) vitamin E consumed by North Americans is the gamma-tocopherol form due to the abundance of soy and corn in our diets. He believes that vitamin E supplements used for disease prevention should be a blend of both tocopherols and tocotrienols. I agree with this view, because these forms are more similar to what we find in food.

One example of a full-spectrum vitamin E product that has a good ratio of tocopherols and tocotrienols is Now Foods' Tru-E BioComplex. To find a health-food store that sells this product, call 888-669-3663 or go to www.nowfoods.com. A good dosage for anyone, healthy or not, is 200 IU daily. Consult with your doctor before using dosages above that—especially if you are taking a blood-thinning medication, such as *warfarin* (Coumadin)—vitamin E can have a blood-thinning effect.

Natural Help for Incontinence

With a grimace, Peter, 79, tugged at his waistband and growled, "It's darned inconvenient trying to get to a bathroom every half hour during the day and four times each night. And I really hate wearing this so-called 'absorbent undergarment.' I feel like a baby wetting his diapers!"

Peter's urinary incontinence had begun three years earlier, after a cancer diagnosis and surgery to remove his prostate gland. He also had Parkinson's disease (a neurological disorder that impairs movement control). Medications helped to ease some of his *Parkinson's symptoms*, but the disease exacerbated his incontinence.

Temporary or chronic urinary incontinence affects one in five adults over age 40, primarily women. It can result from pelvic injury or surgery… pregnancy, childbirth or menopause… and/or neurological diseases, infection or aging.

For Peter, I prescribed a liquid formula of extracts from six safe herbs that I have used with a number of my patients—male and female—over the past several years. It is called Bladder Tonic by Wise Woman Herbals (541-895-5172, www.wisewomanherbals.com). All these herbs have a long history of successful use by naturopathic doctors and herbalists.

• **Lady's mantle** is believed to strengthen the muscles of the bladder (so it is better able to hold urine) and of the sphincter that controls the *urethra* (the tube that drains urine out of the body).

• **Partridge berry** also helps to improve the bladder's muscular tone.

• **Gotu kola** (a perennial plant native to Asia) may strengthen the bladder's connective tissue.

• **St. John's wort** (known for its antidepressant effect) may soothe irritated nerves of the urinary tract. (It should not be used by people who take antidepressant drugs or birth control pills.)

• **Witch hazel** eases inflammation and tightens lax (loose) tissues of the bladder.

• **Corn silk** soothes tissues and reduces urinary tract inflammation.

Formulas similar to the one I prescribe for my incontinent patients are sold at health-food stores or through herbalists and naturopathic physicians.

Recommended: One teaspoonful twice daily, mixed with water. Other than very occasional and mild stomach upset from the corn silk, side effects are rare, and these herbs are safe for everyone (except pregnant and nursing women, who should avoid them as a general precaution).

After six weeks on this regimen, Peter returned for a follow-up visit feeling extremely encouraged. He was urinating only half as often during the day, so he could pursue his activities with fewer interruptions, and his nighttime need for the toilet was somewhat improved. Although he still wore a protective undergarment as a precaution, Peter was satisfied. "No more wet baby," he laughed. "I feel like a man again."

Eleven Things You Never Knew

1. Moderate to severe depression could increase your death risk by 400 percent. Even mild depression can increase it by 60 percent.

2. Ashwaganda was shown in a study to reduce stress hormone (cortisol) levels by 28 percent.

3. Stress can cause inflammation levels to soar contributing to diseases like heart disease, cancer, and diabetes.

4. Women who take multivitamins were found to have a 65 percent lower risk of stress and a 68 percent lower risk of anxiety.

5. Soda drinkers (diet or regular) are nearly a third more likely to suffer depression than people who avoid sodas and soft drinks.

6. Common anxiety drugs benzodiazepines could increase your risk of pneumonia by 54 percent and risk of death by up to a third.

7. SSRI drugs may slow down your heart, increasing your chances of an abnormal heart rhythm or sudden cardiac death.

8. Poor sleep may cause genetic damage to your DNA in as little as five days.

9. Too much overtime at work could bump up your risk of a major depression by two and half times.

10. A steady junk-food habit can boost your risk of depression by up to 51 percent.

11. Stress can shoot your heart attack risk up by 27 percent.

Banishing the Red Face of Rosacea Naturally

It's never a good idea to trade one health problem for another (or even worse, one for many), but that's exactly what conventional medicine doctors ask rosacea sufferers to do every single day.

"Dr. Stengler, I want to get off these antibiotics for my rosacea, I know they are messing my body up!" These were the desperate words of Kim, a middle-aged woman, who, without make up, looked like her nose and cheeks were chronically sunburned. Kim, like more than 16 million other Americans, has a condition called acne rosacea.

Rosacea causes redness of the cheeks, nose, chin, or forehead. You may also have visible blood vessels, pimples, or bumps on the face. Irritated and watery eyes affect half of those with the disease. And, my patients tell me that their face blushes more easily than before, making an already embarrassing problem even more embarrassing.

Rosacea occurs most commonly in fair-skinned women between the ages of 30 and 60, and it often makes its first appearance during menopause. But if you're a guy you're not off the hook because it can also occur in middle-aged men.

Mainstream medicine has some heavy-duty blinders on when it

comes to treating acne rosacea. And those blinders have them dashing off prescriptions for antibiotics with the belief that there's no other choice.

While it's true that the antibiotics might, in fact, help reverse some of the inflammation and accompanying redness that comes with rosacea, they also come with their own slew of nasty, gut-busting side effects. Fortunately, I happen to know of a natural treatment that's incredibly effective, simple to use, and inexpensive. And I can assure you that you'll never hear about it from your dermatologist.

I'll share all the details on that safe alternative with you in just a moment, but first let's take a closer look at what we know about the cause of rosacea (hint… it's not a whole lot) and the havoc that the mainstream's treatment of choice can play with your health.

The mysteriously-frustrating face of rosacea

There are various theories about what causes rosacea, but the truth is we don't really know for sure. Factors like sun exposure, exercise, stress, alcohol, spicy foods, and genetics all may play a part in causing blood vessels in the face to dilate too easily. Links have also been made between a bacterial infection of the stomach with Helicobacter pylori as well as an increased number of mites on the face known as Demodex folliculorum.

As is typical with chronic skin conditions, conventional medicine's approach can be very frustrating for patients with rosacea. Treatment usually consists of antibiotics applied topically to the face or taken internally. Interestingly, they aren't used however to kill bacteria that's been linked to rosacea, but rather for their anti-inflammatory effect. Of course we have far better—not to mention safer—natural ways to reduce inflammation, and one that's particularly effective for rosacea, but more on that in a bit.

When the "cure" is as bad as the disease

The most obvious problem with antibiotics is, of course, the digestive upset that comes with them which can include nausea, gas, bloating, and loose stool. Mainstream medicine doctors will be quick to tell you that a low dose antibiotic regimen will not have these gastric side effects. But I can assure you this is nonsense. Rosacea patients who are frustrated with the conventional antibiotic approach come to my office reporting these side effects all the time. And really it's no wonder, when you consider that they may have been on antibiotics for months or even years before they come to me.

The fact is long term antibiotic use… even at low doses… destroys friendly gut bacteria and sets the stage for the overgrowth of fungal organisms like candida albicans. Next thing you know you have a chronic fungal infection and instead of digesting your food properly your body starts essentially fermenting it. This creates havoc with your digestive tract and ultimately your immune system.

The topical application of antibiotics may seem like a safer option since you're not swallowing them. But the truth is they're bad news too, carrying their own unwelcome side effects. You see we have friendly flora as well as naturally occurring fungal organisms inhabiting the surface of our skin. And once you destroy the healthy bacteria the door is opened for an overgrowth of fungus and, ironically, more inflammation of the skin.

Powerful antioxidant fights flare-ups

If you're suffering with rosacea you deserve a reliable treatment that controls the redness and inflammation of your skin without all the antibiotic side effects. Fortunately there's a safe, natural, and phenomenally effective solution. In fact, I've been using it successfully with my own patients.

You've probably heard of alpha lipoic acid (ALA) before. The supplement is used to help reduce blood sugar levels, control neuropathies, combat chronic hepatitis, and ward off the effects of aging. But it turns out that when it's used topically it's also an incredibly effective treatment for rosacea.

I've used a variety of topical nutraceuticals with rosacea patients over the years. I've found that ALA is by far and away the most effective natural agent for reducing the redness and inflammation.

Within just two weeks of being on ALA my patients typically notice a great improvement in their rosacea and within six weeks their skin is as good as… or even better than… it was when they were using antibiotics. No doubt ALA has a natural anti-inflammatory effect when applied to the skin.

While I'm unaware of any formal studies with ALA to treat rosacea, a study in the *British Journal of Dermatology* found the topical use of the antioxidant was effective in the treatment of facial sun damage.[1] In other words, it has an anti-inflammatory and regenerative effect on the skin. And this finding, of course, backs up the great results I've already been seeing in my own practice.

Ban the blush with natural supplements

The best way to use ALA is a five percent concentrated facial cream. You can find alpha lipoic acid cream in stores and on the internet, However, you need to be careful when choosing one because few actually contain the five percent concentration that they need to be effective. Many skin products contain ALA but it's usually in a non-therapeutic concentration mixed with other antioxidants. These combination formulas often don't even bother to list the amounts of the topical nutrients, so there's really no way to know what you're getting.

The best way to be sure your getting the right amount of ALA in a facial cream is to simply have your doctor prescribe you a formulation to fill at your local compounding pharmacy. You'll want to start with a small amount on your skin to make sure you're not sensitive to it. I find a small percentage of patients experience some minor skin irritation and need a weaker concentration. In these cases I reduce the concentration to three percent.

Apply the ALA to your face nightly and watch your skin redness dramatically decrease over the following weeks. Continue applying the cream every night for four months and then you may be able to drop back to using it every other night.

While you are getting non-toxic relief for your rosacea it's also important to treat your body internally. I recommend you start by getting yourself tested for food sensitivities, which can often contribute to your symptoms.

Next, since there's almost always some connection between skin conditions and the inside of your body… particularly the digestive tract… you should start taking a daily probiotic to fortify your friendly flora. And to improve your stomach function and help with the breakdown of food and nutrients try taking betaine hydrochloride—which mimics your own stomach acid—with meals.

For general skin support you should also be taking a daily B complex, and a fish or krill oil supplement. And finally, if you are menopausal have your holistic doctor check your hormone levels and if they are low then consider using natural progesterone and natural estrogen, which can help normalize blood vessel dilation and reduce inflammation.

A Homeopathic Remedy
for Bruises

The homeopathic remedy *Arnica montana* (also known as leopard's bane) can significantly reduce bruising. In a double-blind clinical trial involving 29 women who were undergoing face-lifts, participants were randomly assigned to receive homeopathic arnica (12C potency) or a placebo beginning the morning of surgery. The treatment was repeated every eight hours for four days. Facial bruising and swelling were evaluated by doctors and nurses, as well as through a computerized digital-image analysis of photographs taken before and after surgery. Subjective symptoms—those observed by the patients and professional staff—and the degree of discoloration were not significantly improved by the arnica. However, the area of bruising was significantly smaller for the group of subjects who took arnica. Although the study was on women, I would expect the same results for men and for other types of bruising.

Arnica preparations have been used in homeopathic medicine for two centuries. *Sesquiterpene lactones*, major active compounds in arnica, are known to reduce inflammation, decrease pain and improve circulation.

I can attest to hundreds of cases in which arnica has reduced pain and swelling. I also have seen this benefit with infants and animals—where a placebo effect is unlikely. You can use arnica for any soft-tissue injury, such as bruising after a fall or a sprained ankle. The most common dose is two pellets of 30C strength taken two to four times daily for two days. Or apply homeopathic arnica cream two to three times daily until healed. Arnica is sold at most health-food stores and some pharmacies.

Caution: Do not use topical arnica on broken skin or open wounds.

Blowing Away the "Expensive Urine" Myth: Why Multivitamins Make Sense

How many times have you heard the so called "medical experts" parrot the old myth that multivitamins just give you expensive urine? How many times have you had to sit through a lecture about how they're a waste of money?

The truth is, there are a stack of studies that say otherwise! And now we can add yet one more to that growing pile. A new study out of Australia found that supplementing with a daily, high-dose, multivitamin helped raise volunteer's energy levels and left them in a better mood.[1]

I'd be willing to bet that those are two things that almost anyone could use more of. Not to mention two things that most of us would be happy to hand over a small fee for in exchange for the vim and vigor to get out there and get more out of life.

The multivitamin, which was provided by the study's sponsor, contained amounts of B vitamins and vitamins C, D, and E that met or exceeded the Recommended Dietary Intakes as well as doses of calcium, magnesium, potassium, iron, and a collection of herbal extracts. After 16 weeks of regular use, the men and women in the study reported a noticeable increase in their mood and energy plus an added bonus: Better sleep.

Of course, I have to admit I wasn't at all surprised by these results. These are the same kinds of benefits I've seen thousands of patients reap over the years when they start taking a high-potency quality multivitamin.

The fact is, multivitamins are a convenient and inexpensive way to boost your mood, energy, and quality of sleep. And if that's all they did they would already be worth taking. But these little powerhouses don't stop there. Multivitamins also support your telomeres, which protect your DNA and play a role in aging. They've even been shown to reduce your risk of the common cold and improve IQ.

So, the next time your doctor tells you to get all your nutrients from your food and stop wasting your money on a multivitamin politely tell him that he should do a little more research on multivitamins. He's clearly missed all the positive studies. Maybe you can even provide him with a copy of this article to get him started. And while you're at it, go ahead and explain to him that you'd much rather have pricy pee than the nutrient deficiencies which predispose you to disease!

References

Part I: Pain

**The Shocking Hidden Cause of Your Chronic Pain and Muscle Weakness…
And the Simple Solution to Feeling Like Yourself Again**

[1] Lowe JC, Yellin J, Honeyman-Lowe G. Female fibromyalgia patients: lower resting metabolic rates that matched healthy controls. *Med Sci Monit.* 2006 Jul;12(7):CR282-9.

[2] Lowe JC, Garrison RL, Reichman AJ, Yellin J, Thompson M, Kaufman D. Effectiveness and safety of T3 (triiodothyronine) therapy for euthyroid fibromyalgia: a double-blind placebo-controlled response-driven crossover study. *Clin Bull Myofascial Ther* 1997;2:31–58.

[3] Teitelbaum JE, Bird B, Greenfield RM ,Weiss A., Muenz L, Gould L. Effective Treatment of CFS and Fibromyalgia: A Randomized, Double-blind, Placebo-controlled, Intent to Treat Study. *The Journal of Chronic Fatigue Syndrome.* 2001; 8(2):3-28.

[4] Abraham GE. The bioavailability of iodine applied to the skin. *The Original Internist.* 2008;15(2):77-79.

This Common Drug—Not Old Age—Could be the REAL Cause of Your Aching Painful Joints

[1] Mansi I, Frei CR, Pugh MJ, Makris U, Mortensen EM. Statins and musculoskeletal conditions, arthropathies, and injuries. *JAMA Intern Med* 2013; DOI:10.1001/jamainternmed.2013.6184

[2] ibid

[3] Estruch R, Ros E, Salas-Salvadó J, et al. Primary prevention of cardiovascular disease with a Mediterranean diet. *N Engl J Med.* 2013 February 25. [Epub ahead of print].

[4] B. Antony,* B. Merina, and V. Sheeba. Amlamax™ in the Management of Dyslipidemia in Humans. *Indian J Pharm Sci.* 2008 Jul-Aug; 70(4): 504–507.

[5] Ehara S, Ueda M, et al., "Elevated levels of oxidized low density lipoprotein show a positive relationship with the severity of acute coronary syndromes," *Circulation.* 2001;103:1955-1960.

[6] Zhao SP, Lu ZL, Du BM, Chen Z, Wu YF, Yu XH, Zhao YC, Liu L, Ye HJ, Wu ZH; China Coronary Secondary Prevention Study (CCSPS). *J Cardiovasc Pharmacol.* 2007 Feb;49(2):81-4.

[7] Mollace V, Sacco I, Janda E, Malara C, Ventrice D, Colica C, Visalli V,

Muscoli S, Ragusa S, Muscoli C, Rotiroti D, Romeo F.Fitoterapia. 2011 Apr;82(3):309-16. doi: 10.1016/j.fitote.2010.10.014. Epub 2010 Nov 4. Hypolipemic and hypoglycaemic activity of bergamot polyphenols: from animal models to human studies.

The Drug-Free Back Pain Solution

[1] Modic MT, Ross JS. Lumbar degenerative disk disease. *Radiology*. Oct 2007;245(1):43-61.

Part II: Cancer

The Seafood Secret to Stopping Cancer and Halting Heart Disease in its Tracks

[1] Yang Y, Lu N, Chen D, Meng L, Zheng Y, Hui R. Effects of n-3 PUFA supplementation on plasma soluble adhesion molecules: a meta-analysis of randomized controlled trials. *Am J Clin Nutr*. 2012 Apr;95(4):972-80. Epub

[2] Touvier M, Kesse-Guyot E, Andreeva VA, Fezeu L, Charnaux N, Sutton A, Druesne-Pecollo N, Hercberg S, Galan P, Zelek L, Latino-Martel P, Czernichow S. Modulation of the association between plasma intercellular adhesion molecule-1 and cancer risk by n-3 PUFA intake: a nested case-control study. *Am J Clin Nutr*. 2012 Apr;95(4):944-50. Epub 2012 Feb 29

Say Goodbye to Chemo and So Long to Those Harsh Drugs… Starve Cancer Cells to Death Instead!

[1] Graham NA, Tahmasian M, Kohli B, Komisopoulou E, Zhu M, Vivanco I, Teitell MA, Wu H, Ribas A, Lo RS, Mellinghoff IK, Mischel PS, Graeber TG. Glucose deprivation activates a metabolic and signaling amplification loop leading to cell death. *Mol Syst Biol*. 2012 Jun 26;8:589. doi: 10.1038/msb.2012.20

[2] Harvard Health Publications. Accessed July 8, 2012 at http://www.health.harvard.edu/newsweek/Glycemic_index_and_glycemic_load_for_100_foods.htm

[3] ibid

[4] Schmidt M, et al. Effects of a ketogenic diet on the quality of life in 16 patients with advanced cancer: A pilot trial. *Nutrition & Metabolism* 2011;8:54.

Fight Cancer Fatigue and Beat Exhaustion with This Native American Herbal Gem

[1] Stengler. Mark. The Natural Physician's Healing Therapies, 2010. *Prentice Hall Press*. Page 222

[2] 2012 American Society of Clinical Oncology Annual Meeting; "Phase III

evaluation of American ginseng (panax quinquefolius) to improve cancer-related fatigue" Debra L. Barton et al. Accessed July 22, 2012 at http://www.asco.org/ASCOv2/Meetings/Abstracts?&vmview=abst_detail_view&confID=114&abstractID=94721

[3] Wang CZ, Aung HH, Zhang B, Sun S, Li XL, He H, Xie JT, He TC, Du W, Yuan CS. Chemopreventive effects of heat-processed Panax quinquefolius root on human breast cancercells. *Anticancer Res.* 2008 Sep-Oct;28(5A):2545-51.

[4] King ML, Murphy LL. American ginseng (Panax quinquefolius L.) extract alters mitogen-activated protein kinase cell signaling and inhibits proliferation of MCF-7 cells. *J Exp Ther Oncol.* 2007;6(2):147-55

Miracle Mineral Could Reduce Your Risk of Prostate Cancer by Forty Percent or More!

[1] Hurst R, et al. Selenium and prostate cancer: systematic review and meta-analysis. *Am J Clin Nutr* 2012;96(1): 111-122

Part III: Heart and Blood

27 Percent Lower Blood Pressure Readings with "Hypertension Soup"

[1] Medina-Remon A, et al., Gazpacho consumption is associated with lower blood pressure and reduced hypertension in a high cardiovascular risk cohort. Cross-sectional study of the PREDIMED trial. *Nutrition, Metabolism & Cardiovascular Diseases.* Epub ahead of print.

[2] Norman RC Campbell, MD and Guanmin Chen, MD PhD Canadian efforts to prevent and control hypertension. *Can J Cardiol.* 2010 Aug-Sep; 26(Suppl C): 14C–17C.

[3] Centers for Disease Control Website. Accessed January 6, 2013 at www.cdc.gov/dhdsp/pubs/docs/SIB_BP_Medication_Use.pdf.

[4] Centers for Disease Control Website. Accessed January 6, 2013 at www.cdc.gov/mmwr/preview/mmwrhtml/mm6004a4.htm?s_cid=mm6004a4_w

Powerful Herb Beats High Blood Pressure without Drug Side Effects

[1] National Institutes of Health: National Institute on Aging. Accessed February 17, 2013 online at http://www.nia.nih.gov/health/publication/high-blood-pressure.

[2] ibid

[3] AARM Reference Review. *Journal of Restorative Medicine* 2012;1: page 98-99.

[4] Shamon SD, Perez MI. Blood pressure lowering efficacy of reserpine for primary hypertension. *Cochrane Database Syst Rev.* 2009 Oct 7;(4)

Pop Painkillers and You Could Raise Your Heart Attack Risk

Olsen AM, et al. Long-term cardiovascular risk of nonsteroidal anti-inflammatory drug use according to time passed after first-time myocardial infarction: a nationwide cohort study. *Circulation.* 2012;126:1955-1963.

The Overlooked Artery Enemy: Knowing Your Levels of This "Hidden Heart Menace" Could Save Your Life!

[1] Mertens A, Holvoet P. Oxidized LDL and HDL: antagonists in atherothrombosis. *FASEB J.* 2001;15:2073-2084.

[2] Itabe H, Takeshima E, Iwasaki H, et al. A monoclonalantibody against oxidized lipoprotein recognizes foam cells in atherosclerotic lesions. Complex formation of oxidized phosphatidylcholines and polypeptides. *J Biol Chem.* 1994;269:15274-15279.

[3] Kaess BM, Vasan RS. Statins are not associated with a decrease in all cause mortality in a high-risk primary prevention setting. *Evidence Based Medicine.* 2011;16:8-9.

[4] Ehara S, Ueda M, et al., "Elevated levels of oxidized low density lipoprotein show a positive relationship with the severity of acute coronary syndromes," *Circulation.* 2001;103:1955-1960.

[5] Johnston N. et al. Improved identification of patients with coronary artery disease by the use of new lipid and lipoprotein biomarkers. *Am J Cardiol.* 2006;97:640-645.

[6] Itabe H, Obama T, Kato R. The dynamics of oxidized ldl during atherogenesis. *J Lipids.* 2011;2011:418313.

[7] Fito M, Guxens M, et al. Effect of a traditional Mediterranean diet on lipoprotein oxidation: a randomized controlled trial. *Arch Intern Med.* 2007;167:1195-1203.

[8] Eklan A-C, Sjoberg B, Kolsrud B, et al. Gluten-free vegan diet induces decreased LDL and oxidized LDL levels and raised atheroprotective natural antibodies against phosphorylcholine in patients with rheumatoid arthritis: a randomized study. *Arthritis Res Ther.* 2008;10:R34.

[9] Aviram M, Dornfeld L, Kaplan M, et al. Pomegranate juice flavonoids inhibit low-density lipoprotein oxidation and cardiovascular diseases: studies in atherosclerotic mice and in humans. *Drugs Exp Clin Res.* 2002;28:49-62.

[10] Gomikawa S, Ishikawa Y, Hayase W, et al. Effect of ground green tea

drinking for 2 weeks on the susceptibility of plasma and LDL to theoxidation ex vivo in healthy volunteers. *Kobe J Med Sci.* 2008;54:E62-E72.

[11] Reaven PD, Khouw A, Bletz WF, et al. Effect of dietary antioxidant combinations in humans. Protection by vitamin E, but not by beta-carotene. 1993;13:590-600.

[12] Tsai KL, Huang YH, Kao CL. A novel mechanism of coenzyme Q10 protects against human endothelial cells from oxidative stress-induced injury by modulating NO-related pathways. *J Nutr Biochem.* 2012;23:458-468.

[13] Earnest CP, Wood KA, Church TS. Complex multivitamin supplementation improves homocysteine and resistance to ldl-c oxidation. *J Am Coll Nutr.* 2003;22:400-407.

[14] Costantini F, Pierdomenico SD, De Cesare D, et al. Effect of thyroid function on LDL oxidation. *Arterioscler Thromb Vasc Biol.* 1998;18:732-737.

Stop the Silent "Thick Blood" Killer That's Putting Your Yeart and Health at Risk—Before it's Too Late!

[1] Sloop GD. A unifying theory of atherogenesis. Med Hypotheses. 1996; 47:321-5. www.ncbi.nlm.nih.gov/pubmed/8910882>

[2] Lowe GD, Lee AJ, Rumley A, et al. Blood viscosity and risk of cardiovascular events: the Edinburgh Artery Study. *Br J Haematol* 1997; 96:168-173.

[3] G. Ciuffetti, et al. Prognostic Impact of Low-Shear Whole Blood Viscosity in Hypertensive Men. *European Journal of Clinical Investigation*, 2005:35(2), 93-98.

[4] Hyperviscosity Syndrome. Accessed February 10, 2013 online at www.emedicine.medscape.com/article/780258-overview#a0104.

[5] Larsen, Pushpa. Earlier, More Accurate Prediction of Cardiovascular Event Risk. Naturopathic Doctor News and Review. Accessed February 10, 2013 online at www.ndnr.com/web-articles/cardiopulmonary-medicine/blood-viscosity.

[6] Clivillé, et al. Hemorheological, coagulative and fibrinolytic changes during autologous blood donation. *Clinical Hemorheology and Microcirculation*, 18 (1998) 265-272.

[7] J. Solonen, et al. Donation of blood is associated with reduced risk of myocardial infarction. *American Journal of Epidemiology*, 148 (1998) 445-451.

[8] Klein BE, Howard KP, Gangnon RE, Dreyer JO, Lee KE, Klein R. Long-term use of aspirin and age-related macular degeneration. *JAMA.* 2012 Dec 19;308(23):2469-78.

The Up-and-Coming Heart Health Superstar That Everyone Will Be Talking About: Put the MEGA into Your OMEGA

[1] Garg ML, et al., Macadamia nut consumption lowers plasma total and LDL cholesterol levels in hypercholesterolemic men, *J Nutr.* 2003; 133: 1060-1063

[2] Baggio E, et al., Italian multicenter study on the safety and efficacy of coenzyme Q10 as adjunctive therapy in heart failure. CoQ10 Drug Surveillance Investigators, *Mol Aspects Med.* 1994; 15 Suppl: s287-294

[3] Coenzyme Q10. Monograph," Altern Med Rev. 2007; 12: 159-168

[4] Antony, et al., Amlamax(TM) in the Management of Dyslipidemia in Humans, *Indian Journal of Pharmacueitcal Sciences*, July-August 2008

[5] Antony, et al., Effect of standardized Amla extract on atheroscleoris and dyslipidmia, *Indian Journal of Pharmaceutical Sciences*, July-August 2006

[6] Katan MB, et al., Efficacy and safety of plant stanols and sterols in the management of blood cholesterol levels, *Mayo Clin Proc.* 2003; 78: 965-978

[7] Acuff RV, et al., The lipid lowering effect of plant sterol ester capsules in hypercholesterolemic subjects, *Lipids Health Dis.* 2007; 6: 11

[8] Abumweis SS, et al.,Plant sterols/stanols as cholesterol lowering agents: A meta-analysis of randomized controlled trials, *Food Nutr Res.*2008; 52

[9] Edirisinghe, et al., Mechanism of the endothelium-dependent relaxation evoked by a grape seed extract, *Clinical Science* (2008) 114, 331–337

[10] Robinson, et al.,Effects of grape seed extract in subjects with pre-hypertension 2007, University of California, Davis, Davis, California, USA

Part V: Weight Loss

The Hormone That May Help You Decrease Belly Fat

Dennis T. Villareal, MD, associate professor, division of geriatrics and nutritional science, Washington University School of Medicine, St. Louis… Roberta Anding, RD, clinical dietitian, Texas Children's Hospital, Houston…*Journal of the American Medical Association.*

How to Safely and Easily Shed 20 to 30 Pounds in Just 3 to 4 Weeks Flat

[1] www.Inchesaway.com/wp-content/uploads/2010/12/dr-simeons-manuscript.pdf

[2] PubMed Health website. Accessed November 22, 2012 at www.ncbi.nlm.nih.gov/pubmedhealth/PMH0000605/.

[3] Belluscio, Daniel. Utility of an oral presentation of HCG Human Cho-

riogonadotropin for the management of obesity: A double blind study. Accessed November 22, 2012 online at www.hcgobesity.org/hcg_obesity_study.htm#RESULTS.

[4] ibid

[5] Bernstein L, Hanisch R, Sullivan-Halley J, Ross RK. Treatment with human chorionic gonadotropin and risk of breast cancer. *Cancer Epidemiol Biomarkers Prev.* 1995 Jul-Aug;4(5):437-40.

[6] Jaak Ph. Janssens et al. Human Chorionic Gonadotropin (hCG) and prevention of breast cancer. "Molecular and Cellular Endocrinology" 269, 1-2 (2007) 93.

Part VI: Diabetes

Test for Diabetes

American Diabetes Association, www.diabetes.org.

New Study Shocker: America's #1 Drug Increases Your Risk of Diabetes by up to 80 Percent

[1] Culver AL, Ockene IS, Balasubramanian R, et al. Statin use and risk of diabetes mellitus in postmenopausal women in the Women's Health Initiative. *Arch Intern Med* 2012; DOI: 10.1001/archinternmed.2011.625

[2] Kwang Kon Koh, MD,* Michael J. Quon, MD, PhD,† Seung Hwan Han, MD,* Yonghee Lee, PhD,‡ Soo Jin Kim, RN,* and Eak Kyun Shin, MD*. Atorvastatin Causes Insulin Resistance and Increases Ambient Glycemia in Hypercholesterolemic Patients. *J Am Coll Cardiol.* 2010 March 23; 55(12): 1209–1216.

[3] Preiss D, Seshasai SR, Welsh P et al. Risk of incident diabetes with intensive-dose compared with moderate-dose statin therapy: a meta-analysis. *JAMA* 2011;305:2556-64.

[4] Earl S. Ford, MD, MPH; Manuela M. Bergmann, PhD; Janine Kröger; Anja Schienkiewitz, PhD, MPH;Cornelia Weikert, MD, MPH; Heiner Boeing, PhD, MSPH. Healthy Living is the Best Revengs. Findings From the European Prospective Investigation Into Cancer and Nutrition–Potsdam Study. *Arch Intern Med.* 169(15): 1355-62.

How an All-Natural "Bean Cure" Can Get You Off Your Diabetes Drug— For Good

[1] "FDA Warns of Bladder Cancer Risk With Actos," Fiore, Kristina, Med-

Page Today, Published: June 15, 2011

[2] World Health Oragnization. Diabetes Fact Sheet N°312, August 2011. www.who.int

[3] "National Diabetes Fact Sheet, 2011" Centers for Disease Control website. www.cdc.gov

[4] Ibid

[5] "Use May Increase Risk for Diabetic Macular Edema." Canavan, Neil. *TZD*, www.medscape.com

[6] Pharmacoepidem. Drug Safe. 2012;doi: 10.1002/pds.3234. "Use of thiazolidinediones and risk of osteoporotic fracture: disease or drugs,"

[7] "ACTOS (pioglitazone hydrochloride)" and AVANDIA (rosiglitazone maleate)". www.rxlist.com

[8] Am J Clin Nutr. 2008 Jan;87(1):162-7. "Legume and soy food intake and the incidence of type 2 diabetes in the Shanghai Women's Health Study."

[9] *Am J Clin Nutr.* 2008 Oct;88(4):1167-75. "Effect of glucomannan on plasma lipid and glucose concentrations, body weight, and blood pressure: systematic review and meta-analysis."

[10] *Journal of Human Nutrition and Dietetics.* Volume 24, Issue 4, pages 351–359, August 2011. "Effects of a 3-month supplementation with a novel soluble highly viscous polysaccharide on anthropometry and blood lipids in non-dieting overweight or obese adults."

"Hidden-in-Plain-Sight" Toxin Rockets Your Risk for Developing Diabetes up by 65 Percent—Read This BEFORE You Take Your Next Bite

[1] K. He, et al. Mercury exposure in young adulthood and incidence of diabetes later in life: the CARDIA trace element study. Diabetes Care. 2013 Feb 19. Epub ahead of print.

[2] The Proceedings from the 13th International Symposium of The Institute of Functional Medicine. Managing Biotransformation: The Metabolic, Genomic, and Detoxification Balance Points. Alternative Therapies website. Accessed online April 20, 2013 at http://www.alternative-therapies.com/at/web_pdfs/ifm_proceedings_low.pdf

[3] Preventing Disease through Heal Thy Environment Exposures to Mercury: A Major Public Health Concern. World Health Organization. Accessed April 24, 2013 online at http://www.who.int/ipcs/features/mercury.pdf

[4] EPA website. Mercury. Accessed April 14, 2013 online at http://www. epa.gov/hg/about.htm.

[5] Ibid

[6] BioDiversity Research Institute website. Global Mercury Hotspots. Accessed online April 14, 2013 at http://www.briloon.org/uploads/documents/hgcenter/gmh/gmhSummary.pdf

[7] CBS Evening News Website. Accessed online April 14, 2013 at http://www.cbsnews.com/8301-18563_162-57563739/study-finds-unsafe-mercury-levels-in-84-percent-of-all-fish/

[8] Vimy MJ, Lorsheider FL. Intra-oral air mercury released from dental amalgams. *J Dent Res* 1985;64(8):1069-1071.

[9] Emedicine health website. Mercury poisoning. Accessed online April 14, 2013 at http://www.emedicinehealth.com/mercury_poisoning/page3_em.htm

America's Secret Poison: Diet Soda's Surprising Hidden Link to Diabetes

[1] G. Fagherazzi, et al. Consumption of artificially and sugar-sweetened beverages and incident type 2 diabetes in the Etude Epidémiologique auprès des femmes de la Mutuelle Générale de l'Education Nationale–European Prospective Investigation into Cancer and Nutrition cohort. *Am J Clin Nutr.* Published online ahead of print January 2013.

Part VII: Alzheimer's Disease and Memory

Protect Your Brain with the Two MUST-HAVE Nutrients for Fighting Alzheimer's

[1] *Arch Intern Med.* 2010;170:1135-1141, 1099-1100.

[2] *Journal of Alzheimer's Disease*, 2012;29:51-62.

[3] *Neurology.* 2001;57:985-989.

[4] *Am J Epidemiol.* 2006;164:898-906.

[5] *Ther Adv Psychopharm.* Published online before print February 24, 2012,.

[6] Alzheimer's Disease International (ADI) 27th International Conference. Abstract P098. Presented March 9, 2012.

How You Can Boost Your Brainpower and Revitalize Memory with a Powerful Nutrient You've Never Heard Of

[1] Fiorvanti M, Yanagi M. The Cochrane Library, Oxford, England. 2006; Issue 4

[2] D'Orlando KJ, Sandage BW. Citicoline (CDP-choline): mechanisms of action and effects in ischemic brain injury. *Neurol Res* 1995;17(4):281-284.

[3] Secades JJ, Lorenzo JL. Citicoline: pharmacological and clinical review, 2006 update. *Methods Find Exp Clin Pharmacol.* 2006; 27(Suppl B): 1–56.

[4] Alvarez XA et al. Citicoline improves memory performance in elderly subjects. *Methods Find Exp Clin Pharmacol.* 1997; 19(3): 201–10.

[5] Spiers PA et al. Citicoline improves verbal memory in aging. *Arch Neurol.* 1996; 53: 441–48.

[6] Franco-Maside A, Caamaño J, Gómez MJ, Cacabelos R. Brain mapping activity and mental performance after chronic treatment with CDP-choline in Alzheimer's disease. *Methods Find Exp Clin Pharmacol.* 1994;16(8):597-607.

[7] Caamaño J, Gómez MJ, Franco A, Cacabelos R. Effects of CDP-choline on cognition and cerebral hemodynamics in patients with Alzheimer's disease. *Methods Find Exp Clin Pharmacol.* 1994;16(3):211-218.

Stop Alzheimer's BEFORE it Starts—With the Breakthrough Brain-Saving "Penny Cure"

[1] Vellas, B., et al., Prevention trials inAlzheimer's disease:An EU-US task force report. Prog. *Neurobiol.* (2011), doi:10.1016/j.pneuro-bio.2011.08.014

[2] Gwenaëlle Douaud, Helga Refsum,Celeste A. de Jager, Robin Jacoby,Thomas E. Nichols, Stephen M. Smith, and A. David Smith, Preventing Alzheimer's disease-related gray matter atrophy by B-vitamin treatment *PNAS* 2013 ; published ahead of print May 20, 2013

[3] Bloomberg website accessed online May 27, 2013 at http://www.bloomberg.com/news/2013-05-20/vitamins-that-cost-pennies-a-day-seen-delaying-dementia.html

Part VIII: Allergies, Digestion and Nutrition

My "Identify and Conquer" Plan for Beating Asthma and Breathing Better

[1] American Academy of Allergy Asthma and Immunology website. Accessed September 15, 2012 at http://www.aaaai.org/about-the-aaaai/newsroom/asthma-statistics.aspx

[2] American Academy of Allergy Asthma and Immunology website. Accessed September 15, 2012 at http://www.aaaai.org/conditions-and-treatments/asthma.aspx

[3] American Academy of Allergy Asthma and Immunology website. Accessed September 15, 2012 at http://www.aaaai.org/conditions-and-treatments/drug-guide.aspx

[4] American Academy of Allergy Asthma and Immunology website. Accessed September 15, 2012 at http://www.aaaai.org/conditions-and-treatments/asthma.aspx

[5] Lau BH, Riesen SK, Truong KP, et al. Pycnogenol as an adjunct in the management of childhood asthma. *J Asthma* 2004;41:825-32.

[6] van Oeffelen AA, Bekkers MB, Smit HA, Kerkhof M, Koppelman GH, Haveman-Nies A, van der A DL, Jansen EH, Wijga AH., Serum micronutrient concentrations and childhood asthma: the PIAMA birth cohort study. *Pediatr Allergy Immunol.* 2011 Dec;22(8):784-93. doi: 10.1111/j.1399-3038.2011.01190.x. Epub 2011 Sep 19.

[7] Schenk P, Vonbank K, Schnack B, et al. Intravenous magnesium sulfate for bronchial hyperreactivity: a randomized, controlled, double-blind study. *Clin Pharmacol Ther* 2001;69:365-71.

[8] Ciarallo L, Brousseau D, Reinert S. Higher-dose intravenous magnesium therapy for children with moderate to severe acute asthma. *Arch Pediatr Adolesc Med* 2000;154:979-83.

[9] Torres S, Sticco N, Bosch JJ, Iolster T, Siaba A, Rocca Rivarola M, Schnitzler E. Effectiveness of magnesium sulfate as initial treatment of acute severe asthma in children, conducted in a tertiary-level university hospital: A randomized, controlled trial. *Arch Argent Pediatr.* 2012 Aug;110(4):291-6.

[10] Brehm JM, Schuemann B, Fuhlbrigge AL, Hollis BW, Strunk RC, Zeiger RS, et al. Childhood Asthma Management Program Research Group Serum vitamin D levels and severe asthma exacerbations in the Childhood Asthma Management Program study. *J Allergy Clin Immunol.* 2010;126:52–8.e5. doi: 10.1016/j.jaci.2010.03.043.

[11] Chinellato I, Piazza M, Sandri M, Peroni D, Piacentini G, Boner AL. Vitamin D serum levels and markers of asthma control in Italian children. *J Pediatr*. 2011;158:437–41. doi: 10.1016/j.jpeds.2010.08.043.

[12] Chinellato I, Piazza M, Sandri M, Peroni DG, Cardinale F, Piacentini GL, et al. Serum vitamin D levels and exercise-induced bronchoconstriction in children with asthma. *Eur Respir J*. 2011;37:1366–70. doi: 10.1183/09031936.00044710

[13] Black PN, Scragg R. Relationship between serum 25-hydroxyvitamin d and pulmonary function in the third national health and nutrition examination survey. *Chest*. 2005;128:3792–8. doi: 10.1378/chest.128.6.3792.

[14] Li F, Peng M, Jiang L, Sun Q, Zhang K, Lian F, et al. Vitamin D deficiency is associated with decreased lung function in Chinese adults with asthma. *Respiration*. 2011;81:469–75. doi: 10.1159/000322008.

[15] Sutherland ER, Goleva E, Jackson LP, Stevens AD, Leung DY. Vitamin D levels, lung function, and steroid response in adult asthma. *Am J Respir Crit Care Med*. 2010;181:699–704. doi: 10.1164/rccm.200911-1710OC.

[16] Stengler, Mark A. The Natural Physician's Healing Therapies, 2nd edition. Pgs 42-44, 2010. Prentice Hall Press, New York, NY, USA.

[17] Neuman I, Nahum H, Ben-Amotz A. Reduction of exercise-induced asthma oxidative stress by lycopene, a natural antioxidant. *Allergy*. 2000 Dec;55(12):1184-9.

The Stomach-Turning Trouble That Could Be Lurking in Your Next Meal

[1] PubMed Health website. Accessed October 24, 2012 at http://www.ncbi.nlm.nih.gov/pubmedhealth/PMH0004978/

[2] ibid

[3] Marianne G. Pedersen, MSc; Preben Bo Mortensen, DrMedSc; Bent Norgaard-Pedersen, Dr MedSc; Teodor T. Postolache, MD. Toxoplasma gondii Infection and Self-directed Violence in Mothers . *Arch Gen Psychiatry*. 2012;():1-8. doi:10.1001/archgenpsychiatry.2012.668.

[4] Hamidinejat H, Ghorbanpoor M, Hosseini H, Alavi SM, Nabavi L, Jalali MH, Borojeni MP, Jafari H, Mohammadaligol S. Toxoplasma gondii infection in first-episode and inpatient individuals with schizophrenia. *Int J Infect Dis*. 2010 Nov;14(11):e978-81. Epub 2010 Sep 16.

[5] Balch, James, Stengler M. Prescription for Natural Cures 2nd Edition, pgs 363-364. Wiley, 2011, Hoboken, NJ, USA.

Part IX: Immune System

Revealing the REAL Truth Behind the Flu Vaccine: How to Dodge the Flu Bullet This Year, and Every Year—Naturally

[1] Centers for Disease Control and Prevention website. Accessed October 14, 2012 at http://www.cdc.gov/flu/about/season/flu-season-2012-2013.htm.

[2] ibid

[3] Centers for Disease Control and Prevention website. Accessed October 14, 2012 at http://www.cdc.gov/flu/protect/keyfacts.htm

[4] Centers for Disease Control and Prevention website: 2011-2012 Flu season draws to a close. Accessed October 14,2012 at: http://www.cdc.gov/flu/spotlights/2011-2012-flu-season-wrapup.htm

[5] Centers for Disease Control and Prevention website. Accessed October 14, 2012 at http://www.cdc.gov/flu/about/qa/disease.htm

[6] Stanford University website. Accessed October 14, 2012 at http://virus.stanford.edu/uda/

[7] Branswell H. Vancouver researcher finds flu shot is linked to H1N1 illness. Vancouver Sun September 10, 2012. Available at: http://www.vancouversun.com/health/Vancouver+researcher+finds+shot+linked+H1N1+illness/7217609/story.html#ixzz27P1gHlZj

[8] ibid

[9] Centers for Disease Control and Prevention website. Accessed October 14, 2012 at http://www.cdc.gov/flu/protect/vaccine/vaccines.htm

[10] Centers for Disease Control and Prevention website. Accessed October 24, 2012 at http://www.cdc.gov/vaccines/pubs/pinkbook/downloads/appendices/B/excipient-table-2.pdf

[11] Centers for Disease Control and Prevention website. Accessed October 24, 2012 at http://www.atsdr.cdc.gov/substances/toxsubstance.asp?toxid=39

[12] Vaccines.gov website Accessed October 24, 2012 at http://www.vaccines.gov/who_and_when/infant/index.html

[13] Urashima, M. Segawa, T. Okazaki, M. Kurihara, M. Wada, Y. Ida, H.Randomized trial of vitamin D supplementation to prevent seasonal influenza A in schoolchildren. *Am J Clin Nutr*. 2010 May; 91 (5): 1255-60.

[14] Boge T, Rémigy M, Vaudaine S, Tanguy J, Bourdet-Sicard R, van der Werf S.A probiotic fermented dairy drink improves antibody response to influenza vaccination in the elderly in two randomised controlled trials.

Vaccine. 2009 Sep 18;27(41):5677-84. Epub 2009 Jul 16.

[15] De Flora S, Grassi C, Carati L. Attenuation of influenza-like symptomatology and improvement of cell-mediated immunity with long-term N-acetylcysteine treatment. *Eur Respir J.* 1997 Jul;10(7):1535-41

[16] (Zakay-Rones Z, Thom E, Wollan T, Wadstein J. Randomized study of the efficacy and safety of oral elderberry extract in the treatment of influenza A and B virus infections. *J Int Med Res.* 2004;32:132-40.)

[17] Zakay-Rones Z, Varsano N, Zlotnik M, et al. Inhibition of several strains of influenza virus in vitro and reduction of symptoms by an elderberry extract (Sambucus nigra L.) during an outbreak of influenza B Panama. *J Alt Complement Med.* 1995;1:361-9.)

The Hydrogen Peroxide "Miracle Cure" That Your Doctor's Never Even Heard Of

[1] Osborne, Virginia; Carter, Dan; Anderson, Paul. IV Nutritional Therapy for Seminars for Physicians. September 2009.

How to Conquer America's Growing Super-Infection Threat—Naturally

[1] Far more could be done to stop the deadly bacteria C. diff. MayoClinic.com Accessed August 19, 2012 at http://www.usatoday.com/news/health/story/2012-08-16/deadly-bacteria-hospital-infections/57079514/1

[2] Emedicine medscape. Accessed August 19, 2012 at http://emedicine.medscape.com/article/186458-overview

[3] Study Shows Cases of C. Diff Increased 12-Fold Among Children. Medscape.com. Accessed August 19, 2012 at http://www.medscape.com/viewarticle/764275

[4] Emedicine medscape. Accessed August 19, 2012 at http://emedicine.medscape.com/article/186458-overview

[5] Emedicine medscape. Accessed August 19, 2012 at http://emedicine.medscape.com/article/186458-overview#a0104

[6] McFarland LV. Meta-analysis of probiotics for the prevention of antibiotic associated diarrhea and the treatment of Clostridium difficile disease. *Am J Gastroenterol.* 2006 Apr;101(4):812-22.

[7] McFarland LV, Surawicz CM, Greenberg RN, et al. A randomized placebo-controlled trial of Saccharomyces boulardii in combination with standard antibiotics for Clostridium difficile disease. *JAMA* 1994;271:1913-8.

[8] Surawicz CM, McFarland LV, Elmer G, et al. Treatment of recurrent clostridium difficile colitis with vancomycin and Saccharomyces boulardii.

Am J Gastroenterol 1989;84:1285-7.

[9] McFarland LV. Meta-analysis of probiotics for the prevention of antibiotic associated diarrhea and the treatment of Clostridium difficile disease. *Am J Gastroenterol* 2006;101:812-22.

[10] Castagliuolo I, Riegler MF, Valenick L, et al. Saccharomyces boulardii protease inhibits the effects of clostridium difficile toxins A and B in human colonic mucosa. *Infection and Immun* 1999;67:302-7.

[11] FDA: "FDA Drug Safety Communication: Clostridium difficile-associated diarrhea can be associated with stomach acid drugs known as proton pump inhibitors (PPIs)." Accessed August 20, 2012 at http://www.fda.gov/drugs/drugsafety/ucm290510.htm

Part X: Men and Women's Health

Don't Let a Dip in This Critical Hormone Doom You to Fuzzy Thinking, Ho-Hum Sex, and an Early Grave

[1] A.B. Araujo, et al. "Prevalence of symptomatic androgen deficiency in men." *J Clin Endrocrinol Metab.* 2007;92:4241-4247.

[2] G. Corona, et al. "Following the common association between testosterone deficiency and diabetes mellitus, can testosterone be regarded as a new therapy for diabetes?" *Int J Androl.* 2009;32:431-441.

[3] This table originally appeared in: S. Bhasin, et al. Testosterone Therapy in Adult Men with Androgen Deficiency Syndromes: An Endocrine Society Clinical Practice Guideline. Chevy Chase, MD: The Endocrine Society; 2010.

[4] E. Wehr, et al. "Low free testosterone is associated with heart failure mortality in older men referred for coronary angioplasty." *Eur J Heart Fail.* 2011;13:482-488.

[5] M. Muller, et al. "Endogenous sex hormones and progression of carotid atherosclerosis in elderly men," *Circulation.* 2004;109:2074-2079.

[6] K.S. Channer, et al. "Low serum testosterone and increased mortality in men with coronary disease," *Heart.* 2010;96:1821-1825.

[7] S. Dhindsa, et al. "Frequent occurrence of hypogonadism in type 2 diabetes." *J Clin Endocrinol Metab.* 2004;89:5462-5468.

[8] H. Jones, et al. "Testosterone improves glycaemic control, insulin resistance, body fat and sexual function in men with the metabolic syndrome and/or type 2 diabetes: A multicenter European Clincal Trial: The

TIMES2 Study". *Endocrine Abstracts.* 2010;21:OC1.6.

[9] F.A. Zarrouf , et al. "Testosterone and depression: systematic review and meta-analysis." *J Psychiatr Pract.* 2009;15:289-305.

[10] American Academy of Orthopaedic Surgeons. OrthoInfo: First fracture may be a warning sign. www.orthoinfo.aaos.org/topic.cfm?topic=A00281.

[11] S. Bhasin, et al. Testosterone Therapy in Adult Men with Androgen Deficiency Syndromes: An Endocrine Society Clinical Practice Guideline. Chevy Chase, MD: The Endocrine Society; 2010:15.

Avoid Mainstream Medicine's Synthetic Hormone Trap: How to Navigate the Maze of Menopause Naturally with Bio-Identical Hormones

[1, 2, 3] The North American Menopause Society website. Accessed online at www.menopause.org/Consumers.aspx April 29, 2012.

[4] RxList.com website. Accessed online at www.rxlist.com/catapres-drug/clinical-pharmacology.htm April 29, 2012.

[5] MedicineNet.com website. Accessed online at http://www.medicinenet.com/gabapentin/article.htm April 29, 2012.

[6] Zhang F, Bolton JL.Chem Res Toxicol. Synthesis of the equine estrogen metabolites 2-hydroxyequilin and 2-hydroxyequilenin.1999 Feb;12(2):200-3.

[7] Pisha E, Lui X, Constantinou AI, Bolton JL. Evidence that a metabolite of equine estrogens, 4-hydroxyequilenin, induces cellular transformation in vitro. *Chem Res Toxicol.* 2001 Jan;14(1):82-90.

[8] Premarin.com website. Accessed online at http://premarin.com/side-effects-safety-info.aspx April 29, 2012.

[9] Agnès Fournier, Alban Fabre, Sylvie Mesrine, Marie- Christine Boutron-Ruault, Franco Berrino, Françoise Clavel-Chapelon. *Journal of Clinical Oncology*, Vol 26, No 8 (March 10), 2008: pp. 1260-126

[10] Leonetti HB, Wilson KJ, Anasti JN. Topical progesterone cream has an anti-proliferative eff ect on estrogen-stimulated endometrium. *Fertil Steril.* 2003 Jan; 79(1):221-2

[11, 12] L'hermite M, Simoncini T, Fuller S, Genazzani AR. Could transdermal estradiol + progesterone be a safer postmenopausal HRT? A review. Maturitas. 2008 Jul Aug;60(3-4):185-201. Epub 2008 Sep 5.

[13] N. L. Rasgon, et al. Diff erences in verbal memory performance in postmenopausal women receiving hormone therapy: 17b-estradiol versus conjugated equine estrogens. *American Journal of Geriatric Psychiatry* (2011).

[14] Experimental benefits of sex hormones on vascular function and the outcome of hormone therapy in cardiovascular disease. *Current Cardiology Reviews.* 2008 November; 4(4): 309-322

[15] Maturitas. 2009;63(1):63-66; Safety of Testosterone Use in Women

Part XI: Dr. Stengler's Urgent Health Warnings

Toxic Toilet Paper: Revealed… How Your Toilet Paper May Be Making You Sick!

[1] Gehring M, et al. Bisphenol A contamination of wastepaper, cellulose and recycled paper products. In: Popov V, et al, eds. Waste Management and the Environment II. Southampton, UK; 2004.

Your Prostate Drug Could Be Killing You! Common Prostate Drugs Given to Millions Linked to Aggressive Prostate Cancer

[1] FDA website. Accessed January 1, 2013 at www.fda.gov/Drugs/Drug Safety/ucm258314.htm

[2] ibid

[3] Medscape Today website. Accessed January 1, 2013 at www.medscape.com/viewarticle/718351

[4] ibid

[5] ibid

[6] Safarinejad M. R. et al. Effects of EPA, gamma-linolenic acid or coenzyme Q10 on serum prostate-specific antigen levels: a randomised, double-blind trial. *British Journal of Nutrition.* Published online December 2012.

[7] Williams CD, Whitley BM, Hoyo C, Grant DJ, Iraggi JD, Newman KA, Gerber L, Taylor LA, McKeever MG, Freedland SJ., A high ratio of dietary n-6/n-3 polyunsaturated fatty acids is associated with increased risk of prostate cancer. *Nutr Res.* 2011 Jan;31(1):1-8. doi: 10.1016/j.nutres.2011.01.002.

[8] Key TJ, Schatzkin A, Willett WC, Allen NE, Spencer EA, Travis RC. Diet, nutrition and the prevention of cancer. *Public Health Nutr.* 2004 Feb;7(1A):193.

[9] Yan L, Spitznagel EL. Soy consumption and prostate cancer risk in men: a revisit of a meta-analysis. *Am J Clin Nutr.* 2009 Apr;89(4):1155-63. doi: 10.3945/ajcn.2008.27029. Epub 2009 Feb 11.

[10] National Cancer Institute website. Accessed January 5, 2013 at

www.cancer.gov/cancertopics/pdq/cam/prostatesupplements/Patient/page7

[11] Seeram NP et al. In vitro antiproliferative, apoptotic and antioxidant activities of punicalagin, ellagic acid and a total pomegranate tannin extract are enhanced in combination with other polyphenols as found in pomegranate juice. *J Nutr Biochem* 2005 Jun; 16(6):360-67.

[12] Sartippour MR et al. Ellagitannin-rich pomegranate extract inhibits angiogenesis in prostate cancer in vitro and in vivo. *Intl J Oncol* 2008; 32:475-80.

[13] Pantuck AJ, et al. Phase II study of pomegranate juice for men with rising prostate-specific antigen following surgery or radiation for prostate cancer. *Clin Cancer Res* 2006; 12:4018-26.

[14] Zhang Q, Radisavljevic ZM, Siroky MB, Azadzoi KM. Dietary antioxidants improve arteriogenic erectile dysfunction. *Int J Androl.* 2011 Jun;34(3):225-35. doi: 10.1111/j.1365-2605.2010.01083.x.

[15] Schwarz S, Obermüller-Jevic UC, Hellmis E, Koch W, Jacobi G, Biesalski HK. Lycopene inhibits disease progression in patients with benign prostate hyperplasia. *J Nutr.* 2008 Jan;138(1):49-53.

[16] Ziglioli F et al. Vanilloid-mediated apoptosis in prostate cancer cells through a TRPV-1 dependent and a TRPV-1-independent mechanism. *Acta Biomed* 2009 Apr; 80(1): 13-20.

[17] Athanasiou A et al. Vanilloid receptor agonists and antagonists are mitochondrial inhibitors: how vanilloids cause non-vanilloid receptor mediated cell death. *Biochem Biophys Res Commun* 2007 Mar 2; 354(1): 50-55.

The Common Household Poison That's Making You and Your Children Dumber

[1] Choi AL, Sun G, Zhang Y, Grandjean P 2012. Developmental Fluoride Neurotoxicity: A Systematic Review and Meta-Analysis. Environ Health Perspect. http://dx.doi.org/10.1289/ehp.1104912.

[2] Harvard School of Public Health website. Accessed August 26, 2012 at http://www.hsph.harvard.edu/news/features/features/fluoride-childrens-health-grandjean-choi.html.

[3] Tang QQ, et al. Fluoride and children's intelligence: a meta-analysis. *Biol Trace Elem Res.* 2008 Winter;126(1-3):115-20. Epub 2008 Aug 10

[4] Centers for Disease Control and Prevention website. Accessed August 26, 2012 at http://www.cdc.gov/nchs/data/databriefs/db53.htm

[5] Turner CH, et al. Fluoride reduces bone strength in older rats. *J Dent*

Res. 1995;74:1475-1481.

[6] Sandhu R, et al. Serum fluoride and sialic acid levels in osteosarcoma. *Biol Trace Elem Res.* 2011 Dec;144(1-3):1-5. Epub 2009 Apr 24.

[7] Karademir S, et al. Effects of fluorosis on QT dispersion, heart rate variability and echocardiographic parameters in children. 2011 Mar;11(2):150-5. doi: 10.5152/akd.2011.038. Epub 2011 Feb 23.

[8] Gutowska I, et al. Fluoride as a pro-inflammatory factor and inhibitor of ATP bioavailability in differentiated human THP1 monocytic cells. *Toxicol Lett.* 2010 Jul 1;196(2):74-9. Epub 2010 Apr 22.

[9] Campus G, et al Six months of high-dose xylitol in high-risk caries subjects-a 2-year randomised, clinical trial. *Clin Oral Investig.* 2012 Jul 13. [Epub ahead of print]

[10] CDC has recognized water fluoridation as one of 10 great public health achievements of the 20th century. Centers For Disease Control and Prevention. Accessed August 26, 2012 at http://www.cdc.gov/fluoridation.

WARNING: These Common Medications Could be Destroying Your Hearing!

[1] Khan AS, Sheikh Z, Khan S, Dwivedi R, Benjamin E. Viagra deafness-sensorineural hearing loss and phosphodiesterase-5 inhibitors. *Laryngoscope.* 2011 May;121(5):1049-54.

[2] Cascella V, Giordano P, Hatzopoulos S, Petruccelli J, Prosser S, Simoni E, Astolfi L, Fetoni AR, Skarżyński H, Martini A. A new oral otoprotective agent. Part 1: Electrophysiology data from protection against noise-induced hearing loss. *Med Sci Monit.* 2012 Jan;18(1):BR1-8.

[3] Guastini L, Mora R, Dellepiane M, Santomauro V, Giorgio M, Salami A.Water-soluble coenzyme Q10 formulation in presbycusis: long-term effects. *Acta Otolaryngol.* 2011 May;131(5):512-7. Epub 2010 Dec 16.

[4] B. Gopinath, V. M. Flood, C. M. McMahon, G. Burlutsky, C. Spankovich, L. J. Hood and Paul Mitchell. Dietary antioxidant intake is associated with the prevalence but not incidence of age-related hearing loss. *The Journal of Nutrition, Health & Aging* Volume 15, Number 10 (2011), 896-900

Is Cancer on Tap in YOUR Kitchen?

[1] Margel D, Fleshner NE. Oral contraceptive use is associated with prostate cancer: an ecological study. *BMJ Open* 2011;1:e000311. doi:10.1136/bmjopen-2011-000311

The Bitter Truth About Artificial Sweeteners and Cancer

[1] Calorie Control Council website Aspartame Information Center. Accessed November 25, 2012 at www.aspartame.org.

[2] Schernhammer ES, Bertrand KA, Birmann BM, Sampson L, Willett WC, Feskanich D. Consumption of artificial sweetener–and sugar-containing soda and risk of lymphoma and leukemia in men and women. *American Journal of Clinical Nutrition* 2012;96:1419–28.

[3] S. Ghanta, el al., Oxidative DNA damage preventive activity and antioxidant potential of Stevia rebaudiana (Bertoni) Bertoni, a natural sweetener. *The Journal of Agricultural and Food Chemistry* (2007)

Part XII: Dr. Stengler's Top 19 Healing Secrets

How to Fight the Hidden "Wasting Disease" that You May Already be Suffering From

[1] Alfonso J et al. Sarcopenia: European Consensus on Definition and Diagnosis: Report of the European Working Group on Sarcopenia in Older People. Age Ageing. 2010;39(4):412-423. Accessed December 16, 2012 at http://www.medscape.com/viewarticle/723929_5

[2] Ibid

[3] The World's Healthiest Foods website. Accessed December 16, 2012 at www.whfoods.com

[4] Coker, R. et al. Whey protein and essential amino acids promote the reduction of adipose tissue and increased muscle protein synthesis during caloric restriction-induced weight loss in elderly, obese individuals. *Nutrition Journal* 2012, 11:105 doi:10.1186/1475-2891-11-105

[5] Cribb PJ, Williams AD, Carey MF, Hayes A. The effect of whey isolate and resistance training on strength, body composition, and plasma glutamine. *It J Sport Nutr Exerc Metab.* 2006 Oct;16(5):494-509

[6] Aguiar AF, er al., Long-term creatine supplementation improves muscular performance during resistance training in older women. *Eur J Appl Physiol.* 2012 Oct 7

[7] Environmental Nutrition. "Losing muscle is a part of aging, but you can minimize the effects." 30:11. November 2007

[8] Kinney, John. "Nutritional frailty, sarcopenia and falls in the elderly." Current Opinion in Clinical Nutrition and Metabolic Care. 7:15-20. 2004

[9] Borst, Stephen. "Interventions for sarcopenia and muscle weakness in older people." *Age and Ageing.* 33:6. British Geriatrics Society. 2004